Nutrient-Drug Interactions

Edited by

Kelly Anne Meckling

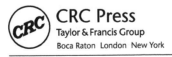

CRC Press
Taylor & Francis Group
Boca Raton London New York

CRC Press is an imprint of the
Taylor & Francis Group, an **informa** business

NUTRITION AND DISEASE PREVENTION

1. Genomics and Proteomics in Nutrition, *edited by Carolyn D. Berdanier and Naima Moustaid-Moussa*

2. Perinatal Nutrition: Optimizing Infant Health and Development, *edited by Jatinder Bhatia*

3. Soy in Health and Disease Prevention, *edited by Michihiro Sugano*

4. Nutrition and Cancer Prevention, *edited by Atif B. Awad and Peter G. Bradford*

5. Cancer Prevention and Management through Exercise and Weight Control, *edited by Anne McTiernan*

6. Nutritional Strategies for the Diabetic/Prediabetic Patient, *edited by Jeffrey I. Mechanick and Elise M. Brett*

7. Nutrient–Drug Interactions, *edited by Kelly Anne Meckling*

Related Volumes

Introduction to Clinical Nutrition: Second Edition, Revised
and Expanded, *edited by V. Sardesai*

Pediatric Gastroenterology and Nutrition in Clinical Practice,
edited by Carlos Lifschitz

Nutrients and Cell Signaling, *edited by Janos Zempleni
and K. Dakshinamurti*

Mitochondria in Health and Disease, *edited by Carolyn D. Berdanier*

Thiamine, *edited by Frank Jordan and Mulchand Patel*

Phytochemicals in Health and Disease, *edited by Yongping Bao
and Roger Fenwick*

Handbook of Obesity: Etiology and Pathophysiology, Second Edition,
edited by George Bray and Claude Bouchard

Handbook of Obesity: Clinical Applications, Second Edition,
edited by George Bray and Claude Bouchard

CRC Press
Taylor & Francis Group
6000 Broken Sound Parkway NW, Suite 300
Boca Raton, FL 33487-2742

First issued in paperback 2019

ISBN-13: 978-1-57444-915-0 (hbk)
ISBN-13: 978-0-367-39065-5 (pbk)

Library of Congress Card Number 2006042561

Library of Congress Cataloging-in-Publication Data

Nutrient drug interactions / edited by Kelly Anne Meckling.
    p. cm. -- (Nutrition and disease prevention)
  Includes bibliographical references and index.
  ISBN 1-57444-915-X (alk. paper)
  1. Drug-nutrient interactions. I. Meckling, Kelly Anne. II. Series.

RM302.4.N85 2006
615'.70452--dc22

2006042561

Visit the Taylor & Francis Web site at
http://www.taylorandfrancis.com

and the CRC Press Web site at
http://www.crcpress.com

Introduction

The idea of food as medicine has been around for millennia. However, the acceptance of specific foods, food components, extracts, herbals and supplements as part of conventional medical practice in industrialized countries is still a highly controversial subject. Western medicine has largely depended on the availability of pharmacologic agents or "drugs" for the prevention and treatment of human disease with lesser emphasis on lifestyle and dietary habits as major contributory factors, particularly with respect to chronic disease prevention. Furthermore, there are many additional tools in the repertoire of complementary medical practitioners that go far beyond what is ingested, inhaled or spread on the skin to ward off disease or treat illness.

The goal of this volume is not to consider the entirety of complementary medicine, but to focus on food, herbals and their chemical constituents as contributors to human health through control of metabolism, primarily as they relate to chronic disease development and treatment. More specifically, we will consider how what is consumed affects response, whether on a population or individual level, to pharmacologic agents that are the mainstay of chronic disease treatment/prevention around the world. Many of these drugs have their history as natural compounds isolated from flora and fauna in our environment; however the public perception has often been that "drugs" come with significant risk and are less safe than "foods" or "natural health products." Promulgating this view are vocal members of the public who perceive a conspiracy by big business and the pharmacologic giants to protect their billion-dollar stocks by presenting alternative medical practice as "flawed." Furthermore, many complementary practitioners themselves will say that they usually do not consider that adverse events may occur in response to their therapies, nor do they ask their patients to report any side effects,[1] which exacerbates the problem.

Regardless of the particular approach that is taken, patients must demand of their practitioners that applied therapies be safe and effective. Thus, evidence-based medical practice must continue to be the cornerstone of health care delivery for the foreseeable future. While testing through phase I, II and III clinical trials following extensive testing in model systems is the standard for determining the safety and efficacy of pharmacologic agents and synthetic food additives, this has not been the case for many "natural products." Assumptions of safety and efficacy for natural health products have often come from demonstration of historical use over many years, or possibly centuries, in specific populations with specific lifestyle and cultural practices. This limited scope of use can hardly be expected to predict the complicated behaviors that could occur in individuals or populations following very different lifestyles or using them in combination with other therapies.

There have been incredible advances in our understanding of how the chemicals in foods and herbs we consume interact with natural and synthetic drugs used to prevent or treat human disease. It is standard practice to examine the effects of food consumption on the absorption and pharmacokinetics of new drugs, but the relevant issues have become much greater than "should this medicine be taken with or without food." Long-term use of many medications has the potential to modify gastrointestinal function and alter the uptake and handling of both macronutrients, micronutrients and many phytochemicals that we now know have impacts on nutritional status and overall health. Manipulating the diet or the administration of supplements, orally or systemically, can help prevent nutritional deficiencies that could develop during chronic drug administration. A much more difficult task is to understand the potential for the thousands of chemical compounds found in food and natural health products to modify drug bioavailability, biodistribution, toxicity, efficacy and metabolism. In some cases a single food or supplement could profoundly increase or decrease the toxicity and/or efficacy of a single drug.

A major emphasis, from a clinical point of view, has been to identify these substances and remove them from the diets or supplement list of patients undergoing drug therapy. The focus, then, has been almost exclusively on simplifying the drug treatment plan. An alternative approach would be to use our knowledge of the mechanisms by which food chemicals modify drug action and to develop adjuvant therapy protocols that use food (functional foods and nutraceuticals) and drugs together to optimize treatment outcome. This could result in a decreased requirement, by the patient, for expensive medications, possibly increased efficacy with decreased toxicity toward normal or uninfected tissues, and the maintenance of a food substance with multiple healthful components.

In this collection of reviews, these major issues will be addressed by experts in their relevant disciplines. The organization of the book will place the focus on the ailment being treated or prevented and, thus, on the targets of therapy. Within each section a comprehensive examination of macronutrient, micronutrient and phytochemical impacts on drug action will be undertaken. Where a given drug affects nutritional status, the appropriate diet modification or supplement will be suggested. The major focus of each section will be on the molecular mechanism(s) by which the food or chemical is thought to modify disease process and drug behavior. Where specific active chemicals have been identified, their precise molecular targets, including regulation of gene expression, will be described. The book will finish with a description of the roles of genetic variation and polymorphism in determining nutrient/drug responses, and how individuals might be "profiled" in future to identify those likely to demonstrate specific interactions and who would benefit most from adjuvant or complementary therapies.

Kelly Anne Meckling, Ph.D.

REFERENCE

1. Abbott, A., Survey questions safety of alternative medicine. *Nature*, 436 (7053): 898, 2005.

The Editor

Kelly Anne Meckling, Ph.D., completed an Honors B.Sc. with Distinction in Biochemistry with a minor in psychology from the University of Calgary in 1984, and her M.Sc. with Dr. Tony Pawson from the University of British Columbia. She then transferred to the University of Toronto to complete her Ph.D. in medical biophysics in 1989, examining the signaling pathways unique to human leukemia and normal blood cell development.

Dr. Meckling's travels took her to the University of Alberta in Edmonton in 1989, where she examined the role of growth factors and cancer development on transport of chemotherapeutic drugs. In 1991, she became a faculty member in the Department of Nutritional Sciences at the University of Guelph, with no formal nutrition training. She rapidly acquired this knowledge through reading, attending undergraduate and graduate lectures and through her teaching activities. Since that time, she has continued as an active researcher in the area of nutrient signaling and the prevention/treatment of chronic diseases, including cancer, cardiovascular disease and obesity.

Dr. Meckling currently is associated with the Natural Sciences Engineering Research Council of Canada and the Breast Cancer Society, where she carries out both *in vitro* studies in model systems and human clinical intervention trials. She teaches undergraduate biology to 2000 students per year as well as advanced courses in nutrition and the metabolic control of disease. Also, Dr. Meckling is academic advisor to students majoring in nutritional and nutraceutical sciences.

Contributors

Marica Bakovic
Department of Human Health and
  Nutritional Sciences
University of Guelph
Guelph, Ontario, Canada

Amir Baluch
Department of Anesthesiology
Louisiana State University
New Orleans, Louisiana

Matthew Chronowic
Department of Human Health and
  Nutritional Sciences
University of Guelph
Guelph, Ontario, Canada

Ennio Esposito
Istituto di Ricerche Farmacologiche
  Mario Negri
Santa Maria Imbaro, Italy

Jason M. Hoover
Department of Anesthesiology
Louisiana State University
New Orleans, Louisiana

Alan D. Kaye
Department of Anesthesiology
Louisiana State University
  Health Sciences Center
New Orleans, Louisiana

James B. Kirkland
Human Health and Nutritional
  Sciences
University of Guelph
Guelph, Ontario, Canada

Alexandre Loktionov
Colonix Ltd.
Babraham Research Campus
Cambridge, United Kingdom

Kelly Anne Meckling
Human Health and Nutritional
  Sciences
University of Guelph
Guelph, Ontario, Canada

André J. Scheen
Division of Diabetes, Nutrition and
  Metabolic Disorders
Department of Medicine
Sart Tilman Hospital
Liège, Belgium

Kevin Wood
Department of Human Health and
  Nutritional Sciences
University of Guelph
Guelph, Ontario, Canada

Contents

Chapter 9

1 Diabetes, Obesity, and Metabolic Syndrome

André J. Scheen

CONTENTS

1.1 INTRODUCTION

Metabolic disorders, such as diabetes mellitus, overweight/obesity, and the so-called metabolic syndrome (including atherogenic dyslipidemia) are rapidly increasing in the westernized world because of poor lifestyle habits favoring fat- and sucrose-enriched meals and low physical activity or sedentariness.[1] Medical nutrition therapy is an integral component of diabetes mellitus,[2] obesity[3] and metabolic syndrome management.[4] Therapy should be individualized, with consideration given to the individual's usual food and eating habits, metabolic profile, treatment goals, and desired outcomes. When diet, associated with regular physical exercise and healthy lifestyle habits, is insufficient to control blood glucose, reduce body weight and/or improve the metabolic profile, pharmacological interventions may be considered to reach these objectives.[5] While insulin therapy is essential in all patients with type 1 diabetes, drug therapy is now a key element in the management of type 2 diabetes mellitus and is becoming more and more sophisticated with the recent launch of new compounds and the increased use of combined therapy.[6,7] In contrast, pharmacological intervention for obesity still remains a controversial issue because of only modest long-term efficacy and/or concern about safety.[8,9] Finally, the recent recognition of the important health problem associated with the metabolic syndrome[10] has stimulated researchers to develop drugs aimed at specifically improving insulin sensitivity and correcting associated metabolic disorders.[4,11]

Because nutrition therapy and pharmacological intervention are major components of the management of metabolic disorders, it is interesting to consider potential food–drug or nutrient–drug interactions in this particular medical field (Figure 1.1). An interaction is said to take place when the effects of one drug are changed by the presence of another drug, food, drink or by some environmental chemical agent.[12] Interactions between food and drugs may inadvertently reduce or increase the effect of the drug, resulting in therapeutic failure (i.e., hyperglycemia in the case of diabetes mellitus) or increased toxicity (i.e., hypoglycemia in the case of diabetes). The majority of clinically relevant food–drug interactions are caused by food-induced changes in the bioavailability of the drug.[13,14] Indeed, since the bioavailability and clinical effect of most drugs are correlated, the bioavailability is an important pharmacokinetic effect parameter. However, in order to evaluate the clinical relevance of a food–drug interaction, the impact of food intake on the clinical effect of the drug has to be quantified as well.[15] This may be particularly relevant as far as food-related metabolic diseases are concerned. Thus, in the field of metabolic disorders, where nutrition plays a major role in the overall treatment, the potential influence of food and nutrient intake on drug therapeutic effect may be crucial.

Pharmacokinetic interferences often occur as a result of a change in drug metabolism. Cytochrome P450 system oxidizes a broad spectrum of drugs by a number of metabolic processes that can be enhanced or reduced by various drugs (known as inducers or inhibitors, respectively).[16] The clinical importance of any drug interaction depends on factors that are drug-, patient- and administration-related. As reviewed extensively,[17] dietary changes can alter the expression and activity of hepatic drug metabolizing enzymes, and dietary components may influence the gastrointestinal metabolism and transports of drugs.[18] Athough this can lead to alterations in the systemic elimination kinetics of drugs metabolized

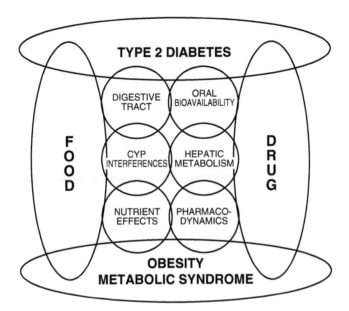

FIGURE 1.1 Potential food–drug or nutrient–drug interactions of clinical interest in patients with metabolic diseases.

by these enzymes, the magnitude of the change is generally small,[13,14] with the exception of the potentially major influence of grapefruit juice.[18] The coadministration of certain drugs with grapefruit juice can markedly elevate drug bioavailability and can alter both pharmacokinetic and pharmacodynamic parameters of the drug.[19–21]

1.2 DIET INTERVENTION

Type 2 diabetes mellitus,[2,22] obesity[3] and metabolic syndrome,[4,11] especially associated dyslipidemia, are clinical entities where diet plays a key role in the overall management.

1.2.1 HEALTHY DIET

The main objective of a healthy diet in patients with metabolic diseases is to prevent weight gain, to limit postprandial glucose excursions and/or to reduce the risk of cardiovascular disease, essentially by improving both lipid profile and antioxidant status. The National Cholesterol Education Program — Adult Treatment Panel III (NCEP-ATP III) recommendations for diet composition in patients with metabolic syndrome are consistent with general dietary recommendations.[11,23] Guidelines for healthy antiatherogenic diet call for (1) low intake of saturated fats, *trans* fats and cholesterol; (2) reduced consumption of simple sugars; and (3) increased intake of fruits, vegetables and whole grains. Such principles also concern diet recommendations for the treatment and prevention of diabetes mellitus and related disorders,[2,22] and of overweight and obesity.[3]

A number of factors influence glycemic responses to foods, including the amount of carbohydrates, type of sugar, nature of the starch, cooking and food processing and food form, as well as other food components. Although it is clear that carbohydrates do have differing glycemic responses, the data reveal no clear trend in outcome benefits. If there are long-term effects on glycemia and lipids, these effects appear to be modest.[22]

In persons with type 2 diabetes (on weight-maintenance diets), replacing carbohydrates with monosaturated fats reduces postprandial glycemia and triglyceridemia. However, there is concern that increased fat intake in *ad libitum* diets may promote weight gain. Therefore, the contributions of carbohydrates and monosaturated fat to energy intake should be individualized based on nutrition assessment, metabolic profiles and treatment goals.[2,22]

Total energy intake remains the most important factor in dietary interventions in obese individuals, but strategies based on emerging factors, such as glycemic index, fiber intake, dietary variety and energy density, may improve efficacy and tolerability of energy restriction.[3]

1.2.2 SPECIAL FOODS AND NUTRIENTS

1.2.2.1 Fibers

People are encouraged to choose a variety of fiber-containing foods, such as whole grains, fruits and vegetables, because they provide vitamins, minerals and other substances important for good health. Diets that include large amounts of natural plant fiber delay gastrointestinal digestion and absorption of sugar and complex carbohydrates, such as starch and dextrins. Early studies show that ingestion of high-fiber foods improves glycemic control in diabetic patients.[24] However, recent studies have reported mixed effects on glycemia and lipids in patients with type 1 diabetes.[22] In subjects with type 2 diabetes, it appears that ingestion of very large amounts of fiber is necessary to confer metabolic benefits on glycemic control, hyperinsulinemia and plasma lipids. It is not clear whether the palatability and the gastrointestinal side effects of fiber in this amount would be acceptable to most people. Dietary fiber, especially soluble fiber, theoretically could influence energy balance by slowing gastric emptying, delaying digestion and absorption of macronutrients, stimulating satiety hormones in the proximal and distal small intestine, and increasing energy excretion. In intervention trials in obese individuals, high fiber intake was associated with decreased body weight, reduced hunger and increased satiety, and decreased short-term food intake.[25]

By binding water, cations and bile acids, or by forming gels that sequester mono- or disaccharides, fiber-containing foods could modify the digestive as well as the absorption process. Reduced absorption of some vitamins and minerals, including iron, has been reported in subjects on high-fiber diets. However, despite the recommendation to increase fiber content in individuals with metabolic diseases, such as obesity, diabetes mellitus and metabolic syndrome, the effects of fiber content on availability of drugs commonly used for treating such patients have not been specifically investigated. One trial showed that guar gum decreases the absorption of metformin in healthy subjects.[26]

1.2.2.2 Dietary Supplements and Herbal Products

Pharmaceutical research conducted over the past 3 decades shows that natural products are a potential source of molecules for drug development, including for diabetes treatment.[27] Moreover, the use of botanical products has increased in recent years. Herbal products are widely used as dietary supplements and are part of complementary or alternative medicine. Importantly, herbal products are often used concurrently with prescribed or over-the-counter medications. The use of herbal products often escapes standard mechanisms for protecting persons from harmful effects of drugs or drug interactions.[28,29] Concurrent use of botanicals with approved prescription drug products can result in therapeutic failures or adverse events.[30] Interactions of herbs with cytochrome P450 have been extensively described.[31] For instance, recent publications have shown that coadministration of St. John's wort (*Hypericum perforatum*) decreases plasma levels of several concomitant drugs (cyclosporin, indinavir, etc.), and the underlying mechanism appears to be induction of the intestinal CYP3A and P-glycoprotein.[29,32]

The potential effects of herbal products on drugs classically used in patients with diabetes, obesity or metabolic syndrome are largely unknown. One Japanese study reported that St. John's wort treatment (300 mg tid [3 times per day] for 14 days) significantly reduced simvastatin area under the curve (AUC) by 50%, but did not interfere with pravastatin pharmacokinetics.[33] Thus, the potential for clinically significant drug interactions between St. John's wort with many CYP3A4 substrates is a real possibility, one that may not be evident from routine "screening" for traditional drug–drug interactions.[29] The potent effects of herbal products coupled with their risk of interactions with other commonly used drugs and the lack of governmental regulation have created a public health dilemma and encouraged the publication of a conference report.

1.2.2.3 Grapefruit Juice

The incidental discovery in a pilot study of a single volunteer demonstrating that grapefruit juice dramatically elevates felodipine bioavailability has led to the publication of numerous articles regarding the interaction between grapefruit juice and various drugs, focusing on different aspects: interaction mechanisms, grapefruit juice constituents that are responsible for the interaction, drugs exhibiting the interaction and the clinical relevance.[19–21,29] An interaction between drug and food or drink might reveal more difficulties than a drug–drug interaction and a major difficulty is the question of who is responsible for warning the public.[34]

The potential interaction of grapefruit juice has been particularly investigated with lipid-lowering agents (see section 1.3.3, Lipid-Lowering Agents). An extensive review of the international literature does not reveal any specific report on potential interactions of glucose-lowering agents with grapefruit juice despite the fact that some recently launched compounds undergo hepatic metabolism at least partially through CYP3A4.

1.3 PHARMACOLOGICAL INTERVENTION

1.3.1 GLUCOSE-LOWERING AGENTS

Various pharmacological classes can be used to lower blood glucose.[6,7,35] Besides classical sulfonylureas (chlorpropamide, glibenclamide, glipizide, gliclazide, glimepiride, etc.) and biguanides (metformin), new agents have been launched during recent years among which α-glucosidase inhibitors (acarbose, miglitol), meglitinide derivatives (repaglinide, nateglinide) and thiazolidinediones — also called glitazones — (pioglitazone, rosiglitazone) are included.[7,36] Numerous drug–drug interactions have been described with these compounds.[37–39] For instance, α-glucosidase inhibitors specifically act in the gastrointestinal tract and potential interferences with intestinal bioavailability of some other drugs have been reported, while meglitinide analogues and thiazolidinediones are metabolized via the cytochrome P450 system and, thus, subject to metabolic interactions.[39] Surprisingly, less is known about the potential influence of food and nutrients on the pharmacokinetic and pharmacodynamic effects of these glucose-lowering agents. In a recent extensive review of food–drug interactions, nothing described effects on oral glucose-lowering agents.[15]

1.3.1.1 Sulfonylureas

Sulfonylureas were the first oral drugs for treatment of type 2 diabetes in clinical practice.[40,41] They act at the pancreatic β-cell membrane by causing closure of adenosine triphosphate (ATP)-sensitive potassium channels, which leads to an enhanced insulin secretion. They are commonly prescribed alone or in combination with metformin, a thiazolidinedione, or an α-glucosidase inhibitor to reach the glucose control targets.[42] Various sulfonylureas have been, or are currently, used in clinical practice. Those with the largest experience are tolbutamide and chlorpropamide (first generation), and glibenclamide, glipizide, gliclazide and glimepiride (second generation).[43]

The kinetic-dynamic relations of sulfonylureas are complex. The timing of food intake, rather than the composition of diet, has been particularly analyzed with the different sulfonylurea compounds. The objective is to accelerate sulfonylurea gut absorption (leading to short t_{max} and high C_{max}), to maximize meal-related, early (first phase) insulin secretion and to reduce postprandial hyperglycemia.[44] The rate of absorption of chlorpropamide or tolbutamide, but not its extent, is decreased by food.[45] Even if concomitant food intake may not delay the absorption of tolbutamide, its efficacy may be improved if the drug is given half an hour before meals rather than with meals.[46] Chlorpropamide is more slowly absorbed than tolbutamide and has the longest elimination half-life of all sulfonylureas. Hence, the timing of the daily dose is less important, and it is irrelevant whether chlorpropamide is ingested before or with breakfast.[43] Prior food intake has no influence on rate and extent of absorption of the classical form of glibenclamide.[47] Although concomitant food intake does not seem to delay the absorption of glibenclamide, its efficacy may be increased if given before meals, at least in the short term. Indeed, 2.5 mg given half an hour before breakfast was more effective than 7.5 mg given together with breakfast.[48]

Food significantly delays absorption of gliclazide and peak concentrations also may be reduced;[49] however, it is not known whether intake before meals makes gliclazide more effective than does intake together with meals.[43] The absorption of glipizide is also retarded by food,[50,51] and is more rapidly absorbed when taken before breakfast than when ingested together with breakfast. Intake before breakfast is also associated with a more appropriate timing of insulin release relative to meal, and with enhanced efficacy of the drug.[51] Food delays the absorption of a tablet of gliquidone only insignificantly.[52] Glimepiride has an absolute bioavailability of 100%,[53] and there were no significant differences in pharmacokinetic and pharmacodynamic responses between glimepiride given 30 min before or immediately after a meal in healthy subjects[54] or between glime-piride given 30 min or directly before breakfast in patients with type 2 diabetes.[55] In clinical practice, glimepiride is usually prescribed once daily in the morn-ing.[56,57]

Gliclazide is a weak acid with a good lipophilicity and a pH-dependent solubility.[58] Gliclazide is practically insoluble in acidic media and its solubility increases as the pH becomes more alkaline. The absorption rate depends upon the gastric emptying time and upon the dissolution rate in the small intestine where the compound is soluble. The variability in absorption of gliclazide could also be related to an early dissolution in the stomach leading to more variability in the absorption in the intestine. From this, it can be anticipated that both delay in gastric emptying and change in pH accompanying food intake might affect the dissolution of the compound in the gastrointestinal tract. In two studies, food altered the pharmacokinetics of gliclazide in type 2 diabetic patients.[49,59] Two mechanisms were thought to be involved: (1) delay in the absorption of gliclazide when given 30 min after breakfast[49] and (2) decrease in the extent of absorption of gliclazide when given 30 min before a meal.[59] Some decrease in gastric emptying is noted; a possible interaction of gliclazide with dietary components, as well as a change in pH, could explain these observations.

A new modified release (MR) formulation containing 30 mg of gliclazide was developed to obtain a better predictable release of the active principle and to allow once-daily dosing regimen at breakfast.[60] In a food-effect study in healthy volunteers, one tablet was given either fasted or 10 min after the start of a standardized breakfast.[61] No significant difference was observed in t_{max}, $t_{1/2}$, C_{max} and AUC of gliclazide after administration of the 30 mg MR tablet under fasted and fed conditions. Thus, the new MR formulation of gliclazide can be given without regard to meals, i.e., before, during or after breakfast.

Chlorpropamide is less commonly used since the launch of second-generation sulfonylureas. One reason for this change results from a specific adverse effect — the chlorpropamide–alcohol flush.[62] Indeed, facial flushing after alcohol occurs much more frequently in type 2 diabetic patients taking chlorpropamide than in those receiving other sulfonylureas. Both alcohol and chlorpropamide concentrations are critical in determining the chlorpropamide–alcohol flush.[63] The mechanism that produces the flush is poorly understood. It has been suggested that chlorpropamide acts as a noncompetitive inhibitor of aldehyde dehydrogenase resulting in increased acetaldehyde concentrations. There is, however, uncertainty whether the flush can be explained solely by a rise in acetaldehyde concentrations. Prostaglandin inhibitors, such as aspirin, have been shown to attenuate the flush in some patients. Thus, alcohol intake should be avoided in diabetic patients treated with chlorpropamide.

1.3.1.2 Metformin

Metformin is a biguanide compound that exerts complex metabolic effects.[64] Biguanides inhibit absorption of various actively transported substances, such as hexoses, amino acids, calcium and bile acids.[65] This effect has been attributed to an interaction with transport systems in the intestinal brush border. Enzyme activities in intestinal epithelium also might be affected.[65] However, the antihyperglycemic activity essentially results from a reduction of hepatic glucose production, which leads to increased insulin action.[66,67] Currently, this molecule is considered as the first-choice drug in obese patients with type 2 diabetes and as the first adjunctive drug to be added to sulfonylurea therapy in case of failure with monotherapy.[68] It may also be prescribed together with a glitazone, leading to a clinically relevant additive, glucose-lowering effect.[39]

The absorption of metformin occurs mainly from the small intestine, and it has been shown that high concentrations (10 to 100 times plasma levels) accumulate in the walls of the gastrointestinal tract (review in Reference 69). Therefore, possible pharmacokinetic interferences with food are not excluded. The oral bioavailability of usual doses of metformin is 50 to 60%.[69] Absorption of metformin is completed within 6 h. There might be a slight delay and decrease after food intake,[70] although this effect does not significantly influence overall metabolic control in clinical practice. Gastrointestinal side effects are rather frequent during metformin therapy, especially diarrhea. Such symptoms may be avoided by gradual dose increases. The symptoms are generally transient and can be reduced by taking the drug with food. One experimental study showed that the absorption of metformin is reduced by concomitant intake of guar gum in healthy subjects.[26]

The effect of metformin on vitamin B_{12} absorption has been demonstrated using conventional Schilling tests, but was not confirmed by a whole-body technique.[64] Serum folic acid concentration might also be affected by metformin,[71] although this effect remains controversial.[72] Vitamin B_{12} malabsorption was found in 30% of diabetic patients during long-term metformin treatment.[72,73] Although it seems to be reversible, it may be persistent.[74] Megalobastic anemia due to vitamin B_{12} malabsorption associated with long-term metformin treatment has been reported, but vitamin B_{12} treatment was successful in correcting such an abnormality.[75] The mechanism of biguanide-induced B_{12} malabsorption remains uncertain, but it may be attributed to direct intestinal effects or bacterial overgrowth with binding of the intrinsic factor B_{12} complex.[74]

Alcohol potentiates the glucose-lowering and hyperlactatemic effect of biguanides and should be limited in patients on chronic treatment with metformin.[67] Alcohol itself decreases lactate oxidation and gluconeogenesis from lactate. The inhibition of gluconeogenesis by alcohol also promotes hypoglycemia, especially in the fasting state.

Diet–metformin interactions deserve further evaluation. In the Diabetes Prevention Program,[76] individuals with impaired glucose tolerance were randomized to one of three intervention groups, which included the intensive nutrition and exercise counseling ("lifestyle") group or either of two masked medication treatment groups — the biguanide metformin group or the placebo group. The latter interventions were combined with standard diet and exercise recommendations. After an average follow-up of 2.8 years, a 58% relative reduction in the progression to diabetes was observed in the lifestyle group, and a 31% relative reduction in the progression to diabetes was observed in the metformin group, compared with controlled subjects (placebo group). Considering these two remarkable protective effects provided by intensive lifestyle intervention on the one hand and by metformin on the other hand, it would be interesting to investigate whether a combination of the two interventions in the same at-risk population is able to provide a further reduction in the incidence of type 2 diabetes.

1.3.1.3 Thiazolidinediones (TZDs)

TZDs are now widely used as part of antidiabetic treatments.[77–79] These agents act by targeting insulin resistance instead of stimulating insulin secretion. They interact with the gamma type of the peroxisome proliferator-activated receptor (PPAR-gamma).[79,80] PPAR-gamma, a member of the nuclear receptor subfamily, stimulates gene expression of proteins involved in glucose metabolism. This results in an increase in insulin sensitivity in skeletal muscle, and adipose and liver tissues. Two TZDs are currently commercialized and widely prescribed — pioglitazone[81,82] and rosiglitazone.[83,84] Unlike sulfonylureas and metformin, TZDs are not used commonly as first-line therapy. However, there is considerable evidence for the incorporation of TZDs into combination regimens, with either sulfonylureas or metformin, particularly in patients who do not achieve glycemic goals with conventional regimens.[85] Pharmacokinetic characteristics of both pioglitazone[86] and rosiglitazone[87] have been described extensively. TZDS are metabolized through the cytochrome P450 system and, thus, are subject to pharmacokinetic interactions.[88] While some drug–drug interactions have been reported,[39] to our knowledge, clinically relevant food–drug interactions have not yet been described.

The effect of food on the pharmacokinetics of rosiglitazone was measured in a single-dose crossover study. Rosiglitazone (2 mg) was administered to healthy male volunteers either in the fasting state or following a standard high-fat breakfast.[89] Overall exposure to rosiglitazone, as assessed by AUC, was unaffected by food. Absorption of rosiglitazone in the fed state was more gradual and sustained than in the fasted state. C_{max} was reduced by approximately 20% and t_{max} was modestly delayed in the fed state. The absence of alterations in the extent of absorption of rosiglitazone when administered with food permits rosiglitazone administration without regard to meals for treatment of type 2 diabetes mellitus.

The effect of food on the pharmacokinetics of pioglitazone was evaluated in a randomized, two-period crossover study in healthy volunteers.[90] Subjects received a single dose of 45 mg pioglitazone after a 10-h fast and 10 min after a standardized meal. For fed and fasted states, the mean AUC for pioglitazone was comparable — the relative bioavailability was 94 to 97% for pioglitazone administered with food compared to a fasted state. The small differences in the absorption rate of pioglitazone with and without food are not considered clinically relevant; pioglitazone, like rosiglitazone, can be taken without regard to meal timing.

1.3.1.4 α-Glucosidase Inhibitors

α-glucosidase inhibitors are pharmacological agents that competitively and reversibly inhibit the α-glucosidase enzymes in the brush border of the small intestine mucosa.[91] There they prevent the hydrolysis of complex carbohydrates, retard the absorption of glucose and limit postprandial hyperglycemia. Acarbose is the most extensively investigated and widely prescribed α-glucosidase inhibitor,[92-94] while miglitol[95] and voglibose are two other compounds belonging to this pharmacological class that are available only in a limited number of countries (Japan for voglibose). While acarbose is an effective monotherapy for type 2 diabetes after diet failure, its distinct and complementary mechanism of action induces a further improvement in glycemic control when it is used in combination with other antidiabetic agents.[91,96,97]

All normal dietary carbohydrates, except for the relatively small amounts of lactose and monosaccharides, are digested by the intestinal α-glucosidases in saliva, pancreatic secretions and the enterocyte brush border. Inhibition of the action of these enzymes by specific inhibitors results in a reduction or even an abolition of hydrolytic activity. This is of great therapeutic importance for three reasons. First, the carbohydrate composition of the diet eaten by patients taking α-glucosidase inhibitors determines the substrate load for the various enzymes. This matters because the degree of inhibition of the various α-glucosidases is different for particular inhibitors and is dose-dependent, and the relationship between the inhibitory profile and the balance of carbohydrate sources in the diet is critical. This must be considered in assessing clinical response to treatment.

Second, if given in excessively high dosage, α-glucosidase inhibitors could result in malabsorption of some carbohydrates through inhibition of digestion. Secondary to carbohydrate malabsorption, there may also be malabsorption of other macro- and micronutrients due to intestinal hurry. Malabsorbed nutrients in any quantity will provoke an osmotic diarrhea and cause associated symptoms. Third, in the case of severe malabsorption induced by an α-glucosidase inhibitor, the only carbohydrate that can be absorbed by the intestine must be in a form in which no enzymatic digestion is required, i.e., monosaccharides and, in particular, glucose. This has important implications for resuscitation in hypoglycemia induced by other glucose-lowering agents given with an α-glucosidase inhibitor. Thus, theoretically, diet composition may influence both the efficacy and tolerability of α-glucosidase inhibitors. Selection of carbohydrates may influence acarbose glucose-lowering activity, while adequate nutrition may lead to a reduction in adverse effects.[98]

Any use of an α-glucosidase inhibitor to improve diabetic control may depend on the composition of the prescribed diet.[98] In clinical trials, a few patients did not benefit from treatment with α-glucosidase inhibitors, while most patients showed a significant reduction in postprandial blood glucose concentrations. When the dietary intake of the patients was analyzed, it could be demonstrated that the nonresponders to α-glucosidase inhibitors had ingested very low amounts of starch and very high amounts of simple sugars. In contrast, the patients who had an appreciable benefit from treatment with acarbose or miglitol had ingested reasonable amounts of complex carbohydrates and had preferred starchy foods to simple sugars. Thus, a diet high in (complex) carbohydrates and low in simple sugars, as recommended by diabetes associations,[2,22] should be maintained by the patients in order to achieve the greatest possible benefit from treatment with α-glucosidase inhibitors. A Japanese study has suggested that to obtain the greatest benefit from acarbose therapy, a strict adherence to high-carbohydrate (>50% of energy intake) diet is required.[99] However, the findings of a Canadian trial do not support this theory, since the glycemic control improved during the treatment despite the rather low carbohydrate intake in the acarbose group.[100] Nevertheless, in using these inhibitors, it is essential that consistent dietary guidelines are used,[98] which should be in keeping with the general dietary recommendations.[2,22]

An appropriate diet can also minimize gastrointestinal symptoms that may occur when fermentable carbohydrates reach the colon. Analysis of individual dietary intake revealed that patients with persistent adverse effects during treatment with α-glucosidase inhibitors had consumed either very high amounts of beer or sweets. During treatment with α-glucosidase inhibitors, a reduction in rapidly absorbable carbohydrates helps to prevent flatulence, abdominal discomfort or diarrhea.[98] With an adequate diet and individualized acarbose doses (starting with a low dose and followed by individualized titration), malabsorption should not usually occur and adverse effects will be markedly reduced.

As diet can influence the gastrointestinal tolerance profile of α-glucosidase inhibitors, one may suspect that the use of these drugs may influence the composition of the diet in treated patients. Apparently, this is not the case. In a double-blind, 24-week Finnish study, no significant differences in nutrient intakes between acarbose-treated and placebo-treated diabetic patients were observed by analyzing 4-d food diaries at 0, 4, 12 and 24 weeks.[101] Also, the energy intake and energy proportion of fat and carbohydrates remained unchanged in both groups. Thus, the improvement in metabolic control in patients treated with acarbose seems not to be a result of concomitant dietary changes. Similar findings were seen in a pilot study of shorter duration[102] and in a Canadian multicenter trial.[103]

Acarbose is administrered to patients to modulate the absorption of sugars and it has caused some degree of compensated carbohydrate malabsorption, especially at higher dosages. There has been some interest to see whether acarbose also affects the absorption and metabolism of other nutrients and minerals. In a double-blind trial involving 24 patients with type 2 diabetes, acarbose 300 mg/d for 10 weeks induced no significant alterations in the concentrations of important electrolytes (including calcium and magnesium), iron, vitamin B_{12} and folic acid.[104] Thus, at least at this point, there is little evidence that acarbose negatively affects other macro- or micronutrient availability.

1.3.1.5 Meglitinide Derivatives

Meglitinide analogues are nonsulfonylurea agents that are insulin secretagogues and have a similar mechanism of action to the sulfonylureas, but with different pharmacokinetic and pharmacodynamic properties.[105] Repaglinide[106,107] and nateglinide[108,109] belong to a new class of oral agents with a specific action on early-phase insulin release, thus targeting postprandial hyperglycemia, and a shorter elimination half-life and duration of action, therefore reducing the risk of late hypoglycemia. The meglitinide derivatives, especially nateglinide, are ideally suited for combination use with metformin or with TZDs. The pharmacokinetics of repaglinide[110,111] and nateglinide[112,113] are well known. Both compounds are metabolized through the P450 cytochrome system, which may lead to potential metabolic interactions. Drug–drug interactions have already been described,[39] but information on possible food–drug interactions is scarce.

Co-administration with food has only minor effects on repaglinide pharmacokinetics. Compared with the fasted state, administration of repaglinide (2 mg) 15 min before a high-fat meal, to 24 healthy men, produced a slight reduction in C_{max} (−20%) and AUC (−12%). Conversely, the mean residence time increased slightly (+21%) and t_{max} remained unchanged at 0.5 h.[114] Therefore, repaglinide may be administered preprandially without changing the rate of absorption. One study investigated the effects of repaglinide, 1 mg before each meal, in maintaining glycemic control in type 2 diabetic patients who either missed a meal or had an extra meal.[115] Meal-associated treatment with repaglinide provided good glycemic control and was well tolerated, without significant hypoglycemic events, irrespective of the number of meals consumed per day.

Results indicate that a synergistic interaction occurs between nateglinide and elevated mealtime plasma glucose concentrations to stimulate insulin secretion.[116]

Significantly greater insulin secretion was observed when nateglinide was taken before a meal compared to when given in the fasted state or in response to merely a meal. When given before meals, nateglinide produced rapid and short-lived insulin secretion, effectively reducing mealtime glucose excursions, yet lowering the risk of hypoglycemic episodes.

When nateglinide was given to healthy subjects 10 min before ingestion of a high-fat meal, the rate of absorption was increased relative to when it was given during a continued fast, as evidenced by a 12% increase in C_{max} and a 52% decrease in t_{max}.[117] However, there was no significant effect on the extent of absorption as assessed by the AUC. Alternatively, when nateglinide was given after the meal, a food effect was observed that was characterized by a decrease in the rate of absorption: a 34% decrease in C_{max} and a 22% increase in t_{max}, but no significant effect on AUC. Regardless of timing, the combination of a meal and nateglinide produced a larger increase in plasma insulin levels than did nateglinide alone.

The influence of timing of administration of nateglinide on the glucose profile and β-cell secretory response to a standardized test meal was studied, as well as the effect of meal composition on the pharmacokinetic and pharmacodynamic profile.[118] Nateglinide administration 10 min before a meal resulted in a more rapid rise and a higher peak nateglinide plasma concentration than when it was given 10 min after the start of the meal, irrespective of the meal composition (i.e., high in carbohydrates, fat or protein). Preprandial administration of nateglinide was more effective in reducing prandial glucose excursions, compared with post-meal dosing, a consequence of the earlier insulin response. Meal composition had no effect on the plasma nateglinide profile, which is of particular importance because nateglinide is a D-phenylalanine derivative and, thus, there was the possibility that its absorption could be influenced by the presence of high amino acid concentrations. The findings of this study clearly demonstrated that, even in the presence of a high-protein meal (32% of calories derived from protein), no effect on absorption of nateglinide was observed.

1.3.2 ANTIOBESITY AGENTS

During recent years, interest has intensified in two unique antiobesity preparations — the pancreatic lipase inhibitor, orlistat, and the noradrenaline and serotonin re-uptake inhibitor, sibutramine.[8,9,119]

1.3.2.1 Orlistat

Orlistat, a semisynthetic derivative of lipstatin, is a potent and selective inhibitor of gastric and pancreatic lipases.[120] When administered with fat-containing foods, it partially inhibits the hydrolysis of triglycerides, thus reducing the subsequent absorption of monoglycerides and free fatty acids. Orlistat treatment results in a dose-dependent reduction in body weight in obese subjects, with an optimal dosage regimen of 120 mg tid, and is generally well tolerated, with some intestinal side-effects during the first few days or weeks of administration.[120] Several 1- and 2-year trials showed that orlistat, when used with a health-promoting, low-fat and moderately energy-restricted diet, confers some advantages in the long-term management of obesity.[121] Clinical trials performed in obese subjects with type 2 diabetes demonstrated that orlistat (120 mg tid) slightly increased weight loss and resulted in a significant reduction in glycated hemoglobin levels in patients treated with sulfonylureas, metformin or even insulin, as compared to a placebo.[122] In all of these cliniical studies, orlistat proved to be effective only when its use was combined with a reduced-calorie diet (600 to 800 kcal/day deficit) containing 30% of calories from fat. Interestingly, treatment with orlistat plus lifestyle changes resulted in early and sustained improvements in cardiovascular risk factors, including waist circumference, glucose/insulin parameters, blood pressure and lipids, all parameters belonging to the metabolic syndrome. A 37% significant reduction in the incidence of new cases of type 2 diabetes was also reported after 4 years of treatment with orlistat as compared to a placebo in obese subjects.[123] The effects of orlistat on weight and on serum lipids in obese patients with hypercholesterolemia were investigated in a randomized, double-blind, placebo-controlled, multicentre study.[124] A 10% additional specific cholesterol-lowering effect of orlistat was demonstrated, independent of weight reduction, in obese patients already on a lipid-lowering hypocaloric diet.

In normal, healthy volunteers consuming 60 g/day of fat, orlistat (360 mg/day) recipients excreted 21.5 g/day more fecal fat than placebo recipients.[125] Approximately 32% of ingested fat was lost in the feces of orlistat recipients vs. 4.4% in placebo recipients, and this percentage does not change significantly when increasing the dosage of orlistat to 600 mg/day or the amount of dietary fat from 60 to 76 g/day. Dietary fiber content (28 vs. 10 g/day) did not influence fecal fat excretion after orlistat (80 mg q3d) in healthy male volunteers.[126] Over an 8-day period, the effect of orlistat (80 mg q3d) on fecal fat excretion was not influenced by administration time relative to meals in an experimental study in which the agent was given to 24 healthy volunteers mid-meal or 1 or 2 h after the meal.[127]

Adverse events observed with orlistat therapy result from the inhibition of fat absorption rather than the drug itself. They include abdominal pain, fatty/oily evacuation and, occasionally, fecal incontinence.[120] Orlistat (75 mg/day) was "better tolerated" by healthy volunteers when the dietary fat content was reduced from 130 to 110 g/day.[125] However, adverse events were similar in placebo and orlistat recipients when dietary fat was reduced from 130 to 45 g/day and the agent was administrered 2 h before food (i.e., with little or no fat content in the stomach).[120]

Orlistat inhibits the absorption of ingested fats. It is possible, therefore, that endogenous levels of fat-soluble vitamins (A, D, E and K vitamins) may become depleted with prolonged use of the agent.[120] Orlistat (360 mg/day) for 9 days, compared with a placebo, decreased the maximum plasma concentrations and the AUC-time curve values of oral vitamin E acetate supplementation (400 IU given on Day 4 of orlistat administration) by 43% and 60%, respectively. This suggests that short-term administration of orlistat may compromise vitamin E absorption from the gut. Conversely, the pharmacokinetic profile of oral vitamin A acetate supplementation (25,000 IU given on Day 4 of orlistat administration) was not significantly affected.[128] Small, clinically insignificant decreases in serum levels of vitamins A and D were seen in obese patients after 12 weeks of treatment with a placebo or orlistat 30 to 360 mg/day.[129] In contrast, vitamin E levels were significantly reduced with orlistat 180 and 360 mg/day and increased with a placebo (all, p <0.01). Approximately 60% of a supplemental dose of β-carotene, a major dietary source of vitamin A, was absorbed when a single 30 to 120 mg dose was given (on Day 4) to healthy volunteers receiving 360 mg/day orlistat.[130] This may be sufficient to achieve physiological levels of β-carotene in obese patients who may develop reduced levels of this vitamin during orlistat therapy. Analysis of biological results in obese patients who received 360 mg/day orlistat or a placebo for up to 2 years in a large European multicenter clinical trial, revealed that plasma levels of vitamins D and E and β-carotene were significantly reduced in orlistat compared with placebo recipients; the levels, however, remained within the normal clinical range.[131] Those results were confirmed in further large, long-term clinical trials performed in Europe and in the U.S. None of the trials reported bone density or bone mineral changes.[121]

1.3.2.2 Sibutramine

Sibutramine, a noradrenaline and 5-hydroxytryptamine re-uptake inhibitor, has been shown to produce a dose-related weight loss in obese subjects, with optimal doses of 10 to 15 mg/day.[132] The multicenter prospective "Sibutramine Trial of Obesity Reduction and Maintenance" (STORM) clinical study showed that almost all obese patients who persisted with the management scheme combining restricted diet and sibutramine (10 mg/day) can achieve at least a 5% weight loss, and over half can lose more than 10% of body weight within 6 months.[133] Furthermore, sustained weight loss was maintained in most patients continuing therapy with sibutramine for 2 years, whereas weight regain was noticed in most patients randomized to a placebo, thus demonstrating that sibutramine (10 to 20 mg/day) favors weight maintenance in the long term. The clinical effectiveness of sibutramine was demonstrated in several other clinical trials in nondiabetic and diabetic obese individuals.[122,134] In all of these trials, patients were prescribed a 600 kcal deficit diet based on a macronutrient content of <30% fat and 15% protein.[133]

Mean total daily energy intake was significantly reduced with sibutramine 10 or 30 mg/day compared with a placebo in obese women who were not attempting to lose weight.[135] After a 2-week treatment period, energy intake was 18.8 and 26.1% lower with sibutramine 10 and 30 mg/day, respectively, than with a placebo. Correspondingly, food intake was 13.9 and 27.7% lower. With respect to individual macronutrients, the total daily intake of both fat and protein was significantly reduced by the two dosages of sibutramine; there was no significant effect on daily carbohydrate intake. Overall, there was no significant effect on the percentage of energy from macronutrients consumed during each treatment phase, although both fat and carbohydrate intake were up to 12.4% lower after sibutramine than after a placebo.

Similar effects were seen in healthy, nonobese males who received 15 mg/day sibutramine or a placebo, in a randomized, double-blind, crossover trial.[136] Sibutramine significantly reduced total energy, protein, fat and carbohydrate intake vs. a placebo. Although the overall proportion of macronutrients did not differ significantly between treatment groups, lunch-time fat and protein, but not carbohydrate, intake were reduced, and dinner-time carbohydrate, but not fat or protein, intake was reduced with sibutramine compared with a placebo. However, in a large group of obese patients on a calorie-reduced diet, carbohydrate and protein intake were increased by 4.8 and 36%, respectively, from baseline, and fat intake was reduced by 7.8% after sibutramine (10 mg/day) for 6 months.[137]

Available published pharmacokinetic data for sibutramine are limited to information from abstracts. The bioavailability of the drug over the dose range of 10 to 30 mg was not altered by the presence of food in healthy volunteers.[138] The drug undergoes extensive first-pass metabolism to form pharmacologically active primary (M1) and secondary (M2) amine metabolites.[132] The influence of food composition on this process remains unknown.

1.3.3 LIPID-LOWERING AGENTS

Most obese individuals (especially those with abdominal adiposity), subjects with the metabolic syndrome and patients with type 2 diabetes have plasma lipid disturbances leading to atherogenic dyslipidemia (moderately elevated total and LDL cholesterol levels, low HDL cholesterol concentration and both fasting and postprandial hypertriglyceridemia) and increased cardiovascular morbidity and mortality. Again, healthy diet is essential to improving lipid profile of these individuals.[23] However, lipid-lowering drugs may also be useful and should be prescribed to numerous high-risk persons in order to reach target lipid levels.[139,140] Statins have proven their efficacy in reducing the incidence of cardiovascular complications in numerous primary and secondary prevention trials.[141] The primary effect of this pharmacological class is a specific inhibition of cholesterol synthesis in the hepatocytes leading to an impressive reduction in total and LDL cholesterol levels, although various pleiotropic effects also appear to play a role in the overall protective cardiovascular effect.[142] A recent clinical guideline from the American College of Physicians recommends lipid-lowering therapy with a statin in almost all patients with type 2 diabetes.[143] Fibric acid derivatives (fibrates) are also widely prescribed in diabetic patients because these drugs have a positive impact on diabetic dyslipidemia characterized by low HDL cholesterol and high triglyceride concentrations.[144]

1.3.3.1 Statins

The hydroxymethylglutaryl coenzyme A (HMG CoA) reductase inhibitors (statins) are well tolerated apart from two uncommon but potentially serious adverse effects: asymptomatic elevation of liver enzymes and skeletal muscle abnormalities, which range from benign myalgias to life-threatening rhabdomyolysis.[139] Adverse effects with statins are frequently associated with drug interactions because of their use in patients who are likely to be exposed to polypharmacy. The cytochome P450 enzyme system plays an important part in the metabolism of most statins (except pravastatin), leading to clinically relevant interactions with other pharmacological agents.[145–148] Alternatively, food interaction may also be suspected, especially an inhibition of metabolism by grapefruit juice, a potent CYP inhibitor.[19–21]

The various HMG CoA reductase inhibitors have very different chemical and pharmacokinetic properties. The bioavailability of lovastatin increases by 50% when taken with a regular meal; this is reflected in an increased drug effect.[149] However, the ingestion of fibers or fruit as part of a lipid-lowering diet may strikingly reduce the absorption of lovastatin and may increase the risk of treatment failure.[150] In contrast to lovastatin, the bioavailability of pravastatin is reduced by 31% when taken with food; however, since its lipid-lowering efficacy is unchanged, the interaction is not clinically important.[151] For atorvastatin[152,153] and fluvastatin,[154] bioavailability and lipid-lowering efficacy are unaffected by food intake. It seems to be also the case with simvastatin and rosuvastatin, although no published study is available to support this statement.

Excessive ingestion of grapefruit juice increases the bioavailability of lovastatin, atorvastatin and simvastatin by 1400, 200 and 1500%, respectively. This may lead to drug accumulation and the possible development of adverse effects.[155–157] Thus, concomitant use of grapefruit juice, at least in large amounts, and lovastatin or simvastatin should be avoided, or the dose of the statin should be greatly reduced. However, daily consumption of a glass of regular-strength grapefruit juice has only a minimal effect on plasma concentrations of lovastatin (30 to 40% increase) after a 40 mg evening dose of lovastatin.[158] The probable mechanism of this interaction is inhibition of CYP3A4-mediated first-pass metabolism of these statins by grapefruit juice in the small intestine and, thus, inhibition of their first-pass metabolism. Pravastatin and fluvastatin are not metabolized by CYP3A4 and, consequently, are not subject to drug–grapefruit juice interactions.[156,159] No study investigating the possible interaction of grapefruit juice with rosuvastatin is available, but such interaction appears to be unlikely as rosuvastatin is only minimally metabolized by the CYP450 enzyme system with no significant involvement of the 3A4 enzyme.[160] Thus, it would be wise to avoid the combination of certain statins (especially simvastatin and lovastatin) with grapefruit juice.[21] Indeed, the concomitant intake of such statins with CYP3A4 inhibitors may exacerbate adverse effects, such as rhabdomyolysis and acute renal failure.[146]

1.3.3.2 Fibrates

The two most commonly used fibric derivatives are gemfibrozil in the U.S.[161,162] and fenofibrate[163–165] in Europe. Fibrates are metabolized by the hepatic cytochrome P450 (CYP) 3A4 and, thus, are subject to drug interactions.[166]

Gemfibrozil is rapidly and completely absorbed when orally administered.[161] *In vitro* results suggest that solubility and dissolution of the drug may be increased in the fed state compared with the fasting state,[167] although clinical studies are needed to verify this. Whereas several important drug–drug interactions have been reported with gemfibrozil, especially with cerivastatin and repaglinide,[39] no one report is available concerning the potential interactions between food and gemfibrozil, especially grapefruit juice that contains inhibitors of the CYP P450 system.[19–21,159]

The C_{max} of fenofibric acid occurs within 6 to 8 h after fenofibrate administration, and the absorption of fenofibrate is increased when administered with food.[168] With the microcoated tablets, the extent of absorption is increased by approximately 35% under fed as compared with fasting conditions.[169] The fat content of a meal eaten at the time of fenofibrate administration does not have a marked effect on pharmacokinetics. When micronized fenofibrate 200 mg capsules were administered with a high-fat meal, the AUC (+15%) and the C_{max} (–2%) were only slightly altered, while the elimination half-life was shortened (–41%), compared when fenofibrate was taken with a low-fat meal.[166] The clinical relevance of these pharmacokinetic changes remains unclear.

1.3.3.3 Resins

Resins (cholestyramine and colestipol) act by binding bile salts in the gastrointestinal lumen.[139] Both compounds are large polymers that are not absorbed systemically. They bind bile acids by exchanging them for chloride ions; binding is irreversible. The bound bile salts are not reabsorbed, which leads to a depletion of the bile acid pool. The liver compensates by increasing synthesis of bile acids, which results in intracellular cholesterol depletion leading to increased expression of LDL receptors on the hepatocyte cell membrane and, thereby, increased LDL clearance. These drugs are given in the form of a powder, which is usually taken with meals as a suspension in juice or water. Compliance is the major problem on the grounds of palatability and adverse gastrointestinal effects. The absorption of several drugs may be impaired by resins, including statins, digoxin, amiodarone, thyroxine, warfarin, thiazide diuretics, and beta blockers. Reduced absorption of folic acid and fat-soluble vitamins may occur, but clinical deficiency is rare. Resins are less commonly used since the expansion of statin prescription and the recent launch of ezetimibe, a selective inhibitor of cholesterol intestinal absorption.

1.3.3.4 Ezetimibe

Ezetimibe is the first of a new class of antihyperlipidemic agents, the cholesterol-absorption inhibitors. It is indicated for use as monotherapy or in combination with a statin as an adjunct to dietary treatment for the reduction of elevated total cholesterol, LDL cholesterol and apo B in patients with primary hypercholesterolemia.[170,171] Although one study found that the oral bioavailability of ezetimibe did not appear to be substantially affected by the intake of high-fat or nonfat meals,[172] other data suggest that the oral bioavailability of ezetimibe may be increased by 25 to 35% with food and that plasma concentrations of ezetimibe may also be increased by up to 38% when the drug is taken with a high-fat meal.[173] Even if food may have a substantial effect on bioavailability of the compound, this effect is not expected to alter the efficacy or safety profile of ezetimibe because the drug is not extensively absorbed.[170,171] The LDL-lowering effect of ezetimibe according to dietary fat and cholesterol intake was investigated in a large multicenter, double-blind, randomized, placebo-controlled study in 1719 men and women (only reported in abstract form, Reference 174). When stratified according to dietary fat intake or daily cholesterol intake, all ezetimibe subgroups had significantly greater reductions in LDL-cholesterol levels compared with the respective placebo subgroups. These results suggest that ezetimibe can reduce LDL-cholesterol levels regardless of dietary fat or cholesterol intake.

1.3.3.5 Sterols and Stanols

Plant sterols have a moderate hypocholesterolemic effect. This is thought to stem from inhibition of the absorption of both exogenous dietary and endogenous biliary cholesterol from the distal small intestine. In recent years, research focus has shifted from plant sterols to plant stanols for reasons of safety and efficacy.[175] Especially, esterification of plant stanols with fatty acids from vegetable oil has made it possible to produce spreads, other foods and supplements containing plant stanols. Food preparations that provide 3.4 to 5.1 g/day of plant stanol esters, of which the plant stanol component is 2 to 3 g/day, significantly reduce serum total and LDL cholesterol levels without affecting HDL cholesterol or serum triglycerides, and are well tolerated. As both stanol esters and statins can be used in combination to accentuate the cholesterol lowering effect, it would be interesting to investigate the potential interactions between these nutrients and the pharmacological agent. Plant stanol esters block the absorption of cholesterol, whereas statins block the synthesis of cholesterol. Both mechanisms work in a complementary or concerted fashion to amplify LDL receptor activity and the clearance of LDL cholesterol from the plasma. A randomized, double-blind, clinical trial compared the effect of plant sterol ester spread (5.1 g/day) with a placebo spread on cholesterol in patients taking statin therapy, but who still had elevated LDL cholesterol.[176] As compared to the placebo, plant stanol ester spread induced a greater reduction in total cholesterol (−7%) and LDL cholesterol (−10%) at 8 weeks. No significant adverse events were noted. Thus, an incremental lowering of LDL cholesterol by about 10% was achieved by adding a stanol ester spread to the daily diet in persons taking a stable dose of a statin, and this effect was seen in all four statins (atorvastatin, lovastatin, pravastatin and simvastatin) included in this study. Preliminary observations confirmed these results in patients after cardiac transplantation.[177] Seventeen stable cardiac transplant recipients, of whom 16 were on statin therapy, used margarine with stanol/sterol esters. Total cholesterol was lowered by 17% and LDL cholesterol was reduced by 22%, allowing a reduction in statin dosages in some patients. The tolerance of the combination was good.

1.4 CONCLUSIONS

Metabolic disorders generally require combined dietary and pharmacological interventions. While food–drug or nutrient–drug interactions might be of particular importance in patients with metabolic diseases, only scarce data are available in the scientific literature, as compared to the overwhelming information regarding drug–drug interactions. Obviously, food composition may influence the efficacy of drugs affecting glucose, lipid and energy metabolism. In addition, since meal-related kinetics is crucial in controlling postprandial blood glucose in diabetic patents, the influence of food on drug bioavailability may also be important, especially for drugs that stimulate insulin secretion. Furthermore, meal content and/or timing may also influence drug gastrointestinal tolerability, as described with metformin, α-glucosidase inhibitors and orlistat. Finally, as food may interfere with CYP P450, potential food–drug interactions may be suspected in using pharmacological agents metabolized via the cytochrome system. A clear interaction with grapefruit juice was described with statins metabolized via CYP3A4, especially lovastatin and simvastatin. From a public health point of view, an interaction between drug and food or drink might reveal more difficulties than a drug–drug interaction. It is important that the awareness for this potential food–drug interaction will increase, and actions must be taken in order to increase the efficacy of diet–drug combination in metabolic diseases and to prevent undesired and harmful clinical consequences.

REFERENCES

1. Zimmet P. Globalization, coca-colonization and the chronic disease epidemic: can the doomsday scenario be averted? *J Intern Med* 2002; 247: 301–310.
2. Franz MJ, Bantle JP, Beebe CA, Brunzell JD, Chiasson J-L, Garg A, Holzmeister LA, Hoogwerf B, Mayer-Davis E, Mooradian AD, Purnell JQ, Wheeler M. Evidence-based nutrition principles and recommendations for the treatment and prevention of diabetes and related complications (Technical review). *Diabetes Care* 2002; 25: 148–198.
3. Hajduk CL, Roberts SB, Saltzman E. Dietary treatment of obesity. *Curr Opin Endocrinol Diabetes* 2001; 8: 240–246.
4. Scheen AJ. Management of the metabolic syndrome. *Minerva Endocrinol* 2004; 29: 31–45.
5. Scheen AJ. Current management of coexisting obesity and type 2 diabetes. *Drugs* 2003; 63: 1165–1184.
6. Scheen AJ, Lefèbvre PJ. Oral antidiabetic agents: a guide to selection. *Drugs* 1998; 55: 225–236.
7. Inzucchi SE. Oral antihyperglycemic therapy for type 2 diabetes: scientific review. *JAMA* 2002; 287: 360–372.

8. Scheen AJ, Lefèbvre PJ. Pharmacological treatment of obesity: present status. *Int J Obes* 1999; 23 (Suppl 1): 47–53.
9. Fernandez-Lopez J-A, Remesar X, Foz M, Alemany M. Pharmacological approaches for the treatment of obesity. *Drugs* 2002; 62: 915–944.
10. Grundy SM, Brewer HB Jr, Cleeman JI, Smith SC, Lenfant C, for Conference Participants. Definition of metabolic syndrome: report of the National Heart, Lung, and Blood Institute/American Heart Association conference on scientific issues related to definition. *Circulation* 2004; 109: 433–438.
11. Grundy SM, Hansen B, Smith SC, Cleeman JI, Kahn RA, for Conference Participants. Clinical management of metabolic syndrome. Report of the American Heart Association/National Heart, Lung, and Blood Institute/American Diabetes Association Conference on scientific issues related to management. *Circulation* 2004; 109: 551–556.
12. Sorensen JM. Herb–drug, food–drug, nutrient–drug, and drug–drug interactions: mechanisms involved and their medical implications. *J Altern Complement Med* 2002; 8: 293–308.
13. Anderson KE. Influences of diet and nutrition on clinical pharmacokinetics. *Clin Pharmacokinet* 1988; 14: 325–346.
14. Walter-Sack I, Klotz U. Influence of diet and nutritional status on drug metabolism. *Clin Pharmacokinet* 1996; 31: 47–64.
15. Schmidt LE, Dalhoff K. Food–drug interactions. *Drugs* 2002; 62: 1481–1502.
16. Dresser GK, Spence JD, Bailey DG. Pharmacokinetic–pharmacodynamic consequences and clinical relevance of cytochrome P450 3A4 inhibition. *Clin Pharmacokinet* 2000; 38: 41–57.
17. Ioannides C. Effect of diet and nutrition on the expression of cytochromes P450. *Xenobiotica* 1999; 29: 109–154.
18. Evans AM. Influence of dietary components on the gastrointestinal metabolism and transport of drugs. *Ther Drug Monit* 2000; 22: 131–136.
19. Bailey DG, Malcolm J, Arnold O, Spence JD. Grapefruit juice–drug interactions. *Br J Clin Pharmacol* 1998; 46: 101–110.
20. Fuhr U. Drugs interactions with grapefruit juice. Extent, probable mechanism and clinical relevance. *Drug Saf* 1998; 18: 251–272.
21. Dahan A, Altman H. Food-drug interaction: grapefruit juice augments drug bioavailability — mechanism, extent and relevance. *Eur J Clin Nutr* 2004; 58: 1–9.
22. American Diabetes Association. Nutrition principles and recommendations in diabetes. *Diabetes Care* 2004; 27 (Suppl 1): S36–46.
23. Krauss RM, Eckel RH, Howard B, Appel LJ, Daniels SR, Deckelbaum RJ, Erdman JW Jr, Kris-Etherton P, Goldberg IJ, Kotchen TA, Lichtenstein AH, Mitch WE, Mullis R, Robinson K, Wylie-Rosett J, St Jeor S, Suttie J, Tribble DL, Bazzarre TL. AHA Dietary Guidelines: Revision 2000: a statement for healthcare professionals from the Nutrition Committee of the American Heart Association. *Circulation* 2000; 102: 2284–2299
24. Anderson JA, Midgley WR, Wedman B. Fiber and diabetes. *Diabetes Care* 1979; 2: 369–379.
25. Howard NC, Saltzman E, Roberts SB. Dietary fiber and weight regulation. *Nutr Rev* 2001; 59: 129–139.
26. Gin H, Orgerie MB, Aubertin J. The influence of guar gum on absorption of metformin from the gut in healthy volunteers. *Horm Metab Res* 1989; 21: 81–83.

27. Oubre AY, Carlson TJ, King SR, Reaven GM. From plant to patient: an ethno-medical approach to the identification of new drugs for the treatment of NIDDM. *Diabetologia* 1997; 40: 614–617.

28. Miller L. Herbal medicinals: selected clinical considerations focusing on known or potential drug–herb interactions. *Arch Intern Med* 1998; 158: 2200–2211.

29. Huang S-M, Hall SD, Watkins P, Love LA, Serabjit-Singh C, Betz JM, Hoffman FA, Honig P, Coates PM, Bull J, Chen ST, Kearns GL, Murray MD. Drug interactions with herbal products and grapefruit juice: A conference report. *Clin Pharmacol Ther* 2004; 75: 1–12.

30. Zhou S, Koh HL, Gao ZY, Lee EJ. Herbal bioactivation: the good, the bad and the ugly. *Life Sci* 2004; 74: 935–968.

31. Zhou S, Gao Y, Jiang W, Huang M, Xu A, Paxton JW. Interactions of herbs with cytochrome P450. *Drug Metab Rev* 2003; 35: 35–98.

32. Wang Z, Gorski JC, Hamman MA, Huang SM, Lesko LJ, Hall SD. The effect of St John's wort (*Hypericum perforatum*) on human cytochrome P450 activity. *Clin Pharmacol Ther* 2001; 70: 317–326.

33. Sugimoto K, Ohmori M, Tsuruoka S, Nishiki K, Kawaguchi A, Harada K, Arakawa M, Sakamoto K, Masada M, Miyamori I, Fujimura A. Different effects of St John's wort on the pharmacokinetics of simvastatin and pravastatin. *Clin Pharmacol Ther* 2001; 70: 518–524.

34. Spence JD. Drug interactions with grapefruit: whose responsibility is it to warn the public? *Clin Pharmacol Ther* 1997; 61: 395–400.

35. Kuhlmann J, Puls W. Oral antidiabetics. *Handbook of Experimental Pharmacology*. Vol. 119. Berlin: Springer, 1996.

36. Scheen AJ. Drug treatment of non-insulin-dependent diabetes mellitus in the 1990s: achievements and future developments. *Drugs* 1997; 54: 355–368.

37. Brian WR. Hypoglycemic agents. In Levy RH, Thummel KE, Trager WF, Hansten PD, Eichelbaum M, Eds. *Metabolic Drug Interactions*. Philadelphia: Lippincott Williams & Wilkins, 2000: 529–543.

38. Scheen AJ, Lefèbvre PJ. Antihyperglycaemic agents. Drug interactions of clinical importance. *Drug Safety* 1995; 12: 32–45.

39. Scheen AJ. Drug interactions of clinical importance with antihyperglycaemic agents: an update. *Drug Safety* 2005; 28: 601–631.

40. Groop LC. Sulfonylureas and NIDDM. *Diabetes Care* 1992; 15: 737–754.

41. Lebovitz HE, Melander A. Sulfonylureas: basic aspects and clinical uses. In Alberti KGMM, Zimmet P, DeFronzo RA, Keen H, Eds. *International Textbook of Diabetes Mellitus*. 2nd ed. Chichester, John Wiley & Sons, 1997: 817–840.

42. Rendell M. The role of sulphonylureas in the management of type 2 diabetes mellitus. *Drugs* 2004; 64: 1339–1358.

43. Groop L, Neugebauer G. Clinical pharmacology of sulfonylureas. In Kuhlmann J, Puls W, Eds. Oral antidiabetics. *Handbook of Experimental Pharmacology*. Vol. 119. Berlin, Springer, 1996: 199–259.

44. Del Prato S, Tiengo A. The importance of first-phase insulin secretion: implications for the therapy of type 2 diabetes mellitus. *Diabetes Metab Res Rev* 2001; 17: 164–174.

45. Sartor G, Melander A, Scherstén B, Wahlin-Boll E. Influence of food and age on the single-dose kinetics and effects of tolbutamide and chlorpropamide. *Eur J Clin Pharmacol* 1980; 17: 285–293.

46. Silins RA, Butcher MA, Marlin GE. Improved effect of tolbutamide when given before food in patients on long-term therapy (letter). *Br J Clin Pharmacol* 1984; 18: 647–648.
47. Sartor G, Melander A, Scherstén B, Wahlin-Boll E. Serum glibenclamide in diabetic patients and influence of food on the kinetics and effects of glibenclamide. *Diabetologia* 1980; 18: 17–22.
48. Sartor G, Lundquist I, Melander A, Schersten B, Wahlin-Boll E. Improved effect of glibenclamide on administration before breakfast. *Eur J Clin Pharmacol* 1982; 21: 403–408.
49. Batch J, Ma A, Bird D, Noble R, Charles B, Ravenscroft P, Cameron D. The effects of ingestion time of gliclazide in relationship to meals on plasma glucose, insulin and C-peptide levels. *Eur J Clin Pharmacol* 1990; 38: 465–467.
50. Sartor G, Melander A, Scherstén B, Wahlin-Boll E. Comparative single-dose kinetics and effects of four sulfonylureas in healthy volunteers. *Acta Med Scand* 1980; 208: 301–307.
51. Wahlin-Boll E, Melander A, Sartor G, Scherstén B. Influence of food intake on the absorption and effect of glipizide in diabetics and healthy subjects. *Eur J Clin Pharmacol* 1980; 18: 279–283.
52. Talaulicar M, Willms B. Investigations on Glurenorm blood levels. *Diab Croat* 1976; 5: 613–622.
53. Rosskamp R, Wernicke-Panten K, Draeger E. Clinical profile of the novel sulphonylurea glimepiride. *Diab Res Clin Pract* 1996; 31 Suppl: S33–S42.
54. Malerczyk V, Badian M, Korn A, Lehr K-H, Waldhäusl W. Dose linearity assessment of glimepriride (Amaryl®) tablets in healthy volunteers. *Drug Metab Drug Interactions* 1994; 11: 341–357.
55. Rosskamp R, Herz M. Effect of the time of ingestion of the sulfonylurea glimepiride on the daily blood glucose profile in NIDDM-patients (abstract). *Proceedings of the 15th International Federation Congress*, Kobe, Japan, 1994, No. 10A5PP1050.
56. Langtry HD, Balfour JA. Glimepiride: a review of its use in the management of type 2 diabetes mellitus. *Drugs* 1998; 55: 563-584.
57. McCall AL. Clinical review of glimepiride. *Expert Opin Pharmacother* 2001; 2: 699-713.
58. Palmer KJ, Brodgen RN. Gliclazide, an update on its pharmacological properties and therapeutic efficacy in non-insulin-dependent diabetes mellitus. *Drugs* 1993; 46: 92–125.
59. Ishibashi F, Takashina S. The effect of timing on gliclazide absorption and action. *Hiroshima J Med Sci* 1990; 39: 7–9.
60. Mc Gavin JK, Perry CM, Goa KL. Gliclazide modified release. *Drugs* 2002; 62: 1357–1364.
61. Delrat P, Paraire M, Jochemsen R. Complete bioavailability and lack of food effect on pharmacokinetics of gliclazide 30 mg modified release in healthy volunteers. *Biopharm Drug Dispos* 2002; 23: 151–157.
62. Fitzgerald MG, Gaddie R, Malins JM, O'Sullivan DJ. Alcohol sensitivity in diabetics receiving chlorpropamide. *Diabetes* 1962; 11: 40–43.
63. Groop L, Eriksson CJP, Huupponen R, Ylikahri R, Pelkonen R. Roles of chlorpropamide, alcohol and acetaldehyde in determining the chlorpropamide-alcohol flush. *Diabetologia* 1984; 26: 34–38.

64. Hermann LS. Metformin: a review of its pharmacological properties and therapeutic use. *Diab Metab* 1979; 5: 233–245.
65. Caspary WF. Biguanides and intestinal absorption function. *Act Hep Gastr* 1977; 24: 473–480.
66. Dunn CJ, Peters DH. Metformin A review of its pharmacological properties and therapeutic use in non-insulin-dependent diabetes mellitus. *Drugs* 1995; 49: 721–749.
67. Cusi K, DeFronzo RA. Metformin: a review of its metabolic effects. *Diabetes Rev* 1998; 6: 89–131.
68. Setter SM, Iltz JL, Thams J, Campbell RK. Metformin hydrochloride in the treatment of type 2 diabetes mellitus: a clinical review with a focus on dual therapy. *Clin Ther* 2003; 25: 2991–3027.
69. Scheen AJ. Clinical pharmacokinetics of metformin. *Clin Pharmacokin* 1996; 30: 359–371.
70. Brookes LG, Sambol NC, Lin ET, Gee W, Benet LZ. Effect of dosage form, dose and food on the pharmacokinetics of metformin (abstract). *Pharm Res* 1991; 8 (Suppl): 32.
71. Berchtold P, Dahlqvist A, Gustafson A, Asp NG. Effects of a biguanide (metformin) on vitamin B_{12} and folic acid absorption and intestinal enzyme activities. *Scand J Gastroenterol* 1971; 6: 751–754.
72. Carpentier J-L, Bury J, Luyckx A, Lefèbvre P. Vitamin B_{12} and folic acid serum levels in diabetics under various therapeutic regimens. *Diab Metab* 1976; 2: 187–190.
73. Tomkin GH, Hadden DR, Weaver JA, Montgomery DAD. Vitamin B_{12} status in patients on long-term metformin therapy. *Br Med J* 1971; 2: 685–687.
74. Adams JF, Clark JS, Ireland JT, Kesson CM, Watson WS. Malabsorption of vitamin B_{12} and intrinsic factor secretion during biguanide therapy. *Diabetologia* 1983; 24: 16–18.
75. Callaghan TS, Hadden DR, Tomkin GH. Megaloblastic anaemia due to vitamin B_{12} malabsorption associated with long-term metformin treatment. *Br Med J* 1980; 280: 1214–1215.
76. Diabetes Prevention Program Research Group. Reduction in the incidence of type 2 diabetes with lifestyle intervention or metformin. *N Engl J Med* 2002; 346: 393–403.
77. Diamant M, Heine RJ. Thiazolidinediones in type 2 diabetes mellitus: current clinical evidence. *Drugs* 2003; 63: 1373–1405.
78. Meriden T. Progress with thiazolidinediones in the management of type 2 diabetes mellitus. *Clin Ther* 2004; 26: 177–190.
79. Yki-Järvinen H. Thiazolidinediones. *N Engl J Med* 2004; 351: 1106–1118.
80. Gurnell M, Savage DB, Chatterjee VKK, O'Rahilly S. The metabolic syndrome: peroxisome proliferator-activated receptor γ and its therapeutic modulation. *J Clin Endocrinol Metab* 2003; 88: 2412–2421
81. Gillies PS, Dunn CJ. Pioglitazone. *Drugs* 2000; 60: 333–343.
82. Chilcott J, Tappenden P, Jones ML, Wight JP. A systematic review of the clinical effectiveness of pioglitazone in the treatment of type 2 diabetes mellitus. *Clin Ther* 2001; 23: 1792–1823.
83. Balfour JA, Plosker GL. Rosiglitazone. *Drugs* 1999; 57: 921–930.
84. Wagstaff AJ, Goa KL. Rosiglitazone. A review of its use in the management of type 2 diabetes mellitus. *Drugs* 2002; 62: 1805–1837.

85. Braunstein S. New developments in type 2 diabetes mellitus: combination therapy with a thiazolidinedione. *Clin Ther* 2003; 25: 1895–1917.
86. Eckland DA, Danhof M. Clinical pharmacokinetics of pioglitazone. *Exp Clin Endocrinol Diab* 2000; 108 (Suppl 2): S234–242.
87. Cox PJ, Ryan DA, Hollis FJ, Harris A-M, Miller AK, Vousden M, Cowley H. Absorption, disposition, and metabolism of rosiglitazone, a potent thiazolidinedione insulin sensitizer, in humans. *Drug Metab Dispos* 2000; 28: 772–780.
88. Sahi J, Black CB, Hamilton GA, Zheng X, Jolley S, Rose KA, Gilbert D, LeCluyse EL, Sinz MW. Comparative effects of thiazolidinediones on *in vitro* P450 enzyme induction and inhibition. *Drug Metab Dispos* 2003; 31: 439–446.
89. Freed MI, Allen A, Jorkasky DK, DiCicco RA. Systemic exposure to rosiglitazone is unaltered by food. *Eur J Clin Pharmacol* 1999; 55: 53–56.
90. Geerlof JS, Lebrizzi R, Carey RA. Effect of food on the pharmacokinetics of pioglitazone (abstract). *Diabetes* 2000; 49 (Suppl 1): A357.
91. Lebovitz HE. α-glucosidase inhibitors as agents in the treatment of diabetes. *Diabetes Rev* 1998; 6: 132–145.
92. Clissold SP, Edwards C. Acarbose. A preliminary review of its pharmacodynamic and pharmacokinetic properties, and therapeutic potential. *Drugs* 1988; 35: 214–243.
93. Balfour JA, McTavish D. Acarbose — an update of its pharmacology and therapeutic use in diabetes mellitus. *Drugs* 1993; 46: 1025–1054.
94. Salvatore T, Giugliano D. Pharmacokinetic–pharmacodynamic relationships of acarbose. *Clin Pharmacokinet* 1996; 30: 94–106.
95. Scott LJ, Spencer CM. Miglitol: a review of its therapeutic potential in type 2 diabetes mellitus. *Drugs* 2000; 59: 521–549.
96. Scheen AJ. Clinical efficacy of acarbose in the treatment of diabetes: a critical review of controlled trials. *Diab Metab* 1998; 24: 311–320.
97. Breuer H-WM. Review of acarbose therapeutic strategies in the long-term treatment and in the prevention of type 2 diabetes. *Int J Clin Pharmacol Ther* 2003; 41: 421–440.
98. Toeller M. Nutritional recommendations for diabetic patients and treatment with α-glucosidase inhibitors. *Drugs* 1992; 44 (Suppl 3): 13–20.
99. Hara T, Nakamura J, Koh N, Sakakibara F, Takeuchi N, Hotta N. An importance of carbohydrate ingestion for the expression of the effect of α-glucosidase inhibitor in NIDDM. *Diabetes Care* 1996; 19: 642–647.
100. Wolever TMS, Chiasson JL, Josse RG, Hunt JA, Palmason C, Rodger NW, Ross SA, Ryan EA, Tan MH. No relationship between carbohydrate intake and effect of acarbose on HbA1c or gastrointestinal symptoms in type 2 diabetic subjects consuming 30–60% of energy from carbohydrate. *Diabetes Care* 1998; 21: 1612–1618.
101. Lindström J, Tuomilehto J, Spengler M, for the Finnish Acarbose Study Group. Acarbose treatment does not change the habitual diet of patients with type 2 diabetes mellitus. *Diabet Med* 2000; 17: 20–25.
102. Tuomilehto J, Pohjola M, Lindström J, Aro A. Acarbose and nutrient intake in non-insulin dependent diabetes mellitus. *Diabetes Res Clin Pract* 1994; 26: 215–222.

103. Wolever TM, Chiasson JL, Josse RG, Hunt JA, Palmason C, Rodger NW, Ross SA, Ryan EA, Tan MH. Small weight loss on long-term acarbose therapy with no change in dietary pattern or nutrient intake of individuals with non-insulin-dependent diabetes. *Int J Obes* 1997; 21: 756–763.

104. Van Gaal L, Nobels F, De Leeuw I. Effects of acarbose on carbohydrate metabolism, electrolytes, minerals and vitamins in fairly well-controlled non-insulin-dependent diabetes mellitus. *Z Gastroenterol* 1991; 29: 642–644.

105. Dornhorst A. Insulinotropic meglitinide analogues. *Lancet* 2001; 358: 1709–1716.

106. Owens DR. Repaglinide — prandial glucose regulator: a new class of oral antidiabetic drug. *Diabetic Med* 1998; 15 Suppl. 4: S28–S36.

107. Cully CR, Jarvis B. Repaglinide: a review of its therapeutic use in type 2 diabetes mellitus. *Drugs* 2001; 61: 1625–1660.

108. Dunn CJ, Faulds D. Nateglinide. *Drugs* 2000; 60: 607–615.

109. Norman P, Rabasseda X. Nateglinide: a structurally novel insulin secretion agent. *Drugs of Today* 2001; 37 Suppl. F: 1–16.

110. Hatorp V. Clinical pharmacokinetics and pharmacodynamics of repaglinide. *Clin Pharmacokinet* 2002; 41: 471–483.

111. Bidstrup TB, Bjornsdottir I, Sidelman UG, Thomsen MS, Hansen KT. CYP2C8 and CYP3A4 are the principal enzymes involved in the human *in vitro* biotransformation of the insulin secretagogue repaglinide. *Br J Clin Pharmacol* 2003; 56: 305–314.

112. Weaver ML, Orwig BA, Rodriguez LC, Graham ED, Chin JA, Shapiro MJ, McLeod JF, Mangold JB. Pharmacokinetics and metabolism of nateglinide in humans. *Drug Metab Dispos* 2001; 29: 415–421.

113. McLeod JF. Clinical pharmacokinetics of nateglinide. A rapidly-absorbed, short-acting insulinotropic agent. *Clin Pharmacokinet* 2004; 43: 97–120.

114. Hatorp V, Bayer T. Repaglinide bioavailability in the fed or fasting state (abstract). *J Clin Pharmacol* 1997; 37: 875.

115. Damsbo P, Marbury TC, Hatorp V, Clauson P, Müller PG. Flexible prandial glucose regulation with repaglinide in patients with Type 2 diabetes. *Diabetes Res Clin Pract* 1999; 45: 31–39.

116. Keilson L, Mather S, Walter YH, Subramanian S, McLeod JF. Synergistic effects of nateglinide and meal administration on insulin secretion in patients with type 2 diabetes mellitus. *J Clin Endocrinol Metab* 2000; 85: 1081–1086.

117. Karara AH, Dunning BE, McLeod JF. The effect of food on the oral bioavailability and the pharmacodynamic actions on the insulinotropic agent nateglinide in healthy subjects. *J Clin Pharmacol* 1999; 39: 172–179.

118. Luzio SD, Anderson DM, Owens DR. Effects of timing of administration and meal composition on the pharmacokinetic and pharmacodynamic characteristic of the short-acting oral hypoglycemic agent nateglinide in healthy subjects. *J Clin Endocrinol Metab* 2001; 86: 4874–4880.

119. Alemani M, Remesar X, Fernandez-Lopez JA. Drug strategies for the treatment of obesity. *Drugs* 2003; 6: 566–572.

120. McNeely W, Benfield P. Orlistat. *Drugs* 1998; 56: 241–249.

121. O'Meara S, Riemsma R, Shirran L, Mather L, ter Riet G. A systematic review of the clinical effectiveness of orlistat used for the management of obesity. *Obesity Rev* 2004; 5: 51–68.

122. Scheen AJ, Ernest PH. Antiobesity treatment in type 2 diabetes: results of clinical trials with orlistat and sibutramine. *Diabetes Metab* 2002; 28: 437–445.

123. Torgerson JS, Hauptman J, Boldrin MN, Sjöström L. Xenical in the Prevention of Diabetes in Obese Subjects (XENDOS) study. A randomized study of orlistat as an adjunct to lifestyle for the prevention of type 2 diabetes in obese patients. *Diabetes Care* 2004; 27: 155–161.

124. Muls E, Kolanowski J, Scheen A, Van Gaal L, for the Obelhyx Study Group. The effects of orlistat on weight and on serum lipids in obese patients with hypercholesterolemia: a randomized, double-blind, placebo-controlled, multicenter study. *Int J Obesity* 2001; 25: 1713–1721.

125. Hauptman JB, Jeunet FS, Hartmann D. Initial studies in humans with the novel gastrointestinal lipase inhibitor ro-18-0647 (tetrahydrolipstatin). *Am J Clin Nutr* 1992; 55 Suppl: 309–313.

126. Guzelhan C, Odink J, Niestijl Jansen-Zuidema JJ, Hartmann D. Influence of dietary composition on the inhibition of fat absorption by orlistat. *J Int Med Res* 1994; 22: 255–265.

127. Hartmann D, Hussain Y, Guzelhan C, Odink J. Effect on dietary fat absorption of orlistat, administered at different times relative to meal intake. *Br J Clin Pharmacol* 1993; 36: 266–270.

128. Melia AT, Koss-Twardy SG, Zhi J. The effect of orlistat, an inhibitor of dietary fat absorption, on the absorption of vitamins A and E in healthy volunteers. *J Clin Pharmacol* 1996; 36: 647–653.

129. Drent ML, Larsson I, William-Olsson T, Quaade F, Czubayko F, von Bergmann K, Strobel W, Sjostrom L, van der Veen EA. Orlistat (RO 18-0647), a lipase inhibitor, in the treatment of human obesity: a multiple dose study. *Int J Obesity* 1995; 19: 221–226.

130. Zhi Zhi J, Melia AT, Guerciolini R, Koss-Twardy SG, Passe SM, Rakhit A, Sadowski JA. The effect of orlistat, an inhibitor of dietary fat absorption, on the pharmacokinetics of beta-carotene in healthy volunteers. *J Clin Pharmacol* 1996; 36: 152–159.

131. Sjostrom L, Rissanen A, Andersen T, Boldrin M, Golay A, Koppeschaar HP, Krempf M, for the European Multicentre Orlistat Study Group. Randomized placebo-controlled trial of orlistat for weight loss and prevention of weight regain in obese patients. *Lancet* 1998; 352: 167–173.

132. McNeely W, Goa KL. Sibutramine. A review of its contribution to the management of obesity. *Drugs* 1998; 56: 1093–1124.

133. James WP, Astrup A, Finer N, Hilsted J, Kopelman P, Rossner S, Saris WH, Van Gaal LF, for the Storm Study Group. Effect of sibutramine on weight maintenance after weight loss: a randomized trial. *Lancet* 2000; 356: 2119–2125.

134. O'Meara S, Riemsma R, Shirran L, Mather L, ter Riet G. The clinical effectiveness and cost-effectiveness of sibutramine in the management of obesity: a technology assessment. *Health Technol Assess* 2002; 6: 1–97.

135. Rolls BJ, Shide DJ, Thorwart ML, Ulbrecht JS. Sibutramine reduces food intake in non-dieting women with obesity. *Obes Res* 1998; 6: 1–11.

136. Chapelot D, Marmonier C, Himaya A, Hanotin C, Thomas F. Modalities of the food intake-reducing effect of sibutramine (abstract). *Int J Obes* 1998; 22 (Suppl 3): S270.

137. Saris WHM, STORM Study Group. Sibutramine trial of obesity reduction and maintenance. Lifestyle and diet during the 6-month run-in phase (abstract). *Int J Obes* 1998; 22 (Suppl 3): S271.

138. Garratt CJ, Hind ID, Haddock RE. Sibutramine metabolite bioavailability: effect of dose level and food (abstract). *J Clin Pharmacol* 1995; 35: 927.

139. Knopp R. Drug treatment of lipid disorders. *N Engl J Med* 1999; 341: 498–511.

140. Evans M, Roberts A, Davies S, Rees A. Medical lipid-lowering therapy: current evidence, ongoing trials and future developments. *Drugs* 2004; 64: 1181–1196.

141. Law MR, Wald NJ, Rudnicka AR. Quantifying effect of statins on low density lipoprotein cholesterol, ischaemic heart disease, and stroke: systematic review and meta-analysis. *BMJ* 2003; 326: 1423–1427.

142. Bonetti PO, Lerman LO, Napoli C, Lerman A. Statin effects beyond lipid lowering —are they clinically relevant? *Eur Heart J* 2003; 24: 225–248.

143. Snow V, Aronson MD, Hornbake ER, Mottur-Pilson C, Weiss KB, for the Clinical Efficacy Assessment Subcommittee of the American College of Physicians. Lipid control in the management of type 2 diabetes mellitus: a clinical practice guideline from the American College of Physicians. *Ann Intern Med* 2004; 140: 644–649.

144. Steiner G. Fibrates in the metabolic syndrome and in diabetes. *Endocrinol Metab Clin North Am* 2004; 33: 545–555.

145. Bays HE, Dujovne CA. Drug interactions of lipid-altering drugs. *Drug Saf* 1998; 9: 355–371.

146. Williams D, Feely J. Pharmacokinetic–pharmacodynamic drug interactions with HMG-CoA reductase inhibitors. *Clin Pharmacokinet* 2002; 41: 343–370.

147. Martin J, Krum H. Cytochrome P450 drug interactions within the HMG-CoA reductase inhibitor class: are they clinically relevant? *Drug Safety* 2003; 26: 13–21.

148. Bellosta S, Paoletti R, Corsini A. Safety of statins. Focus on clinical pharmaco-kinetics and drug interactions. *Circulation* 2004; 109 (Suppl. III): III50–57.

149. Dobrinska MR, Stubbs RJ, Gregg MH, et al. Effects of dose and food on HMG-CoA reductase inhibitor profiles after lovastatin (mevacor) (abstract). *Pharm Res* 1988; 5: S182.

150. Richter WO, Jacob BG, Schwandt P. Interaction between fibre and lovastatin (letter). *Lancet* 1991; 338: 706.

151. Pan HY, DeVault AR, Brescia D, Willard DA, McGovern ME, Whigan DB, Ivashkiv E. Effect of food on pravastatin pharmacokinetics and pharmacodynam-ics. *Int J Clin Pharmacol Ther Toxicol* 1993; 31: 291–294.

152. Radulovic LL, Cilla DD, Posvar EL, Sedman AJ, Whitfield LR. Effect of food on the bioavailability of atorvastatin, an HMG-CoA reductase inhibitor. *J Clin Phar-macol* 1995; 35: 990–994.

153. Whitfield LR, Stern RH, Sedman AJ, Abel R, Gibson DM. Effect of food on the pharmacodynamics and pharmacokinetics of atorvastatin, an inhibitor of HMG-CoA reductase. *Eur J Drug Metab Pharmacokinet* 2000; 25: 97–101.

154. Dujovne CA, Davidson MH. Fluvastatin administration at bedtime versus the evening meal: a multicenter comparison of bioavailability, safety, and efficacy. *Am J Med* 1994; 96 (Suppl 6A): S37–40.

155. Kantola T, Kivisto KT, Neuvonen PJ. Grapefruit juice greatly increases serum concentrations of lovastatin and lovastatin acid. *Clin Pharmacol Ther* 1998; 63: 397–402.

156. Lilja JJ, Kivisto KT, Neuvonen PJ. Grapefruit juice increases serum concentrations of atorvastatin and has no effect on pravastatin. *Clin Pharmacol Ther* 1999; 66: 118–127.

157. Lilja JJ, Kivisto KT, Neuvonen PJ. Grapefruit juice–simvastatin interaction: effect on serum concentrations of simvastatin, simvastatin acid, and HMG-CoA reductase inhibitors. *Clin Pharmacol Ther* 1998; 64: 477–483.

158. Rogers JD, Zhao J, Liu L, Amin RD, Gagliano KD, Porras AG, Blum RA, Wilson MF, Stepanavage M, Vega JM. Grapefruit juice has minimal effects on plasma concentrations of lovastatin-derived 3-hydroxy-3-methylglutaryl coenzyme A reductase inhibitors. *Clin Pharmacol Ther* 1999; 66: 358–366.

159. Kane GC, Lipsky JJ. Drug-grapefruit juice interactions. *Mayo Clin Proc* 2000; 75: 933–942.

160. Rosenson RS. Rosuvastatin: a new inhibitor of HMG-coA reductase for the treatment of dyslipidemia. *Expert Rev Cardiovasc Ther* 2003; 1: 495–505.

161. Todd PA, Ward A. Gemfibrozil. A review of its pharmacodynamic and pharmacokinetic properties, and therapeutic use in dyslipidaemia. *Drugs* 1988; 36: 314–339.

162. Spencer CM, Barradell LB. Gemfibrozil. A reappraisal of its pharmacological properties and place in the management of dyslipidaemia. *Drugs* 1996; 51: 982–1018.

163. Balfour JA, McTavish D, Heel RC. Fenofibrate. A review of its pharmacodynamic and pharmacokinetic properties and therapeutic use in dyslipidemia. *Drugs* 1990; 40: 260–290.

164. Adkins JC, Faulds D. Micronized fenofibrate: A review of its pharmacodynamic properties and clinical efficacy in the management of dyslipidaemia. *Drugs* 1997; 54: 615–633.

165. Najib J. Fenofibrate in the treatment of dyslipidemia: a review of the data as they relate to the new suprabioavailable tablet formulation. *Clin Ther* 2002; 24: 2022–2050.

166. Miller DB, Spence JD. Clinical pharmacokinetics of fibric acid derivatives (fibrates). *Clin Pharmacokinet* 1998; 34: 155–162.

167. Luner PE, Babu SR, Radebaugh GW. The effects of bile salts and lipids on the physicochemical behavior of gemfibrozil. *Pharm Res* 1994; 11: 1755–1760.

168. Keating GM, Ormrod D. Micronized fenofibrate. An updated review of its clinical efficacy in the management of dyslipidaemia. *Drugs* 2002; 62: 1909–1944.

169. Abbott Laboratories. TricorR (fenofibrate capsules) prescribing information [on line]. Available from URL: http://www.tricorx.com [Accessed 2002 March 5].

170. Bays H. Ezetimibe. *Expert Opin Invest Drugs* 2002; 11: 1587–1604.

171. Jeu LA, Cheng JWM. Pharmacology and therapeutics of ezetimibe (SCH 58235), a cholesterol-absorption inhibitor. *Clin Ther* 2003; 25: 2352–2387.

172. Courtney RD, Kosoglou T, Statkevich P, et al. Effect of food on the oral bioavailability of ezetimibe (abstract). *Clin Pharmacol Ther* 2002; 71: 80.

173. Punwani N, Pai S, Bach C, et al. Effect of food on oral bioavailability of SCH 58235 in healthy male volunteers (abstract). *AAPS Pharm Sci* 1998; 1: 2147.

174. Dujovne C, Held J, Lipka L, et al. Does cholesterol and/or fat intake affect plasma lipid efficacy of ezetimibe? (abstract). *J Am Coll Cardiol* 2002; 39 (Suppl A): 227A.

175. Cater NB. Historical and scientific basis for the development of plant stanol ester foods as cholesterol-lowering agents. *Eur Heart J* 1999; 1: S36–44.

176. Blair SN, Capuzzi DM, Gottlieb SO, Nguyen T, Morgan JM, Cater NB. Incremental reduction of serum total cholestrol and low-density lipoprotein cholesterol with the addition of plant stanol ester-containing spread to statin therapy. *Am J Cardiol* 2000; 86: 46–52.

177. Vorlat A, Conraads VM, Vrints CJ. Regular use of margarine-containing stanol/ste-
     rol esters reduces total and low-density lipoprotein (LDL) cholesterol and allows
     reduction of statin therapy after cardiac transplantation: preliminary observations.
     J Heart Lung Transplant 2003; 22:1059–1062.

2 Hypolipidemic Therapy: Drugs, Diet, and Interactive Effects

Alexandre Loktionov

CONTENTS

2.1 INTRODUCTION

In the past, the relationship between dietary factors and cardiovascular disease (CVD) was often regarded as primarily and almost exclusively dependent on lipid (especially saturated fat and cholesterol) consumption and metabolism leading to increased serum cholesterol; in particular, low density lipoprotein (LDL) levels resulting in atherosclerotic vascular changes. This idea constituted the core of the traditional "diet–heart" hypothesis.[1] With the development of scientific knowledge on both CVD pathogenesis and bioactive properties of nutrients, the field is rapidly becoming more and more complicated. The range of known pathways and mechanisms contributing to the development of atherosclerosis and CVD has considerably expanded.[2–5] Indeed, the term CVD is now equally applied to different vascular events occurring in different vascular locations (coronary heart disease, cerebrovascular disease, peripheral vascular disorders).[5] Consequently, there is a definite trend to regard a complex of multiple factors and conditions predisposing to atherosclerosis development and its cardiovascular manifestations (lipid-related and general metabolic disorders, inflammation, high blood pressure, increased blood coagulation, etc.) as an extended area of active CVD prevention and treatment. The metabolic syndrome, which is defined as a combination of such common disorders as obesity, insulin resistance, glucose intolerance, hypertension, and dyslipidemia manifested by hypertriglyceridemia and low high density lipoprotein (HDL) cholesterol levels,[6–8] has already become highly prevalent in the U.S.[9] and is regarded as a warning sign of a forthcoming new CVD epidemic.[7,8]

In addition to known links between nutrition and atherosclerosis, it became clear that all conditions constituting the metabolic syndrome are diet-dependent; therefore, assessment of CVD risk modulation by food ingredients requires a thorough consideration of multiple overlapping effects of nutritional influences at the level of different mechanisms contributing to the development of CVD. Additional emerging factors in CVD pathogenesis, such as hyperhomocysteinemia,[5,10,11] inflammation,[5,12,13] oxidative stress,[5,14–16] and others,[5,10] are also affected by diet, thus the area of dietary modulation of CVD risk looks extremely complex. The complexity becomes even higher when problems of CVD treatment with pharmaceutical agents, nutritional preventive/therapeutic approaches, and drug–diet interactions are considered. For this reason, separate analysis of different aspects of the problem appears to be justified.

This chapter is going to be devoted mostly to the analysis of hyperlipidemia and dyslipidemia treatment using both medicamentous therapy and dietary modifications. Emerging problems associated with the introduction of combined problems are also addressed.

2.2 THERAPY OF CVD WITH HYPOCHOLESTEROLEMIC AND HYPOLIPIDEMIC DRUGS

Persistent hyperlipidemia and dyslipidemia is regarded as the leading pathogenetic factor in the development of atherosclerosis and CVD. Recent progress in the field of therapeutic management of hyperlipidemia has resulted in the emergence of a number of potent hypolipidemic agents. Currently several main groups of drugs employed for dyslipidemia treatment can be defined as:

1. 3-hydroxy-3-methylglutaryl coenzyme A (HMG-CoA) reductase inhibitirs (statins)
2. Fibric acid derivatives (fibrates)
3. Bile acid transport inhibitors

4. Niacin (nicotinic acid)
5. Cholesterol absorption inhibitors[17]

Their mechanisms of action and clinical characteristics are briefly considered below.

2.2.1 HMG-CoA Reductase Inhibitors (Statins)

Suppression of cholesterol biosynthesis by HMG-CoA reductase inhibitors derived from fungal metabolites was discovered in 1976.[18] Since that time, the family of statins has expanded and now includes natural products of fungal origin (lovastatin, pravastatin), a semisynthetic derivative (simvastatin), and entirely synthetic drugs (fluvastatin, atorvastatin, rosuvastatin, pitavastatin).[17,19,20] Cerivastatin was withdrawn from clinical practice in 2001 because of adverse effect risk.[21]

The main hypolipidemic effect of statins is exerted through competitive inhibition of the binding of HMG-CoA at the catalytic site of HMG-CoA reductase, the enzyme catalyzing the conversion of HMG-CoA to mevalonate, a sterol precursor important for cholesterol synthesis.[19] Reduced cholesterol biosynthesis results in up-regulation of LDL receptors in the liver and stimulation of LDL clearance from the plasma.[22] It has also been reported that statins decrease hepatic production of very low density lipoproteins (VLDL) and increase catabolism of VLDL remnants.[23] It is, however, apparent now that in addition to direct suppression of lipid biosynthesis, statins influence multiple pathogenetic mechanisms involved in the development of atherosclerosis, CVD, and other chronic conditions, especially those related to the metabolic syndrome.[23] Figure 2.1 schematically presents pleiotropic beneficial effects of statins. Detailed consideration of mechanisms involved in such effects is beyond the scope of this chapter. Interested readers can be addressed to several recent reviews in the field.[15,17,24–26]

Statins are presently the most widely used hypolipidemic drugs. Several clinical trials confirmed their efficiency in both blood lipid lowering and cardiovascular risk reduction with regard to coronary heart disease (CHD),[27–31] cerebrovascular disease,[30–33] and cardiovascular complications of diabetes mellitus.[30,31,34,35] Decrease of the progression of atherosclerosis and even regression of atherosclerotic arterial changes have also been reported.[19,26]

Drugs of this group are usually well tolerated, although such side effects as hepatotoxicity, myotoxicity, and nephrotoxicity have been described.[19] Among other statins, cerivastatin was associated with much higher risk of rhabdomyolysis, especially when applied in combination with gemfibrozil.[21] Carcinogenicity of statins in experimental rodents has been described;[36] however, no evidence of this effect in humans is available. Statins are metabolized by enzymes of the cytochrome P450 (CYP) family. Among them, CYP3A4 is especially important for several statins. As this enzyme is known to be involved in the metabolism of many other drugs and some dietary components, a background for interactive

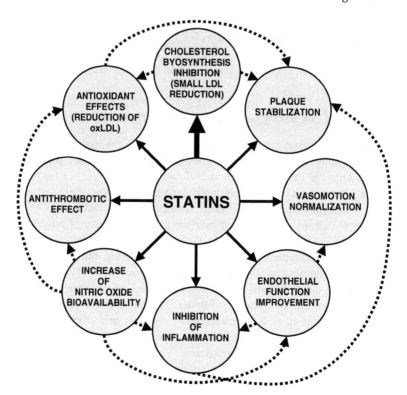

FIGURE 2.1 Pleiotropic beneficial effects of statin therapy. (Dotted arrows indicate interactive links between different mechanisms.)

effects exists.[17] Dietary influences on statin effects are possible and will be considered later in this chapter.

2.2.2 Fibric Acid Derivatives (Fibrates)

The clinical benefit of the use of fibrates is related primarily to the reduction of triglyceride levels and, to some extent, the elevation of blood HDL cholesterol concentration.[37–39] The principal mechanism of fibrate action is defined by their ability to mimic the biological function of free fatty acids (FA) through the specific binding to peroxisome proliferator-activated receptor α (PPARα). PPARα activation affects expression of multiple genes, products of which are involved in lipid metabolism. Hypolipidemic action of fibrate-activated PPARα is exerted through several regulatory pathways, predominantly acting in the liver, including stimulation of FA uptake, their cellular retention, and modulation of the expression of coenzyme A synthetase catalyzing the esterification of FAs. Also, activated PPARα induces mitochondrial FA uptake and catabolism as well as the activity of lipoprotein lipase (LPL), while inhibiting the expression of its antagonist apoC-III.[39,40]

The role of activated PPARα in HDL level modulation is less clear; however, it is believed that induction of the transcription of ApoA-I and Apo A-II lipoproteins in hepatocytes may contribute to the increase of plasma HDL concentrations and a more efficient reverse cholesterol transport.[39,40] Given that PPARs are known to exert multiple biological effects, it is not surprising that a growing body of information regarding pleiotropic effects of fibrates now emerges. Antiinflammatory action and favorable effects on both blood coagulation and fibrinolysis system[40] look especially interesting from a clinical point of view. It is also important to stress that other members of the PPAR family, especially PPARγ, are deeply involved in lipid metabolism regulation. PPARγ agonists of the thiazolidinedione family are already in use for the treatment of diabetes mellitus; however, their hypolipidemic potential has recently emerged as a promising sign for the development of new approaches to CVD treatment.[41] Perspectives of developing new drugs combining PPARα and PPARγ agonist activity[39] may provide a new step in this direction.

Four members of the fibrate family are now in wide clinical use: bezafibrate, ciprofibrate, fenofibrate, and gemfibrosil.[37] Drugs of this group are especially efficient in combination with statins or as monotherapy in patients with normal LDL cholesterol levels, in particular for the treatment of cardiovascular manifestations of the metabolic syndrome.[37,42–44] Although fibrates are demonstrated to be well tolerated in most cases, a few side effects, including changes of hepatic function (hepatic transaminase level elevation), gastrointestinal side effects, and myopathy have been reported.[45,46] Some effects have been associated with particular members of the fibrate family, like rhabdomyolysis with gemfibrozil[35,47] or hyperhomocysteinemia with fenofibrate.[48] Like statins, fibrates have been shown to be carcinogenic in rodents;[36] however, there is no clinical information on this potential problem. It has also been repeatedly stressed that combined hypolipidemic therapy with statins and fibrates may be associated with drug interactions and higher risk of adverse effects.[35,49] Dietary influences should be taken into account in this context and will be discussed later in this chapter.

2.2.3 BILE ACID TRANSPORT INHIBITORS

This heterogenous group of drugs' principle of action is based on the fact that blocking the intestinal reuptake of bile acids substantially increases the loss of bile acids with feces. The loss is compensated in the liver through conversion of cholesterol to bile, which results in the depletion of hepatocyte cholesterol and upregulation of LDL receptors with hypocholesterolemic effect.[17]

Bile acid-binding resins/sequestrants represent the only clinically important group of drugs inhibiting bile acid reuptake. Initially introduced agents, cholestyramine and colestipol, had gastrointestinal side effects, such as bloating, flatulence, heartburn, and nausea.[50–52] For this reason their use is presently restricted to application of low doses in multidrug treatment schemes. A new member of this family, colesevelam, is much better tolerated and is now recommended as an effective alternative to the two older drugs.[51–53] Colesevelam, which forms nonabsorbable complexes with bile acids in the gastrointestinal tract, has been reported four to six times more potent than other bile acid sequestrants, and especially recommended for combination therapy with statins.[53]

Another family of new drugs affecting bile acid transport is represented by agents inhibiting ileal sodium-dependent bile acid transporter (IBAT), which reduce serum cholesterol level by suppressing the reuptake of bile acids in the ileum. Results from animal experiments with a few synthetic compounds have provided encouraging results;[54–56] however, drugs of this family have not hitherto been introduced into clinical practice.

2.2.4 NIACIN (NICOTINIC ACID)

Niacin (nicotinic acid) is one of the oldest hypolipidemic agents in clinical use; however, its mechanisms of action are still partially unknown. The remarkable feature of niacin is that it acts beneficially on practically all lipoprotein abnormalities.[57–59] It is the most effective medication for increasing HDL cholesterol levels, lowering at the same time atherogenic apolipoprotein B.[59] It has been shown that niacin directly inhibits the activity of hepatic diacylglycerol acyltransferase-2 (DGAT2), which is involved in the synthesis of triglycerides and apolipoprotein B.[60] The HDL cholesterol-elevating effect of niacin is probably caused by selective inhibition of the hepatic removal/uptake of lipoprotein AI particles leading to their increased retention in the circulation.[61] Investigation of the mechanisms of niacin action has recently been stimulated by the identification of nicotinic acid receptors[62–65] apparently mediating suppression of adipocyte lypolisis by niacin.[62,65]

Another recently discovered pathway involves stimulation of prostaglandin D2 (PDG2) formation by niacin, which interacts with PPAR-controlled processes through PPAR activation by a major PDG2 metabolite.[66] It is also interesting to note that several single nucleotide polymorphisms (SNPs) have been identified in the coding regions of niacin receptors defining the five major haplotypes,[67] which well may have potential of modifying biological effects of niacin.

Niacin is currently available in three formulations (immediate-release, extended-release, and long-acting).[58] Immediate-release niacin has well known side effects, including flushing, gastrointestinal symptoms, and hyperglycemia. Long-acting drugs may cause hepatotoxicity, while extended-release niacin is associated with fewer flushing and gastrointestinal manifestations without seriously increasing the risk of hepatotoxicity. Lower doses of niacin are often applied in combinations with other hypolipidemic agents, especially statins.[59] Nevertheless, recent progress in nicotinic acid receptor identification raises hopes of developing new specific drugs mimicking the beneficial action of niacin, but free of its adverse effects.

2.2.5 CHOLESTEROL ABSORPTION INHIBITORS

Wide introduction of statins into clinical practice has resulted in the development of multiple schemes of combined therapy designed to complement the hypolipidemic effects governed by different molecular mechanisms. It became obvious that one potential way to improving statin therapy efficiency would be to reduce intestinal cholesterol absorption, which results in upregulation of statin-inhibited HMGCoA reductase expression.[17]

Ezetimibe, a synthetic 2-azetidinone, is the first of a new class of drugs that selectively inhibits the absorption of cholesterol in the intestine without affecting the absorption of triglycerides. The agent is believed to inhibit a putative cholesterol transporter of enterocytes located within the brush-border membrane of the small intestine.[68] Ezetimibe reduces overall cholesterol delivery to the liver, thus stimulating the expression of LDL receptors and increasing the removal of LDL cholesterol from the serum.

Clinical trials have provided promising results demonstrating efficient cholesterol reduction with the use of the drug as a single agent[69] or as a part of combined therapy with statins[17,70,71] or fibrates.[72] No serious adverse effects associated with the use of ezetimibe have been observed,[17,68–72] making the drug a very attractive component of various schemes of dyslipidemia management.

2.2.6 EMERGING AND FUTURE DIRECTIONS IN HYPOLIPIDEMIC THERAPY

New approaches to hypolipidemic therapy are being developed along several directions that often derive from investigation of mechanisms of action of the clinically approved drugs considered above. Whereas covering this rapidly progressing area is not among the purposes of this chapter, briefly highlighting some of the emerging directions appears to be justified.

Active search is going on in the field of lipid metabolism and transport modulation. It is believed that employment of acyl-coenzyme A cholesterol acyltransferase (ACAT) inhibitors affecting two ACAT subtypes may reduce foam cell formation as well as cholesterol absorption;[17,73] however, initial testing of the first agent of this group (avasimibe) in humans has produced inconsistent results.[17,74] Microsomal triglyceride transport protein (MTP) inhibitors, which should affect the assembly of VLDL, have been successfully tested in animal experiments,[75,76] but have not reached human trials so far. Human studies are being performed on cholesteryl ester transfer protein (CETP) inhibitors, which block the transfer of cholesteryl esters from HDL to apoB-containing lipoproteins, thus elevating HDL levels. Although promising results have been obtained with CETP inhibitors JTT-705 and torcetrapib,[17,77,78] additional clinical studies are needed to evaluate both the safety and efficacy of this therapeutic strategy. Another experimentally tested HDL elevation-directed approach is based upon the use of adenosine triphosphate (ATP)-binding cassette transporter A1 (ABCA1) agonists affecting the initial step in reverse cholesterol transport.[17,73]

Finally, the use of nuclear receptor signaling involved in cholesterol homeostasis control is starting to attract increasing attention with regard to the development of hypolipidemic therapy approaches. PPARs have already been discussed
in this chapter; however, several other transcription regulators, such as sterol
regulatory element-binding proteins (SREBPs), liver X receptors (LXRs), farnesoid X receptor (FXR),[73,79] are considered as probable targets for new drugs.

Brief consideration of therapeutic strategies applied to provide efficient management of CVD-related hyperlypidemia and dyslipidemia has shown considerable diversity of drugs applied for this purpose. The second part of the chapter
is devoted to the analysis of the role of dietary factors in lipid homeostasis
regulation and interactions between diet and hypolipidemic drugs.

2.3 DIETARY FACTORS IN LIPID HOMEOSTASIS AND THEIR INTERACTIONS WITH HYPOLIPIDEMIC DRUGS

Lipid homeostasis directly depends on dietary lipid supply. Consumption of
food rich in cholesterol and saturated fatty acids of animal origin, a typical
feature of traditional Western diets, is a generally recognized atherogenic factor
constituting the cornerstone of the classic "diet–heart" hypothesis.[1] Reduced
intake of saturated fat and cholesterol is regarded as the first element of lifestyle
changes recommended for primary prevention of coronary heart disease (CHD)
and is commonly combined with the use of hypolipidemic drugs for secondary
CHD prevention.[80,81] However, these "restrictive" dietary aspects of lipid-lowering strategies constitute a separate important area and will not be analyzed
here.

Consideration of the effects of drugs and dietary factors as well as interactions
between food and drugs with regard to hypolipidemic treatment in humans is the
principal subject of this chapter. Beneficial biological effects of numerous food
components can be (and are) used for therapeutic purposes, so sometimes the
boundary at which a food ingredient becomes a drug is not well defined.[82]
Furthermore, it should be understood that relationships between dietary and
medicamentous treatment of hyperlipidemia comprise at least two dimensions.
Firstly, both pharmaceutical agents and food constituents may have lipid-lowering
properties, thus their combined effects can constitute synergistic interactions of
the "first type." It is obvious that only those food components that possess natural
hypolipidemic properties will be discussed from this point of view. Secondly,
dietary factors can interfere with the effects of drugs by influencing drug metabolism or regulatory pathways important for proper drug action, therefore causing
either synergistic or antagonistic effects — interactions of the "second type."
These two situations will be considered below.

2.3.1 DIETARY INGREDIENTS POSSESSING NATURAL HYPOLIPIDEMIC AND CARDIOPROTECTIVE PROPERTIES

Description of dietary ingredients naturally possessing hypolipidemic properties is not an easy task since the field is extremely dynamic and still full of controversy. Food constituents with reported hypolipidemic properties are listed in Table 2.1, but in many instances beneficial action of nutrients, in terms of reducing CVD risk, has multiple endpoints and involves physiological pathways unrelated to lipid transport and metabolism. Numerous natural products contain complex combinations of biologically active components simultaneously acting through different interacting mechanisms, so comprehensive analysis of such complicated situations is difficult and sometimes prone to simplistic conclusions. Nevertheless, several major groups of important dietary factors can be easily identified (see Table 2.1).

Over the past several decades, the main feature of nutritional recommendations developed to decrease CVD risk was to limit intake of total fat and saturated fat.[132] It is, however, becoming evident that types of fat consumed rather than total dietary fat are important in determining CVD risk.[80,133,134] Indeed, some human populations have relatively low CVD risk levels despite traditional consumption of meat-based diets rich in fat.[135,136] While there is no doubt in the association between saturated fat intake and elevated serum LDL levels, increased consumption of polyunsaturated fatty acids (PUFA) and to some extent monounsaturated fatty acids (MUFA) has been shown to exert beneficial effects (see Table 2.1). Substitution of unsaturated fatty acids for saturated fat appears to be a logical way to follow with the purpose of developing cardioprotective diets. At the same time, there is little clarity regarding the optimal amounts of MUFA and PUFA in the diet.[80,133] One desirable target is achieving a higher ratio between ω-3 PUFA and ω-6 PUFA by encouraging consumption of foods rich in ω-3 PUFA, such as fish, shellfish, and some plant oils.[80,86,87,133]

The hypothesis suggesting LDL oxidation as a major mechanism involved in the development of atherosclerosis[137] has led to the idea that antioxidants can prevent atherosclerosis by limiting this process. Numerous natural antioxidants have been identified, predominantly in foods of plant origin. Flavonoids and antioxidant vitamins constitute two main groups of dietary antioxidants. Flavonoids are bioactive plant polyphenols exerting various physiologic effects (see Table 2.1). Several studies have demonstrated inverse relationship between flavonoid intake and CVD risk;[95,96,138] however, other groups failed to detect any effect.[93,139,140] Although hypolipidemic properties of distinct flavonoids are being actively investigated, it should be noted that disentangling specific action of each of numerous bioactive components present in most natural foods is hardly possible at the present level of scientific knowledge.

Attempts to find a simple solution to this problem are well illustrated by the use of antioxidant vitamin supplements for CVD prevention. Experimental and epidemiological studies suggested that dietary intake of antioxidant vitamins (vitamin E, vitamin C, β-carotene) may be associated with the decrease in CVD

TABLE 2.1
Dietary Ingredients Exerting Beneficial Influences on Hyperlipidemic and Dyslipidemic Conditions

Active Ingredients	Dietary Sources	Physiological Effects	Refs.
Fatty Acids			
Monounsaturated fatty acids (MUFA): oleic acid (OA)	Canola, olive, safflower, sunflower oils, and nuts, olives, avocado	Mild hypocholesterolemic effect, possible reduction of oxLDL (additional nonlipid beneficial effects possible)	83–85
Omega-6 polyunsaturated fatty acids (ω-6 PUFA): linoleic acid (LA)	Corn, safflower, sunflower oils	Mild hypocholesterolemic effect (downregulation of LDL production and enhancement of its clearance); adverse effects on cytokines and platelet aggregation are not excluded	86–88
Omega-3 polyunsaturated fatty acids (ω-3 PUFA): linoleic acid (ALA)	Canola, flaxseed, soybean oils, walnuts	Mild hypocholesterolemic effect, serum triglyceride lowering effect; additional (nonlipid) beneficial effects include antiarrhythmic (especially EPA and DHA) and probably antithrombotic action.	81, 86, 88, 89–92
Eicosapentaenoic acid (EPA) and docosahexaenoic acid (DHA)	Fish, shellfish		
Flavonoids			
Flavonols: quercetin, kaemprefol, myrocetin, fisetin	Apple, onion, kale, broccoli, cabbage, cherries, berries, tea, red wine	Mild hypocholesterolemic effect; atioxidant action is believed to protect from oxLDL accumulation; additional (nonlipid) effects include antiinflammatory action, reduction of platelet aggregation, improved vascular reactivity, weak estrogenic activity (only isoflavones)	93–98
Flavanols (catechins): catechin, epicatechin, epicatechin 3-gallate, epigallocatechin, epigallocatechin 3-gallate, gallocatechin	Green and black tea, red wine, apples, black chocolate, cocoa		
Flavones: apigenin, luteolin	Parsley, celery, thyme		

TABLE 2.1 (CONTINUED)
Dietary Ingredients Exerting Beneficial Influences on Hyperlipidemic and Dyslipidemic Conditions

Active Ingredients	Dietary Sources	Physiological Effects	Refs.
Flavanones: naringenin, hesperetin, eriodictyol	Oranges, grapefruit, and their juices		
Anthocyanins: (anthocyanidins) Cyanidin, pelargonidin, delphinidin, peonidin, petunidin, malvinidin	Berries, cherries, red wine		
Isoflavones: genistein, daidzein, dihydro-daidzein, O-desmethy-langolensin, equol	Soy and soy-containing foods, chick peas		
Antioxidant Vitamins			
α-Tocopherol (vitamin E)	Vegetable oils (sunflower, olive), nuts, seeds	Experimental evidence of lipid peroxidation inhibition: controversial results regarding protection against CVD in humans	99–105
Ascorbic acid (vitamin C)	Fruit (especially citrus), vegetables	Experimental evidence of lipid peroxidation inhibition: controversial results regarding protection against CVD in humans	99, 100, 102, 104–106
Carotenoids: β-carotene	Green leafy, root, and fruiting vegetables	Antioxidant action was suggested as a protective factor against oxLDL accumulation; antiinflammatory effect possible; controversial results regarding protection against CVD in humans	99, 102–105, 107
Lycopene	Tomatoes, tomato products, watermelon	Antioxidant action may provide lipid peroxidation inhibition; protective effect against CVD reported	108–112
Lutein	Leafy vegetables, fruit	Antioxidant effect may influence lipid peroxidation; protective effect against CVD requires confirmation	113

TABLE 2.1 (CONTINUED)
Dietary Ingredients Exerting Beneficial Influences on Hyperlipidemic and Dyslipidemic Conditions

Active Ingredients	Dietary Sources	Physiological Effects	Refs.
Sulfur-Containing Compounds			
Allicin, ajoene, S-allylcysteine, diallyl disulfide, S-methylcysteine sulfoxide, S-allylcysteine sulfoxide	Allium vegetables, especially garlic and its preparations	Mild hypocholesterolemic effect repeatedly described in experimental and small human studies, but needs further confirmation; possible mechanisms may involve inhibition of hepatic cholesterol synthesis and antioxidant effect; possible additional (nonlipid) effects include enhancement of fibrinolytic activity, inhibition of platelet aggregation, blood pressure lowering	114–117
Fiber			
Soluble fiber (psyllium, pectins, guar gum, some hemicelluloses)	Cereals, legumes	Well-documented mild hypocholesterolemic effect; LDL reduction might be related to intestinal binding of bile acids and/or cholesterol followed by LDL receptor upregulation and increased LDL clearance; additional (nonlipid) effects include C-reactive protein reduction and normalization of blood pressure	(118–123)
Protein			
Legume protein	Soy, legumes	Legume proteins, especially those derived from soy, appear to have hypocholesterolemic effects; mechanisms are not clear, difficult to separate from isoflavone effects	124–127
Plant Sterols and Stanols			
Sitosterol, campesterol, stigmasterol, sitostanol, campestanol	Tall (pine tree) oil, soybean oil, seeds, nuts (especially macadamia nut), sterol/stanol-enriched margarines.	Well-documented hypocholesterolemic effect due to cholesterol absorption inhibition	128–131

risk.[99–101] The idea has been tested in a number of controlled trials investigating the effects of antioxidant vitamin supplements on CVD risk. It is remarkable that the results of these studies have been largely disappointing,[101,103–105,141] leading to the conclusion that there is no basis for recommending that patients take vitamin C or E supplements or other antioxidants for the express purpose of preventing or treating coronary artery disease.[141,142]

Likewise, there is some controversy regarding the use of garlic as a potential lipid-lowering and cardioprotective food component. Commonly used garlic preparations and supplements have varying amounts of allicin, which is believed to be at the core of garlic bioactivity (see Table 2.1), so making a definite conclusion on their lipid-reducing efficiency is difficult.[114–117] Nevertheless, despite all problems discussed above, beneficial effects of antioxidant-rich diets based on fruit, vegetables, and products derived from these sources are evident,[97,143–145] and such diets are widely recommended to reduce CVD risk.[141] It appears to be very likely that consumption of natural products containing different antioxidant components acting synergistically may be much more efficient in providing cardiovascular protection than isolated action of food supplements.[97]

Mild hypocholesterolemic effect of dietary soluble fiber is well documented; however, precise mechanisms of this phenomenon are not clear and may be partially related to other components of fiber-rich cereals and legumes.[118] Promotion of increased fiber consumption, especially with whole grains, should be considered as one of the strategic ways of changing overall Western dietary patterns towards CVD prevention.

The amount and type of dietary protein is closely related to the problem of fat intake. It was repeatedly shown that substitution of soy for animal protein results in LDL and triglyceride reduction.[124–127] At the same time, the mechanism of this reduction is unknown and, especially in the case of soy, it is difficult to exclude an impact of isoflavones.[124,126] Overall food composition rather than protein type appears to be more important for serum lipid balance. It has been suggested that consumption of animal protein *per se* may not be harmful, but is commonly associated with an increased intake of saturated fat.[146] To avoid this unhealthy association, it can be recommended to shift the main sources of dietary protein by replacing red meat with nuts, soybeans, legumes, poultry, and fish.[80]

The use of natural cholesterol-lowering properties of plant sterols and stanols inhibiting intestinal cholesterol absorption has emerged as an attractive strategy for serum lipid level correction, especially in mildly hypercholesterolemic subjects.[130] New polyunsaturated margarines with added sterols and stanols have recently been made available for wide consumption.[129] It should be noticed, however, that the use of these products can also reduce the absorption of fat soluble vitamins.[129] Possible consequences of long-term sterol/stanol intake are not entirely known, so caution is needed in the use of this approach.

Food components discussed above are widely used as ingredients of different diets directed on both CVD prevention and attenuation of hyperlipidemia in CVD patients. The search for new natural substances with hypolipidemic properties continues, and such agents as policosanol (a mixture of alcohols isolated from sugar cane),[147] guggulipid (*Commiphora mucul* extract),[148,149] or red yeast rice (embryonic rice fermented with *Monascus ruber* yeast)[150] are now being tested. However, further studies are needed to assess their efficiency.

The analysis of food components possessing natural hypolipidemic properties shows that only mild effects of such dietary treatments can be expected. Nutritional counseling certainly constitutes a major element of healthy lifestyle forming the basis of primary CVD prevention. Specifically composed diets can be successfully combined with the use of hypolipidemic drugs; however, it should be noted that interactions between bioactive food components and medicines are sometimes difficult to predict. These interactions are discussed below.

2.3.2 INTERACTIONS BETWEEN DIETARY COMPONENTS AND HYPOLIPIDEMIC DRUGS

It is well known that simultaneous treatment of a patient with more than one pharmaceutical agent has potential risk of altering expected results of the treatment and even producing some adverse consequences. Such situations usually occur when drugs interact at the level of common regulatory, metabolic, or transport pathways involved in the realization of their action. Certain dietary components can behave in a similar way when taken together with drugs. Foods of plant origin that contain complex mixtures of phytochemicals are especially likely to produce such inadvertent effects.[151–153]

The small intestine is the main site for absorption of both nutrients and orally ingested medicines. Over the past 20 years, it has become obvious that this organ also has complex metabolic functions hosting Phase I and Phase II xenobiotic-metabolizing enzymes as well as associated molecular transporters,[154,155] which, acting together, determine oral bioavailability of drugs. It has been established that enzymes of the CYP3A subfamily are especially important for oxidative reactions of Phase I xenobiotic metabolism, CYP3A4 being the dominant P450 form expressed in human enterocytes.[154,156,157] Numerous drugs are known to be CYP3A4 substrates and several members of the statin family (see Section 2.2.1 of this chapter) are among them. Expression of some other enzymes of the CYP superfamily in the small intestine has been reported[154]; however, information regarding their significance for drug and dietary component metabolism in the human gut is limited.

Phase II metabolic reactions in the small intestine provide conjugation of xenobiotics and their Phase I metabolites resulting in generation of nontoxic and easily excretable products. These reactions are mostly exerted by enzymes of glutathione *S*-transferase (GST), uridine diphosphate glucuronosyltransferase (UGT), and, to some extent, sulfotransferase families.[154] Phase II glucuronidation reactions have been shown to be important for the metabolism of statins and fibrate-statin interactions in human hepatocytes;[158] however, it is not known whether such interactions occur in enterocytes as well. In addition to Phase I and Phase II metabolic pathways, the function of transport proteins greatly contributes to the protection from exogenous xenobiotics by both preventing harmful substances from entering the cell and eliminating products of xenobiotic detoxi-fication reactions.[155] Intestinal P-glycoprotein (a member of the multidrug resis-tance transporter family) expressed in the apical membrane of enterocytes appears to exert its transporter functions in concert with the metabolic role of CYP3A4, thus constituting a dynamic subsystem controlling xenobiotic metabolism/elim-ination rate.[159] Even from the brief description given above, it becomes apparent that disruption of proper functioning of this complex system can have hazardous consequences.

The problem of diet–drug interactions was suddenly highlighted by an unfore-seen discovery in 1989 of the effect of grapefruit juice (GJ) on bioavailability of felodipine, a calcium channel blocker used for hypertension treatment.[160] Since then, multiple studies have shown GJ interactions with various drugs of different families often lead to enhanced adverse effects (see References 153, 161). GJ interactions with hypolipidemic drugs (statins) and some other medicines often prescribed to CVD patients are listed in Table 2.2. Investigation of the mecha-nisms of GJ–drug interaction has revealed that oral intake of GJ selectively inhibits CYP3A4 in the small intestine,[176–178] resulting in a considerable reduction of oxidative metabolism of the substrates of CYP3A4, including numerous drugs. Only intestinal enzyme inhibition was observed, whereas liver CYP3A4 activity appeared to be unaffected[177] as well as pharmacodynamics of drugs metabolized by this enzyme after their intravenous administration.[170,179,180]

However, it has recently been reported that consumption of large amounts of GJ can inhibit hepatic CYP3A4 as well[181]; thus the effect may be dose-dependent with a much higher threshold for the enzyme in the liver. The search for the active GJ ingredients was focused on furanocoumarins (psoralens) and isoflavones as contributors to CYP3A4 inhibition. GJ furanocoumarins, especially bergamottin and 6′,7′-dihydroxybergamottin are regarded as major CYP3A4 inhibi-tors,[178,182–184] but binding properties and enzyme inhibition kinetics of the two furanocoumarins are different,[185] suggesting that different inhibition mechanisms can be involved. In addition, it has been shown that grapefruit flavonoids, in particular, naringin and its derivative naringenin, can act as competitive inhibitors of CYP3A4.[186] The influence of GJ on the intestinal drug metabolism appears to be even more complex since it is not limited by the effects on CYP3A4. GJ components have also been shown to suppress the P-glycoprotein transporter activity,[153,161,187,188] thus further increasing ingested drug bioavailability.

From the point of view of hypolipidemic therapy, interactions between GJ and HMG-CoA reductase inhibitors are especially important since consumption of the juice by individuals taking statins predominantly metabolized by CYP3A4 (atorvastatin, lovastatin or simvastatin) can significantly increase the risk of adverse effects.[161,164,166] Interactions are much less likely with fluvastatin, which is mainly metabolized by CYP2C9,[162] or pravastatin, rosuvastatin, and pitavasta-tin, which are largely metabolized through P450-independent pathways.[163–165,189] It is also apparent that considerable interindividual variation in responses to statin therapy strongly depends on genetic heterogeneity of human populations. Indeed, numerous polymorphic variants of the CYP3A4 gene have been identified,[190–193]

TABLE 2.2
Grapefruit Juice Interactions with Drugs Used for the Treatment of Hyperlipidemia and Other Manifestations of Cardiovascular Disease

Drug Classes, Individual Drugs	Conditions Treated	Reported Adverse Effects	Refs.
HMG-CoA Reductase Inhibitors (Statins)			
Simvastatin, lovastatin, atorvastatin	Hyperlipidemia	Myopathy, rhabdomyolysis, acute renal failure	161–166
Pravastatin, fluvastatin, rosuvastatin, pitavastatin		Little or no influence	
Calcium Channel Blockers (Dihydropyridines)			
Felodipine, nicardipine, nifedipine, nimoldipine, nisoldipine, pranidipine, nitrendipine, verapamil	Hypertension, angina pectoris treatment with verapamil	Excessive vasodilatation, hypotension, tachycardia	153, 161, 167–171
Amlodipine, barnidipine, diltiazem		Little or no influence	
Angiotensin II Receptor 1 Antagonists[a]			
Losartan	Hypertension	Reduced therapeutic effect	161, 172
Beta-Blockers[a]			
Carvedilol	Hypertension, heart failure treatment	Increased drug toxicity	161, 172
Celiprolol		Decreased drug bioavailability	
Antiarrhythmic Agents[a]			
Amiodarone, quinidine, disopyramide, propafenone	Arrhythmias	Increased drug toxicity	161, 174, 175

[a] No information on interactions with other drugs of this group.

and some of them have already been shown to affect lipid profiles in patients receiving statin therapy.[194,195] Moreover, potential influence of multiple polymorphisms of MDR1 gene encoding P-glycoprotein[196,197] or other transporter-encoding genes is impossible to exclude. Interestingly, it has recently been reported that polymorphisms of organic anion transporting polypeptide C have been associated with plasma pravastatin concentrations.[198] At the same time, organic anion-transporting polypeptides may be inhibited by GJ,[161,199] constituting another interaction area.

Although GJ effects on bioavailability of statins are relatively well documented, little is known about potential interactions of this dietary factor with other hypolipidemic drugs. Among them, fibrates present particular interest since their metabolism and transport can be related to the systems discussed above. Fenofibrate has recently been shown to inhibit P-glycoprotein-mediated transport,[200] so some pathways can present background for both drug–drug and diet–drug interactions. Cases of severe adverse effects of statin–fibrate combined therapy, especially associated with the use of gemfibrozil,[21,201] are well known; however, interaction mechanisms causing these effects are still obscure. Although there is no information about GJ–fibrate interactions, it is difficult to be sure that potential risk does not exist, especially in situations of combined therapy.

Presented information highlights the complexity of GJ–drug interactions, which are not necessarily harmful. On the one hand, citrus flavonoids, especially naringenin, are believed to be antiatherogenic.[202,203] On the other hand, in many situations dietary modulation of drug bioavailability might be an advantage on the condition that the consequences of the interaction are perfectly predictable.

Identification of GJ–drug interactions has stimulated interest to possible effects of other fruit juices. Although the information is less abundant, there are reports indicating that either CYP3A4 or multidrug transporter proteins can be affected. Several citrus juices (lime, orange, lemon, pummelo), apple juice, and juices of several exotic fruits have been shown to influence drug pharmacokinetics.[188,199,204–207] As some of the observed effects are attributed to fruit flavonoids, it is difficult to exclude that other flavonoid-containing products can emerge as potential causes of food–drug interactions.

It is often difficult to set strict limits between nutrition and consumption of some natural products for health-related reasons. Health-promoting properties of numerous herbs have been known for centuries, and herbal remedies rich in bioactive compounds are traditionally used for unconventional therapy of various diseases including CVD.[208] At the same time, many herbs, widely regarded as "natural health products," are easily available over the counter and consumed without proper medical control. St. John's wort (*Hypericum perforatum*) is a popular herbal product used for the treatment of depression. It has been shown that St. John's wort affects both intestinal and hepatic xenobiotic metabolism and transport, and action of its bioactive substances (hypericin and hyperforin) appears to be opposite to that of GJ. St. John's wort induces both CYP3A4 and P-glycoprotein expression,[209–211] thereby reducing bioavailability of drugs dependent on this metabolic/transport system. This action may be potentially important for the efficiency of hypolipidemic therapy with statins. It has already been reported that St. John's wort significantly decreases plasma concentrations of simvastatin, but not of pravastatin.[212]

These results are not surprising in view of the metabolic differences between the two drugs described earlier in this chapter. Although no information regarding other interactions between herbal medicines and hypolipidemic drugs is available, such interactions are not excluded since the problem of consequences of simultaneous intake of herbal and conventional medicines has attracted close attention only recently. Potentially harmful effects of natural remedies (echinacea, ephedra, garlic, ginkgo, ginseng, kava, St. John's wort, valerian) interfering with the action of preoperative anesthetics have already been described,[213] and several of these natural agents have been shown to be associated with modulation of drug transport systems.[214] Herb–drug interactions in a wider aspect of cardiovascular pharmacotherapy have been discussed in a recent review.[215]

Examples discussed above show that the problem of possible interactions between food components and hypolipidemic drugs certainly needs further investigation. Nevertheless, many situations when adverse drug effects are provoked by consumption of certain foods, food supplements or natural health products are easily preventable by appropriate medical advice. Moreover, both efficiency of hypolipidemic therapy and the potential of adverse effects of different therapeutic schemes can potentially be individualized if more information is available on individual genetic backgrounds. The latter option is not immediately available; however, rapid growth of understanding of genetic influences on the relationship between nutrition, CVD pathogenesis, and action of hypolipidemic drugs[216–218] allows one to expect significant progress in this direction.

2.4 CONCLUSION

Serum lipid lowering is a pivotal component among measures applied in order to prevent CVD or delay its progression. Dietary approaches can be successfully used for primary prevention of cardiovascular conditions, especially coronary heart disease. General dietary strategy should include recommendations to change fat intake habits (substitute polyunsaturated and monounsaturated fats for saturated fats, increase intake of ω-3 PUFA) and to consume food rich in fruits, vegetables, nuts, and whole grains (i.e., products rich in natural antioxidants, soluble fiber, vegetable protein). It appears that natural products containing complex mixtures of bioactive ingredients acting synergistically provide more beneficial effects compared to most presently available artificial dietary supplements and additives.

Secondary CVD prevention directed to delaying disease progress in individuals with existing conditions is now based upon application of combined therapeutic strategies including hypolipidemic drug therapy and additional dietary measures. The development of new lipid-lowering agents is progressing very fast through introduction of new potent drugs often providing beneficial pleiotropic effects affecting different mechanisms involved in CVD pathogenesis. HMG-CoA reductase inhibitors (statins) have emerged as the central element of hypolipidemic therapy, especially in cases with seriously increased LDL levels. Availability of other types of hypolipidemic medicines that can be combined with statins considerably widens therapeutic options, allowing development of individualized treatment schemes. Successful combination of statin therapy with the use of fibrates, bile acid transport inhibitors, niacin, and cholesterol absorption inhibitors provides an expanding arsenal of therapeutic approaches. Dietary recommendations, which are generally similar to those used for primary CVD prevention, should be specifically adapted for each individual case. This requirement is especially important in view of accumulating evidence of possible interactions between food components and medicines, especially orally ingested drugs. It appears that in many cases food–drug interactions, if properly assessed and understood, can potentially be employed to enhance beneficial therapeutic effects. This understanding, however, requires much better knowledge of individual characteristics of each patient determined by genetic background. "Genetic profiling" of individuals subjected to hypolipidemic therapy can greatly reduce the risk of adverse effects and facilitate determination of optimal therapeutic and dietary schemes applied for CVD treatment.

REFERENCES

1. Gordon T. The diet-heart idea. Outline of a history. *Am J Epidemiol* 1988; 127: 220–225.
2. Lusis AJ. Atherosclerosis. *Nature* 2000; 407: 233–241.
3. Glass CK, Witztum JL. Atherosclerosis: the road ahead. *Cell* 2001; 104: 503–516.
4. Libby P. Inflammation in atherosclerosis. *Nature* 2002; 420: 868–874.
5. Maas R, Böger RH. Old and new cardiovascular risk factors: from unresolved issues to new opportunities. *Atherosclerosis* 2003; Suppl. 4: 5–17.
6. Haffner S, Taegtmeyer H. Epidemic obesity and the metabolic syndrome. *Circulation* 2003, 108: 1541–1545.
7. Deedwania PC. Metabolic syndrome and vascular disease: is nature or nurture leading the new epidemic of cardiovascular disease? *Circulation* 2004; 109: 2–4.
8. Moller DE, Kaufman KD. Metabolic syndrome: a clinical and molecular perspective. *Ann Rev Med* 2005; 56: 45–62.
9. Ford ES, Giles WH, Dietz WH. Prevalence of the metabolic syndrome among U.S. adults: findings from the third National Health and Nutrition Examination Survey. *JAMA* 2002; 287: 356–359.
10. Fruchart JC, Nierman MC, Stroes ES, Kastelein JJ, Duriez P. New risk factors for atherosclerosis and patient risk assessment. *Circulation* 2004; 109; III15–III19.
11. Splaver A, Lamas GA, Hennekens CH. Homocysteine and cardiovascular disease: biological mechanisms, observational epidemiology, and the need for randomized trials. *Am Heart J* 2004; 148: 34-40.
12. Ross R. Atherosclerosis — an inflammatory disease. *N Engl J Med* 1999; 340: 115–126.
13. Shishehbor MH, Hansen SL. Inflammatory and oxidative markers in atherosclerosis: relationship to outcome. *Curr Atheroscler Rep* 2004; 6: 243–250.
14. Diaz MN, Frei B, Vita JA, Keaney JF Jr. Antioxidants and atherosclerotic heart disease. *N Engl J Med* 1997; 337: 408–416.
15. Rosenson RS. Statins in atherosclerosis: lipid-lowering agents with antioxidant capabilities. *Atherosclerosis* 2004; 173: 1–12.
16. Stocker R, Keaney JF Jr. Role of oxidative modifications in atherosclerosis. *Physiol Rev* 2004; 84: 1381–1478.
17. Evans M, Roberts A, Davies S, Rees A. Medical lipid-regulating therapy: current evidence, ongoing trials and future developments. *Drugs* 2004; 64: 1181–1196.

18. Endo A, Tsujita Y, Kuroda M, Tanzawa K. Inhibition of cholesterol synthesis *in vitro* and *in vivo* by ML-236A and ML-236B, competitive inhibitors of 3-hydroxy-3-methylglutaryl-coenzyme A reductase. *Eur J Biochem* 1977; 77: 31–36.

19. Farnier M, Davignon J. Current and future treatment of hyperlipidemia: the role of statins. *Am J Cardiol* 1998; 82: 3J–10J.

20. Wierzbicki AS. Synthetic statins: more data on newer lipid-lowering agents. *Curr Med Res Opin* 2001; 17: 74–77.

21. Psaty BM, Furberg CD, Ray WA, Weiss NS. Potential for conflict of interest in the evaluation of suspected adverse drug reactions: use of cerivastatin and risk of rhabdomyolysis. *JAMA* 2004; 292: 2622–2631.

22. Grundy SM. HMG-CoA reductase inhibitors for treatment of hypercholesterolemia. *N Engl J Med* 1988; 319: 24–33.

23. Slater EE, MacDonald JS. Mechanism of action and biological profile of HNG-CoA reductase inhibitors: a new therapeutic alternative. *Drugs* 1988; 36 (Suppl 3): 72–82.

24. Davignon J. Beneficial cardiovascular pleiotropic effects of statins. *Circulation* 2004; 109 (Suppl III): III39–III43.

25. Miida T, Hirayama S, Nakamura Y. Cholesterol-independent effects of statins and new therapeutic targets: ischemic stroke and dementia. *J Atheroscl Thromb* 2004; 11: 253–264.

26. Balk EM, Karas RH, Jordan HS, Kupelnick B, Chew P, Lau J. Effects of statins on vascular structure and function: a systematic review. *Am J Med* 2004; 117: 775–790.

27. Heart Protection Study Collaborative Group. MRC/BHF Heart Protection Study of cholesterol lowering with simvastatin in 20,536 high-risk individuals: a randomized placebo-controlled trial. *Lancet* 2002; 360: 7–22.

28. Shepherd J, Blauw GJ, Murphy MB, Bollen ELEM, Buckley BM, Cobbe SM, Ford I, Gaw A, Hyland M, Jukema JW, Kamper AM, Macfarlane PW, Meinders AE, Norrie J, Packard CJ, Perry IJ, Stott DJ, Sweeney BJ, Twomey C, Westendorp RGJ, PROSPER study group. Pravastatin in elderly individuals at risk of vascular disease (PROSPER): a randomized controlled trial. *Lancet* 2002; 360: 1623–1630.

29. Nissen SE, Tuzcu EM, Schoenhagen P, Brown BG, Ganz P, Vogel RA, Crowe T, Howard G, Cooper CJ, Brodie B, Grines CL, DeMaria AN, REVERSAL Investigators. Effect of intensive compared with moderate lipid-lowering therapy on progression of coronary atherosclerosis: a randomized controlled trial. *JAMA* 2004; 291: 1071–1080.

30. Cheung BM, Lauder IJ, Lau CP, Kumana CR. Meta-analysis of large randomized controlled trials to evaluate the impact of statins on cardiovascular outcomes. *Br J Clin Pharmacol* 2004; 57: 640–651.

31. Grundy SM, Cleeman JI, Merz CN, Brewer HB, Clark LT, Hunninghake DB, Pasternak RC, Smith SC, Stone NJ; National Heart, Lung, and Blood Institute; American College of Cardiology Foundation; American Heart Association. Implications of recent clinical trials for the National Cholesterol Education Program Adult Treatment Panel III guidelines. *Circulation* 2004; 110: 227–239.

32. Collins R, Armitage J, Parish S, Sleight P, Peto R; Heart Protection Study Collaborative Group. Effects of cholesterol-lowering with simvastatin on stroke and other major vascular events in 20,536 people with cerebrovascular disease or other high-risk condition. *Lancet* 2004; 363: 757–767.

33. Amarenco P, Lavallee P, Touboul PJ. Stroke prevention, blood cholesterol, and statins. *Lancet Neurol* 2004; 3: 271–278.

34. Collins R, Armitage J, Parish S, Sleight P, Peto R; Heart Protection Study Collaborative Group. MRC/BHF Heart Protection Study of cholesterol-lowering with simvastatin in 5963 people with diabetes: a randomised placebo-controlled trial. *Lancet* 2003; 361:2005–2016.

35. Keech A, Colquhoun D, Best J, Kirby A, Simes RJ, Hunt D, Hague W, Beller E, Arulchelwam M, Baker J, Tonkin A; Lipid Study Group. Secondary prevention of cardiovascular events with long-term pravastatin in patients with diabetes or impaired fasting glucose: results from the LIPID trial. *Diabetes Care* 2003; 26: 2713–2721.

36. Newman TB, Hulley SB. Carcinogenicity of lipid-lowering drugs. *JAMA* 1996; 275: 55–60.

37. Chapman MJ. Fibrates in 2003: therapeutic action in atherogenic dyslipidemia and future perspectives. *Atherosclerosis* 2003; 171: 1–13.

38. Rader DJ. Effects of nonstatin lipid drug therapy on high-density lipoprotein metabolism. *Am J Cardiol* 2003; 91: 18E–23E.

39. Staels B, Dallongeville J, Auwerx J, Schoonjans K, Leitersdorf E, Fruchart JC. Mechanism of action of fibrates on lipid and lipoprotein metabolism. *Circulation* 1998; 98: 2088–2093.

40. Barbier O, Pineda Torra I, Duguay Y, Blanquart C, Fruchart JC, Glineur C, Staels B. Pleiotropic actions of peroxisome proliferator-activated receptors in lipid metabolism and atherosclerosis. *Arterioscler Thromb Vasc Biol* 2002; 22: 717–726.

41. Blaschke F, Bruemmer D, Law RE. Will the potential of peroxisome proliferators-activated receptor agonists be realized in the clinical setting? *Clin Cardiol* 2004; 27 (Suppl 4): IV3–IV10.

42. Robins SJ. Cardiovascular disease with diabetes or the metabolic syndrome: should statins or fibrates be first line lipid therapy? *Curr Opin Lipidol* 2003; 14: 575–583.

43. Fazio S, Linton MF. The role of fibrates in managing hyperlipidemia: mechanisms of action and clinical efficacy. *Curr Atheroscler Rep* 2004; 6: 148–157.

44. Maki KC. Fibrates for treatment of the metabolic syndrome. *Curr Atheroscler Rep* 2004; 6: 45–51.

45. Tomlinson B, Chan P, Lan W. How well tolerated are lipid-lowering drugs? *Drugs Aging* 2001; 18: 665-683.

46. Muscari A, Puddu GM, Puddu P. Lipid-lowering drugs: are adverse effects predictable and reversible? *Cardiology* 2002; 97: 115–121.

47. Layne RD, Sehbai AS, Stark LJ. Rhabdomyolysis and renal failure associated with gemfibrozil monotherapy. *Ann Pharmacother* 2004; 38: 232–234.

48. Dierkes J, Westphal S, Luley C. Fenofibrate-induced hyperhomocysteinaemia: clinical implications and management. *Drug Safety* 2003; 26: 81–91.

49. Graham DJ, Staffa JA, Shatin D, Andrade SE, Schech SD, La Grenade L, Gurwitz JH, Chan KA, Goodman MJ, Platt R. Incidence of hospitalized rhabdomyolysis in patients treated with lipid-lowering drugs. *JAMA* 2004; 292: 2585–2590.

50. Ast M, Frishman WH. Bile acid sequestrants. *J Clin Pharmacol* 1990; 30: 99–106.

51. Davidson MH, Dillon MA, Gordon B, Jones P, Samuels J, Weiss S, Issacsohn J, Toth P, Burke SK. Colesevelam hydrochloride (cholestagel): a new, potent bile acid sequestrant associated with a low incidence of gastrointestinal side effects. *Arch Intern Med* 1999; 159: 1893–1900.

52. Melian EB, Plosker GL. Colesevelam. *Am J Cardiovasc Drugs* 2001; 1: 141–146.

53. Steinmetz KL. Colesevelam hydrochloride. *Am J Health Syst Pharmacol* 2002; 59: 932–939.

54. Higaki J, Hara S, Takasu N, Tonda K, Miyata K, Shike T, Nagata K, Mizui T. Inhibition of ileal Na+/bile acid cotransporter by S-8921 reduces serum cholesterol and prevents atherosclerosis in rabbits. *Arterioscler Thromb Vasc Biol* 1998; 18: 1304–1311.

55. Root C, Smith CD, Sundseth SS, Pink HM, Wilson JG, Lewis MC. Ileal bile acid transporter inhibition, CYP7A1 induction, and antilipemic action of 264 W94. *J Lipid Res* 2002; 43: 1320–1330.

56. Li H, Xu G, Shang Q, Pan L, Shefer S, Batta AK, Bollineni J, Tint GS, Keller BT, Salen G. Inhibition of ileal bile acid transport lowers plasma cholesterol levels by inactivating hepatic farnesoid X receptor and stimulating cholesterol 7 alpha-hydroxylase. *Metabolism* 2004; 53: 927–932.

57. Rosenson RS. Antiatherothrombotic effects of nicotinic acid. *Atherosclerosis* 2003; 171: 87–96.

58. McKenney J. New perspectives on the use of niacin in the treatment of lipid disorders. *Arch Intern Med* 2004; 164: 697–705.

59. Meyers CD, Kamanna VS, Kashyap ML. Niacin therapy in atherosclerosis. *Curr Opin Lipidol* 2004; 15: 659–665.

60. Ganji SH, Tavintharan S, Zhu D, Xing Y, Kamanna VS, Kashyap ML. Niacin noncompetitively inhibits DGAT2 but not DGAT1 activity in HepG2 cells. *J Lipid Res* 2004; 45: 1835–1845.

61. Sakai T, Kamanna VS, Kashyap ML. Niacin, but not gemfibrozil, selectively increases LP-AI, a cardioprotective subfraction of HDL, in patients with low HDL cholesterol. *Arterioscler Thromb Vasc Biol* 2001; 21: 1783–1789.

62. Wise A, Foord SM, Fraser NJ, Barnes AA, Elshourbagy N, Eilert M, Ignar DM, Murdock PR, Steplewski K, Green A, Brown AJ, Dowell SJ, Szekeres PG, Hassall DG, Marshall FH, Wilson S, Pike NB. Molecular identification of high and low affinity receptors for nicotinic acid. *J Biol Chem* 2003; 278: 9869–9874.

63. Soga T, Kamohara M, Takasaki J, Matsumoto S, Saito T, Ohishi T, Hiyama H, Matsuo A, Matsushime H, Furuichi K. Molecular identification of nicotinic acid receptor. *Biochem Biophys Res Commun* 2003; 303: 364–369.

64. Tunaru S, Kero J, Schaub A, Wufka C, Blaukat A, Pfeffer K, Offermans S. PUMA-G and HM 74 are receptors for nicotinic acid and mediate its anti-lipolytic effect. *Nature Med* 2003; 9: 352–355.

65. Karpe F, Frayn KN. The nicotinic acid receptor — a new mechanism for an old drug. *Lancet* 2004; 363: 1892–1894.

66. Rubic T, Trottmann M, Lorenz RL. Simulation of CD36 and the key effector of reverse cholesterol transport ATP-binding cassette A1 in monocytoid cells by niacin. *Biochem Pharmacol* 2004; 67: 411–419.

67. Zellner C, Pullinger CR, Aouizerat BE, Frost PH, Kwok PY, Malloy MJ, Kane JP. Variations in human HM74 (GPR109B) and HM74A (GPR109A) niacin receptors. *Hum Mutat* 2005; 25: 18–21.

68. Darkes MJ, Poole RM, Goa KL. Ezetimibe. *Am J Cardiovasc Drugs* 2003; 3: 67–76.
69. Sudhop T, Lutjohann D, Kodal A, Igel M, Tribble DL, Shah S, Perevozskaya I, von Bergmann K. Inhibition of intestinal cholesterol absorption by ezetimibe in humans. *Circulation* 2002: 106: 1943–1948.
70. Gagne C, Gaudet D, Bruckert E, Ezetimibe Study Group. Efficacy and safety of ezetimibe coadministered with atorvastatin or simvastatin in patients with homozygous familial hypercholesterolemia. *Circulation* 2002; 105: 2469–2475.
71. Murdoch D, Scott LJ. Ezetimibe/Simvastatin: a review of its use in the management of hypercholesterolemia. *Am J Cardiovasc Drugs* 2004; 4: 405–422.
72. Reyderman L, Kosoglou T, Statkevich P, Pember L, Boutros T, Maxwell SE, Affrime M, Batra V. Assessment of a multiple-dose drug interaction between ezetimibe, a novel selective cholesterol absorption inhibitor and gemfibrozil. *Int J Clin Pharmacol Ther* 2004; 42: 512–518.
73. Bays H, Stein EA. Pharmacotherapy for dyslipidaemia — current therapies and future agents. *Expert Opin Pharmacother* 2003; 4: 1901–1938.
74. Tardif JC, Gregoire J, L'Allier PL, Anderson TJ, Bertrand O, Reeves F, Title LM, Alfonso F, Schampaert E, Hassan A, McLain R, Pressler ML, Ibrahim R, Lesperance J, Blue J, Heinonen T, Rodes-Cabau J, Avisimibe and Progression of Lesions on UltraSound (A-PLUS) Investigators. Effects of the acyl coenzyme A:cholesterol acyltransferase inhibitor avasimibe on human atherosclerotic lesions. *Circulation* 2004; 110: 3372–3377.
75. Robl JA, Sulsky R, Sun CQ, Simpkins LM, Wang T, Dickson JK Jr, Chen Y, Magnin DR, Taunk , Slusarchyk WA, Biller SA, Lan SJ, Connolly F, Kunselman LK, Sabrah T, Jamil H, Gordon D, Harrity TW, Wetterau JR. A novel series of highly potent benzimidazole-based microsomal triglyceride transfer protein inhibitors. *J Med Chem* 2001; 44: 851–856.
76. Magnin DR, Biller SA, Wetterau J, Rohl JA, Dickson JK Jr, Taunk P, Harrity TW, Lawrence RM, Sun CQ, Wang T, Logan J, Fryszman O, Connolly F, Jolibois K, Kunselman L. Microsomal triglyceride transfer protein inhibitors: discovery and synthesis of alkyl phosphonates as potent MTP inhibitors and cholesterol lowering agents. *Bioorg Med Chem Lett* 2003; 13: 1337–1340.
77. Brousseau ME, Schaefer EJ, Wolfe ML, Bloedon LT, Digenio AG, Clark RW, Mancuso JP, Rader DJ. Effects of an inhibitor of cholesteryl ester transfer protein on HDL cholesterol. *N Engl J Med* 2004; 350: 1491–1494.
78. Doggrell SA. Raising high-density lipoprotein cholesterol with inhibitors of cholesteryl ester transfer protein — a new approach to coronary artery disease. *Expert Opin Investig Drugs* 2004; 13: 1365–1368.
79. Ory DS. Nuclear receptor signaling in the control of cholesterol homeostasis: have the orphans found a home? *Circ Res* 2004; 95: 660–670.
80. Hu WB, Willett WC. Optimal diets for prevention of coronary heart disease. *JAMA* 2002; 2569–2578.
81. Expert Panel on Detection, Evaluation, and Treatment of High Blood Cholesterol in Adults. Executive summary of the third report of the National Cholesterol Education Program (NCEP) expert panel on detection, evaluation, and treatment of high blood cholesterol in adults (Adult Treatment Panel III). *JAMA* 2001; 2486–2497.
82. Zeisel S. Regulation of "nutraceuticals." *Science* 1999; 285: 1853–1855.

83. Gardner CD, Kraemer HC. Monounsaturated versus polyunsaturated dietary fat and serum lipids. A meta-analysis. *Arterioscler Thromb Vasc Biol* 1995; 15: 1917–1927.

84. Kris-Etherton PM. Monounsaturated fatty acids and risk of cardiovascular disease. *J Nutr* 1999; 129: 2280–2284.

85. Perez-Jimenez F, Lopez-Miranda J, Mata P. Protective effect of dietary monounsaturated fat on arteriosclerosis: beyond cholesterol. *Atherosclerosis* 2002; 163: 385–398.

86. Simopoulos AP. Essential fatty acids in health and chronic disease. *Am J Clin Nutr* 1999; 70 (Suppl): 560S–569S.

87. Wijendran V, Hayes KC. Dietary n-6 and n-3 fatty acid balance and cardiovascular health. *Annu Rev Nutr* 2004; 24: 597–615.

88. Kris-Etherton PM, Hecker KD, Binkoski AE. Polyunsaturated fatty acids and cardiovascular health. *Nutr Rev* 2004; 62: 414–426.

89. Albert CM, Hennekens CH, O'Donnell CJ, Ajani UA, Carey VJ, Willett WC, Ruskin JN, Manson JE. Fish consumption and risk of sudden cardiac death. *Jama* 1998; 279: 23–28.

90. Simopoulos AP. The importance of the ratio of omega-6/omega-3 essential fatty acids. *Biomed Pharmacother* 2002; 56: 365–379.

91. Din JN, Newby DE, Flapan AD. Omega 3 fatty acids and cardiovascular disease — fishing for a natural treatment. *BMJ* 2004; 328: 30–35.

92. de Lorgeril M, Salen P. Alpha-linolenic acid and coronary heart disease. *Nutr Metab Cardiovasc Dis* 2004; 14: 162–169.

93. Rimm EB, Katan MB, Ascherio A, Stampfer MJ, Willett WC. Relation between intake of flavonoids and risk for coronary heart disease in male health professionals. *Ann Intern Med* 1996; 125: 384–389.

94. Scalbert A, Williamson G. Dietary intake and bioavailability of polyphenols. *J Nutr* 2000; 130 (Suppl): 2073S–2085S.

95. Arts ICW, Hollman PCH, Feskens EJM, Bueno de Mesquita HB, Kromhout D. Catechin intake might explain the inverse relation between tea consumption and ischemic heart disease: the Zutphen Elderly Study. *Am J Clin Nutr* 2001; 74: 227–232.

96. Knekt P Kumpulainen J, Jarvinen R, Rissanen H, Heliovaara M, Reunanen A, Hakulinen T, Aromaa A. Flavonoid intake and risk of chronic diseases. *Am J Clin Nutr* 2002; 76: 560–568.

97. Liu RH. Health benefits of fruit and vegetables are from additive and synergistic combinations of phytochemicals. *Am J Clin Nutr* 2003; 78 (Suppl): 517S–520S.

98. Park D, Huang T, Frishman WH. Phytoestrogens as cardioprotective agents. *Cardiol Rev* 2005; 13: 13–17.

99. Diaz MN, Frei B, Vita JA, Keaney JF Jr. Antioxidants and atherosclerotic heart disease. *N Engl J Med* 1997; 337: 408–416.

100. Carr AC, Zhu BZ, Frei B. Potential antiatherogenic mechanisms of ascorbate (vitamin C) and alpha-tocopherol (vitamin E). *Circ Res* 2000; 87: 349–354.

101. Heinecke JW. Is the emperor wearing clothes? Clinical trials of vitamin E and the LDL oxidation hypothesis. *Arterioscler Thromb Vasc Biol* 2001; 21: 1261–1264.

102. Gale CR, Ashurst HE, Powers HJ, Martyn CN. Antioxidant vitamin status and carotid atherosclerosis in the elderly. *Am J Clin Nutr* 2001 74: 402–408.

103. Clarke R, Armitage J. Antioxidant vitamins and risk of cardiovascular disease. Review of large-scale randomized trials. *Cardiovasc Drugs Ther* 2002; 16: 411–415.

104. Brown BG, Cheung MC, Lee AC, Zhao XQ, Chait A. Antioxidant vitamins and lipid therapy: end of a long romance? *Arterioscler Thromb Vasc Biol* 2002; 22: 1535–1546.

105. Heart Protection Study Collaborative Group. MRC/BHF Heart Protection Study of antioxidant vitamin supplementation in 20,536 high-risk individuals: a randomized placebo-controlled trial. *Lancet* 2002; 360: 23–33.

106. Padayatty SJ, Katz A, Wang Y, Eck P, Kwon O, Lee JH, Chen S, Corpe C, Dutta A, Dutta SK, Levine M. Vitamin C as an antioxidant: evaluation of its role in disease prevention. *J Am Coll Nutr* 2003; 22: 18–35.

107. Chew BP, Park JS. Carotenoid action on the immune response. *J Nutr* 2004; 134 (Suppl) 257S–261S.

108. Klipstein-Grobusch K, Launer LJ, Geleijnse JM, Boeing H, Hofman A, Witteman JC. Serum carotenoids and atherosclerosis. The Rotterdam study. *Atherosclerosis* 2000; 148: 49–56.

109. Arab L, Steck S. Lycopene and cardiovascular disease. *Am J Clin Nutr* 2000; 71 (Suppl): 1691S–1695S.

110. Rao AV. Lycopene, tomatoes, and the prevention of coronary heart disease. *Exp Biol Med* 2002; 227: 908–913.

111. Visioli F, Riso P, Grande S, Galli C, Porrini M. Protective activity of tomato products on *in vivo* markers of lipid oxidation. *Eur J Nutr* 2003; 42: 201–206.

112. Sesso HD, Buring JE, Norkus EP, Gaziano JM. Plasma lycopene, other carotenoids, and retinol and the risk of cardiovascular disease in women. *Am J Clin Nutr* 2004; 79: 47–53.

113. Granado F, Olmedilla B, Blanco I. Nutritional and clinical relevance of lutein in human health. *Br J Nutr* 2003; 90: 487–502.

114. Stevinson C, Pittler MH, Ernst E. Garlic for treating hypercholesterolemia. A meta-analysis of randomized clinical trials. *Ann Intern Med* 2000; 133: 420–429.

115. Lau BH. Suppression of LDL oxidation by garlic. *J Nutr* 2001; 13 (Suppl): 985S–988S.

116. Yeh YY, Liu L. Cholesterol-lowering effect of garlic extracts and organosulfur compounds: human and animal studies. *J Nutr* 2001; 13 (Suppl): 989S–993S.

117. Banerjee SK, Maulik SK. Effect of garlic on cardiovascular disorders: a review. *Nutr J* 2002; 1: 4.

118. Brown L, Rosner B, Willett WW, Sacks FM. Cholesterol-lowering effects of dietary fiber: a meta-analysis. *Am J Clin Nutr* 1999; 69: 30–42.

119. Mozaffarian D, Kumanyika SK, Lemaitre RN, Olson JL, Burke GL, Siscovick DS. Cereal, fruit, and vegetable fiber intake and the risk of cardiovascular disease in elderly individuals. *JAMA* 2003; 289: 1659–1666.

120. Bazzano LA, He J, Ogden LG, Loria CM, Whelton PK, National Health and Nutrition Examination Survey I Epidemiologic Follow-up Study. Dietary fiber intake and reduced risk of coronary heart disease in U.S. men and women: the National Health and Nutrition Examination Survey I Epidemiologic Follow-up Study. *Arch Intern Med* 2003; 163: 1897–1904.

121. Ajani UA, Ford ES, Mokdad AH. Dietary fiber and C-reactive protein: findings from national health and nutrition examination survey data. *J Nutr* 2004; 134: 1181–1185.

122. Jensen MK, Koh-Banerjee P, Hu FB, Franz M, Sampson L, Gronbaek M, Rimm EB. Intakes of whole grains, bran, and germ and the risk of coronary heart disease in men. *Am J Clin Nutr* 2004; 80: 1492–1499.
123. Streppel MT, Arends LR, van't Veer P, Grobbee DE, Geleijnse JM. Dietary fiber and blood pressure: a meta-analysis of randomized placebo-controlled trials. *Arch Intern Med* 2005; 165: 150–156.
124. Anderson JW, Johnstone BM, Cook-Newell ME. Meta-analysis of the effects of soy protein intake on serum lipids. *N Engl J Med* 1995; 333: 276–282.
125. Anderson JW, Smith BM, Washnock CS. Cardiovascular and renal benefits of dry bean and soybean intake. *Am J Clin Nutr* 1999; 70 (Suppl) 464S–474S.
126. Sagara M, Kanda T, NJelekera M, Teramoto T, Armitage L, Birt N, Birt C, Yamori Y. Effects of dietary intake of soy protein and isoflavones on cardiovascular disease risk factors in high risk, middle-aged men in Scotland. *J Am Coll Nutr* 2004; 23: 85–91.
127. Wang Y, Jones PJ, Ausman LM, Lichtenstein AH. Soy protein reduces triglyceride levels and triglyceride fatty acid fractional synthesis rate in hypercholesterolemic subjects. *Atherosclerosis* 2004; 173: 269–275.
128. Moghadasian MH, Frohlich JJ. Effects of dietary phytosterols on cholesterol metabolism and atherosclerosis: clinical and experimental evidence. *Am J Med* 1999; 107: 588–594.
129. Law M. Plant sterol and stanol margarines and health. *BMJ* 2000; 320: 861–864.
130. de Jong A, Plat J, Mensink RP. Metabolic effects of plant sterols and stanols (Review). *J Nutr Biochem* 2003; 14: 362–369.
131. Miettinen TA, Gylling H. Plant stanol and sterol esters in prevention of cardio-vascular diseases. *Ann Med* 2004; 36: 126–134.
132. Lichtenstein AH, Kennedy E, Barrier P, Danford D, Ernst ND, Grundy SM, Leveille GA, Van Horn L, Williams CL, Booth SL. Dietary fat consumption and health. *Nutr Rev* 1998; 56: S3–S19.
133. Hu FB, Manson JE, Willett WC. Types of dietary fat and risk of coronary heart disease: a critical review. *J Am Coll Nutr* 2001; 20: 5–19.
134. Kris-Etherton PM, Binkoski AE, Zhao G, Coval SM, Clemmer KF, Hecker KD, Jacques H, Etherton TD. Dietary fat: assessing the evidence in support of a moderate diet: the benchmark based on lipoprotein metabolism. *Proc Nutr Soc* 2002; 61: 287–298.
135. Dewailly E, Blanchet C, Lemieux S, Sauve L, Gingras S, Ayotte P, Holub BJ. n-3 Fatty acids and cardiovascular disease risk factors among the Inuit of Nunavik. *Am J Clin Nutr* 2001; 74: 464–473.
136. Cordain L, Eaton SB, Miller JB, Mann N, Hill K. The paradoxical nature of hunter-gatherer diets: meat-based, yet non-atherogenic. *Eur J Clin Nutr* 2002; 56 (Suppl 1): S42–S52.
137. Witztum JL, Steinberg D. Role of oxidized low density lipoprotein in atheroscle-rosis. *J Clin Invest* 1991; 88: 1785–1792.
138. Geleijnse JM, Launer LJ, Van der Kuip DA, Hofman A, Witteman JC. Inverse association of tea and flavonoid intakes with incident myocardial infarction: the Rotterdam study. *Am J Clin Nutr* 2002; 75: 880–886.
139. Hertog MG, Sweetnam PM, Fehily AM, Elwood PC, Kromhout D. Antioxidant flavonoids and ischemic heart disease in a Welsh population of men: the Caerphilly Study. *Am J Clin Nutr* 1997; 65: 1489–1494.

140. Sesso HD, Gaziano JM, Liu S, Buring JE. Flavonoid intake and the risk of cardiovascular disease in women. *Am J Clin Nutr* 2003; 77: 1400–1408.

141. Kris-Etherton PM, Lichtenstein AH, Howard BV, Steinberg D, Witztum JL; for the Nutrition Committee of the American Heart Association Council on Nutrition, Physical Activity, and Metabolism. Antioxidant vitamin supplements and cardiovascular disease. *Circulation* 2004; 110: 637–641.

142. Gibbons RJ, Abrams J, Chatterjee K, Daley J, Deedwania PC, Douglas JS, Ferguson TB Jr, Fihn SD, Fraker TD Jr, Gardin JM, O'Rourke RA, Pasternak RC, Williams SV, Gibbons RJ, Alpert JS, Antman EM, Hiratzka LF, Fuster V, Faxon DP, Gregoratos G, Jacobs AK, Smith SC Jr; American College of Cardiology; American Heart Association Task Force on Practice Guidelines. Committee on the Management of Patients with Chronic Stable Angina. ACC/AHA 2002 guideline update for the management of patients with chronic stable angina – summary article: a report of the American College of Cardiology/American Heart Association Task Force on Practice Guidelines (Committee on the Management of Patients with Chronic Stable Angina). *Circulation* 2003; 107: 149–158.

143. Joshipura KJ, Hu FB, Manson JE, Stampfer MJ, Rimm EB, Speizer FE, Golditz G, Ascherio A, Rosner B, Spiegelman D, Willett WC. The effect of fruit and vegetable intake on risk for coronary heart disease. *Ann Intern Med* 2001; 134: 1106–1114.

144. Hu FB. Plant-based foods and prevention of cardiovascular disease: an overview. *Am J Clin Nutr* 2003; 78 (Suppl) 544S–551S.

145. Boyer J, Liu RH. Apple phytochemicals and their health benefits. *Nutr J* 2004; 3: 5.

146. Hu FB, Stampfer MJ, Manson JE, Rimm E, Colditz GA, Speier FE, Hennekens CH, Willett WC. Dietary protein and risk of ischemic heart disease in women. *Am J Clin Nutr* 1999; 70: 221–227.

147. Janikula M. Policosanol: a new treatment for cardiovascular disease? *Altern Med Rev* 2002; 7: 203–217.

148. Urizar NL, Moore DD. Gugulipid: a natural cholesterol-lowering agent. *Annu Rev Nutr* 2003; 23: 303–313.

149. Szapary PO, Wolfe ML, Bloedon LT, Cucchiara AJ, DerMarderosian AH, Cirigliano MD, Rader DJ. Guggulipid for the treatment of hypercholesterolemia: a randomized controlled trial. *JAMA* 2003; 290: 765–772.

150. Journoud M, Jones PJ. Red yeast rice: a new hypolipidemic drug. *Life Sci* 2004; 74: 2675–2683.

151. Bailey DG, Malcolm J, Arnold O, Spence JD. Grapefruit juice–drug interactions. *Br J Clin Pharmacol* 1998; 46: 101–110.

152. Harris RZ, Jang GR, Tsunoda S. Dietary effects on drug metabolism and transport. *Clin Pharmacokinet* 2003; 42: 1071–1088.

153. Dahan A, Altman H. Food-drug interaction: grapefruit juice augments drug bioavailability — mechanism, extent and relevance. *Eur J Clin Nutr* 2004; 58: 1–9.

154. Kaminsky LS, Zhang QY. The small intestine as a xenobiotic-metabolizing organ. *Drug Metab Dispos* 2003; 31: 1520–1525.

155. Dietrich CG, Geier A, Oude Elferink RP. ABC of oral bioavailability: transporters as gatekeepers in the gut. *Gut* 2003; 52: 1788–1795.

156. Zhang QY, Dunbar D, Ostrowska A, Zeisloft S, Yang J, Kaminsky LS. Characterization of human small intestinal cytochromes P-450. *Drug Metab Dispos* 1999; 27: 804–809.

157. Koch I, Weil R, Wolbold R, Brockmöller J, Hustert E, Burk O, Nuessler A, Neuhaus P, Eichelbaum M, Zanger U, Wojnowski L. Interindividual variability and tissue-specificity in the expression of cytochrome P450 3A mRNA. *Drug Metab Dispos* 2002; 30: 1108–1114.

158. Prueksaritatont T, Tang C, Qiu Y, Mu L, Subramanian R, Lin JH. Effects of fibrates on metabolism of statins in human hepatocytes. *Drug Metab Dispos.* 2002; 30: 1280–1287.

159. Cummins CL, Jacobsen W, Benet LZ. Unmasking the dynamic interplay between intestinal P-glycoprotein and CYP3A4. *J Pharmacol Exp Ther* 2002; 300: 1036–1045.

160. Bailey DG, Spence JD, Edgar B, Bayliff CD, Arnold JM. Ethanol enhances the hemodynamic effects of felodipine. *Clin Invest Med* 1989; 12: 357–362.

161. Bailey DG, Dresser GK. Interactions between grapefruit juice and cardiovascular drugs. *Am J Cardiovasc Drugs* 2004; 4: 281–297.

162. Scripture CD, Pieper JA. Clinical pharmacolinetics of fluvastatin. *Clin Pharmacokinet* 2001; 40: 263–281.

163. Kajinami K, Takekoshi N, Saito Y. Pitavastatin: efficacy and safety profiles of a novel synthetic HMG-CoA reductase inhibitor. *Cardiovasc Drug Rev* 2003; 21: 199–215.

164. Fukazawa I, Uchida N, Uchida E, Yasuhara H. Effects of grapefruit juice on pharmacokinetics of atorvastatin and pravastatin in Japanese. *Br J Clin Pharmacol* 2004; 57: 448–455.

165. Scott LJ, Curran MP, Figgit DP. Rosuvastatin: a review of its use in the management of dyslipidemia. *Am J Cardiovasc Drugs* 2004; 4: 117–138.

166. Lilja JJ, Neuvonen M, Neuvonen PJ. Effects of regular consumption of grapefruit juice on the pharmacokinetics of simvastatin. *Br J Clin Pharmacol* 2004; 58: 56–60.

167. Hashimoto K, Shirafuji T, Sekino H, Matsuoka O, Sekino H, Onnagawa O, Okamoto T, Kudo S, Azuma J. Interaction of citrus juices with pranidipine, a new 1,4-dihydropyridine calcium antagonist, in healthy subjects. *Eur J Clin Pharmacol* 1998; 54: 753–760.

168. Vincent J, Harris SI, Foulds G, Dogolo LC, Willavize S, Friedman HL. Lack of effect of grapefruit juice on the pharmacokinetics and pharmacodynamics of amlodipine. *Br J Clin Pharmacol* 2000; 50: 455–463.

169. Beudeker HJ, van der Velden JW, van der Aar EM. Interaction profile and tolerability of barnidipine. *Int J Clin Pract* 2000; 114 (Suppl): 36–40.

170. Uno T, Ohkubo T, Sugawara K, Higashiyama A, Motomura S, Ishizaki T. Effects of grapefruit juice on the stereoselective disposition of nicardipine in humans: evidence for dominant presystemic elimination at the gut site. *Eur J Clin Pharmacol.* 2000; 56: 643–649.

171. Fuhr U, Müller-Peltzer H, Kern R, Lopez-Rojas P, Junemann M, Harder S, Staib AH. Effects of grapefruit juice and smoking on verapamil concentrations in steady state. *Eur J Clin Pharmacol.* 2002; 58: 45–53.

172. Zaidenstein R, Soback S, Gips M, Avni B, Dishi V, Weissgarten Y, Golik A, Scapa E. Effect of grapefruit juice on the pharmacokinetics of losartan and its active metabolite E3174 in healthy volunteers. *Ther Drug Monit* 2001; 23: 369–373.

173. Lilja JJ, Backman JT, Laitila J, Luurila H, Neuvonen PJ. Itraconazole increases but grapefruit juice greatly decreases plasma concentrations of celiprolol. *Clin Pharmacol Ther* 2003; 73: 192–198.

174. Damkier P, Hansen LL, Brosen K. Effect of diclofenac, disulfiram, itraconazole, grapefruit juice and erythromycin on the pharmacokinetics of quinidine. *Br J Clin Pharmacol* 1999; 48: 829–838.

175. Libersa CC, Brique SA, Motte KB, Caron JF, Guedon-Moreau LM, Humbert L, Vincent A, Devos P, Lhermitte MA. Dramatic inhibition of amiodarone metabolism induced by grapefruit juice. *Br J Clin Pharmacol* 2000; 49: 373–378.

176. Edwards DJ, Bellevue FH III, Woster PM. Identification of 6′,7′-dihydrobergamottin, a cytochrome P450 inhibitor, in grapefruit juice. *Drug Metab Dispos.* 1996; 24: 1287-1290.

177. Lown KS, Bailey DG, Fontana RJ, Janardan SK, Adair CH, Fortlage LA, Brown MB, Guo W, Watkins PB. Grapefruit juice increases felodipine oral availability in humans by decreasing intestinal CYP3A protein expression. *J Clin Invest* 1997; 99: 2545–2553.

178. Schmiedlin-Ren P, Edwards DJ, Fitzsimmons ME, He K, Lown KS, Woster PM, Rahman A, Thummel KE, Fisher JM, Hollenberg PF, Watkins PB. Mechanism of enhanced oral availability of CYP 3A4 substrates by grapefruit constituents. Decreased enterocyte CYP 3A4 concentration and mechanism-based inactivation by furanocoumarins. *Drug Metab Dispos* 1997; 25: 1228–1233.

179. Ducharme MP, Warbasse LH, Edwards DJ. Disposition of intravenous and oral cyclosporine after administration with grapefruit juice. *Clin Pharmacol Ther* 1995; 57: 485–491.

180. Lundahl J, Regardh CG, Edgar B, Johansson G. Effects of grapefruit juice ingestion-pharmacokinetics and haemodynamics of intravenously and orally administered felodipine in healthy men. *Eur J Clin Pharmacol* 1997; 52: 139–145.

181. Veronese ML, Gillen LP, Burke JP, Dorval EP, Hauck WW, Pequignot E, Waldman SA, Greenberg HE. Exposure-dependent inhibition of intestinal and hepatic CYP3A4 *in vivo* by grapefruit juice. *J Clin Pharmacol* 2003; 43: 831–839.

182. Guo LQ, Fukuda K, Ohta T, Yamazoe Y. Role of furanocoumarin derivatives on grapefruit juice-mediated inhibition of human CYP3A activity. *Drug Metab Dispos* 2000; 28: 766–771.

183. Wen YH, Sahi J, Urda E, Kulkarni S, Rose K, Zheng X, Sinclair Jf, Cai H, Strom SC, Kostrubsky VE. Effects of bergamottin on human and monkey drug-metabolizing enzymes in primary cultured hepatocytes. *Drug Metab Dispos* 2002; 30: 977–984.

184. Goosen TC, Cillie D, Bailey DG, Yu C, He K, Hollenberg PF, Woster PM, Cohen L, Williams JA, Rheeders M, Dijkstra HP. Bergamottin contribution to the grapefruit juice-felodipine interaction and disposition in humans. *Clin Pharmacol Ther* 2004; 76: 607–617.

185. Paine MF, Criss AB, Watkins PB. Two major grapefruit juice components differ in intestinal CYP3A4 inhibition kinetic and binding properties. *Drug Metab Dispos* 2004; 32: 1146–1153.

186. Bailey DG, Dresser GK, Kreeft JH, Munoz C, Freeman DJ, Bend JR. Grapefruit–felodipine interaction: effect of unprocessed fruit and probable active ingredients. *Clin Pharmacol Ther* 2000; 68: 468–477.

187. Wang EJ, Casiano CN, Clement RP, Johnson WW. Inhibition of P-glycoprotein transport function by grapefruit juice psoralen. *Pharm Res* 2001; 18: 432–438.

188. Honda Y, Ushigome F, Koyabu N, Moritomo S, Shoyama Y, Uchiumi T, Kuwano M, Ohtani H, Sawada Y. Effects of grapefruit and orange juice components on P-glycoprotein- and MRP2-mediated drug efflux. *Br J Pharmacol* 2004; 143: 856–864.

189. Schachter M. Chemical, pharmacokinetic and pharmacodynamic properties of statins: an update. *Fundam Clin Pharmacol* 2005 19: 117–125.

190. Sata F, Sapone A, Elizondo A, Stocker P, Miller VP, Zheng W, Raunio H, Crespi CL, Gonzalez FJ. *CYP3A4* allelic variants with amino acid substitutions in exons 7 and 12: evidence for an allelic variant with altered catalytic activity. *Clin Pharmacol Ther* 2000 67; 67: 48–56.

191. Lamba JK, Lin YS, Thummel K, Daly A, Watkins PB, Strom S, Zhang J, Scuetz EG. Common allelic variants of cytochrome P4503A and their prevalence in different populations. *Pharmacogenetics* 2002; 12: 121–132.

192. Schuetz EG. Lessons from the *CYP3A4* promoter. *Mol Pharmacol* 2004; 65: 279–281.

193. Matsumura K, Saito T, Takahashi Y, Ozeki T, Kiyotani K, Fujieda M, Yamazaki H, Kunitoh H, Kamataki T. Identification of a novel polymorphic enhancer of the human *CYP3A4* gene. *Mol Pharmacol* 2004; 65: 326–334.

194. Kajinami K, Brousseau ME, Ordovas JM, Schaefer EJ. *CYP3A4* genotypes and plasma lipoprotein levels before and after treatment with atorvastatin in primary hypercholesterolemia. *Am J Cardiol* 2004; 93: 104–107.

195. Wang A, Yu BN, Luo CH, Tan ZR, Zhou G, Wang LS, Zhang W, Li Z Liu J, Zhou HH. *Ile118Val* genetic polymorphism of *CYP3A4* and its effects on lipid-lowering efficacy of simvastatin in Chinese hyperlipidemic patients. *Eur J Clin Pharmacol* 2005; 60: 843–848.

196. Schwab M, Eichelbaum M, Fromm MF. Genetic polymorphisms of the human MDR1 drug transporter. *Annu Rev Pharmacol Toxicol* 2003; 43: 285–307.

197. Sakaeda T, Nakamura T, Okumura K. Pharmacogenetics of MDR1 and its impact on the pharmacokinetics and pharmacodynamics of drugs. *Pharmacogenomics* 2003; 4: 397–410.

198. Niemi M, Schaeffeler E, Lang T, Fromm MF, Neuvonen M, Kyrklund C, Backman JT, Kerb R, Schwab M, Neuvonen PJ, Eichelbaum M, Kivisto KT. High plasma pravastatin concentrations are associated with single nucleotide polymorphisms and haplotypes of organic anion transporting polypeptide-C (OATP-C, SLCO1B1). *Pharmacogenomics* 2004; 14: 429–440.

199. Dresser GK, Bailey DG, Leake BF, Schwarz UI, Dawson PA, Freeman DJ, Kim RB. Fruit juices inhibit organic anion transporting polypeptide-mediated drug intake to decrease the oral availability of fexofenadine. *Clin Pharmacol Ther* 2002; 71: 11–20.

200. Ehrhardt M, Lindenmaier H, Burhenne J, Haefeli WE, Weiss J. Influence of lipid lowering fibrates on P-glycoprotein activity *in vitro*. *Biochem Pharmacol* 2004; 67: 285–292.

201. Chang JT, Staffa JA, Parks M, Green L. Rhabdomyolysis with HMG-CoA reductase inhibitors and gemfibrozil combination therapy. *Pharmacoepidemiol Drug Saf* 2004; 13: 417–426.

202. Borradaile NM, de Dreu LE, Barrett PH, Huff MW. Inhibition of hepatocyte apoB secretion by naringenin: enhanced rapid intracellular degradation independent of reduced microsomal cholesteryl esters. *J Lipid Res* 2002; 43: 1544–1554.

203. Gorinstein S, Caspi A, Libman I, Katrich E, Lerner HT, Trakhtenberg S. Preventive effects of diets supplemented with sweetie fruits in hypercholesterolemic patients suffering from coronary artery disease. *Prev Med* 2004; 38: 841–847.
204. Takanaga H, Ohnishi A, Yamada S, Matsuo H, Morimoto S, Shoyama Y Ohtani H, Sawada Y. Polymethoxylated flavones in orange juice are inhibitors of P-glycoprotein but not cytochrome P450 3A4. *Pharmacol Exp Ther* 2000; 293: 230–236.
205. Xu J, Go ML, Lim LY. Modulation of digoxin transport across Caco-2 cell monolayers by citrus fruit juices: lime, lemon, grapefruit, and pummelo. *Pharm Res* 2003; 20: 169–176.
206. Lilja JJ, Juntti-Patinen L, Neuvonen PJ. Orange juice substantially reduces the bioavailability of the beta-adrenergic-blocking agent celiprolol. *Clin Pharmacol Ther* 2004; 75: 184–190.
207. Hidaka M, Fujita K, Ogikubo T, Yamasaki K, Iwakiri T, Okumura M, Kodama H, Arimori K. Potent inhibition by star fruit of human cytochrome P450 3A (CYP3A) activity. *Drug Metab Dispos.* 2004; 32: 581–583.
208. Craig WJ. Health-promoting properties of common herbs. *Am J Clin Nutr* 1999; 70 (3 Suppl): 491S–499S.
209. Moore LB, Goodwin B, Jones SA, Wisely GB, Serabjit-Singh CJ, Willson TM, Collins JL, Kliewer SA. St. John's wort induces hepatic drug metabolism through activation of the pregnane X receptor. *Proc Natl Acad Sci USA* 2000; 97: 7500–7502.
210. Dürr D, Stieger B, Kullak-Ublick GA, Rentsch KM, Steinert HC, Meier PJ, Fattinger K. St. John's wort induces intestinal P-glycoprotein/MDR1 and intestinal and hepatic CYP3A4. *Clin Pharmacol Ther* 2000; 68: 598–604.
211. Markowitz JS, Donovan JL, DeVane CL, Taylor RM, Ruan Y, Wang J-S, Chavin KD. Effect of St. John's wort on drug metabolism by induction of cytochrome P450 3A4 Enzyme. *JAMA* 2003; 290: 1500–1504.
212. Sugimoto K, Ohmori M, Tsuruoka S, Nishiki K, Kawaguchi A, Harada K, Arakawa M, Sakamoto K, Masada M, Miyamori I, Fujimura A. Different effects of St. John's wort on the pharmacokinetics of simvastatin and pravastatin. *Clin Pharmacol Ther* 2001; 70: 518–524.
213. Ang-Lee MK, Moss J, Yuan C-S. Herbal medicines and perioperative care. *JAMA* 2001; 286: 208–216.
214. Zhou S, Lim LY, Chowbay B. Herbal modulation of P-glycoprotein. *Drug Metab Rev* 2004; 36: 57–104.
215. Izzo AA, Di Carlo G, Borrelli F, Ernst E. Cardiovascular pharmacotherapy and herbal medicines: the risk of drug interaction. *Int J Cardiol* 2005; 98: 1–14.
216. Loktionov A. Common gene polymorphisms and nutrition: emerging links with pathogenesis of multifactorial chronic diseases (review). *J Nutr Biochem* 2003; 14: 426–451.
217. Cascorbi I, Paul M, Kroemer HK. Pharmacogenetics of heart failure — focus on drug disposition and action. *Cardiovasc Res* 2004; 64: 32–39.
218. Masson LF, McNeill G. The effect of genetic variation on the lipid response to dietary change: recent findings. *Curr Opin Lipidol* 2005; 16: 61–67.

3 Phytochemicals, Xenobiotic Metabolism, and Carcinogenesis

James B. Kirkland

CONTENTS

3.1 INTRODUCTION

Nitrite preservatives in processed meats lead to the formation of carcinogenic nitrosamines (NAs), while smoking and cooking of meats leads to the formation of polycyclic aromatic hydrocarbons (PAHs) and heterocyclic amines (HCAs). Cigarette smoke is also a potent source of NA, PAH, and HCA carcinogens. Conversely, consumption of vegetables, spices, and green tea are associated with decreased cancer risk, and many phytochemicals from these sources are proven chemoprotective agents in animal models. NAs, PAHs, and HCAs are stable secondary carcinogens, which are "bioactivated" by P450-based Phase I metabolism to form reactive, ultimate carcinogens. This is also required for effective metabolism, as it allows them to be conjugated (Phase II metabolism) and excreted, preventing the accumulation of parent compounds in areas like the adipose and brain tissue. Thus, the goal in cancer prevention is to find the optimal balance between Phase I and II activities, which allow clearance, while minimizing the accumulation of reactive intermediates. Smoking and regular consumption of cooked meats are negative influences, as P450 enzymes are induced and bioactivation becomes too rapid for Phase II reactions to keep pace. Chemoprotective phytochemicals improve the metabolic balance by antagonizing P450 induction, by competitively inhibiting P450 enzymes, and by inducing the expression of Phase II enzymes. Thus, phytochemical intake can dramatically alter the carcinogenicity of a given exposure to dietary carcinogens.

3.2 DIETARY CARCINOGENS AND XENOBIOTIC METABOLISM

Many of our common cancers are responsive to diet and lifestyle habits, leading to popular estimates that around 60% of cancers are "avoidable" if the ideal diet and lifestyle were to be followed.[1] The most common cancers in men (worldwide) are lung, colorectal, stomach, liver, prostate, esophageal, bladder, and oral cavity.[2] This pattern is also present in women, with the addition of breast, cervical, and ovarian cancers as important sites. Many of the common cancers have well-established negative diet and lifestyle risk factors. Lung and oral cancers are strongly associated with smoking, chewing of tobacco, and alcohol consumption.[1] Colorectal, esophageal, larynx, gastric, bladder, prostate, and breast cancer risks have been associated with a high intake of cooked meat.[3–5] The relationship between meat intake and increased risk of colorectal cancer is greatly strengthened with the use of doneness level as a factor. Sinha et al. found that the enhanced risk of colorectal cancer increased from 10 to 29% per 10 g/d red meat intake when the analysis was restricted to well-done meat.[6] Knize et al. have reviewed epidemiological studies on the consumption of well-done meat and cancer risk, finding that over 80% of studies find significant associations.[3] Hematopoietic,[7] oral,[8] nasopharageal,[8,9] esophageal,[8,10] stomach,[11] colorectal,[8] and prostate[12] cancers have also been linked to preserved meats. Maternal exposure to preserved meats has been associated with childhood brain tumors as well.[13] The association of cancer risk with cooking and preserving of meats is quite controversial, with varied research findings in human and animal studies.

Epidemiological studies present difficulties in estimating not only meat intake, but also cooking methods and the extent of cooking. Survey tools need to be improved, including databases for carcinogen content by meat type and cooking method, and visual aids to maximize the accuracy of collected data.[14,15] Diets rich in cooked and processed meats tend to have more saturated and higher

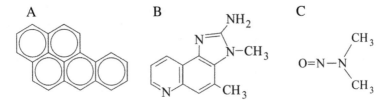

FIGURE 3.1 Examples of the three major classes of dietary secondary carcinogens: (A) Benzo(a)pyrene (BaP), example of a polycyclic aromatic hydrocarbon (PAH), formed through condensation of small radicals during the incomplete combustion of any burnable substrate, requiring temperatures above 250°C. (B) 2-amino-3,4-methylimidazo[4,5-f]quinoline (MeIQ), example of a heterocyclic amine (HCA), formed through condensation of creatinine, amino acids, and sugars, across a broad range of meat cooking conditions, enhanced by drying, as seen in the formation of gravy and jerky products. (C) Dimethylnitrosamine (DMN), example of a nitrosamine (NA), formed through reaction of nitrite with secondary amines found in preserved meats and seafoods, also central to cigarette smoke carcinogenesis in the formation nicotine/nitrite reaction products (e.g., NNK).

levels of fat. Animal models making use of practical foods, rather than single purified carcinogens, will eventually provide unbiased data on these factors. Liver cancer is associated with alcohol abuse in developed countries and hepatitis B and aflatoxin exposure in developing countries.

Many of these negative risk factors can be explained by the exposure to secondary carcinogens. Our major dietary carcinogens are all secondary carcinogens, which are very stable, lipophilic compounds, generally formed during food processing and cooking.[16] The main categories of carcinogens in cooked and preserved meats are polycyclic aromatic hydrocarbons (PAHs), heterocyclic amines (HCAs) and nitrosamines (NAs)[16] (Figure 3.1). PAHs, like benzo(a)pyrene (BaP), are formed when material is partially burned, during smoking, grilling, and barbequing. PAHs will form from any substrate, but flame grilling of high fat foods is an excellent example.[17] PAHs are also formed in the smoke of burning wood chips and they dissolve into meats during the smoking process.[17,18] BaP is the main focus of regulatory efforts, limited to 5 µg/kg in smoked meats in the European Community. This is despite the fact that BaP is a relatively small and variable proportion of total PAH load in cooked or smoked food.[18]

HCAs are formed when meats are cooked at below carbonization temperatures, as creatinine reacts with various amino acids to form products like 2-amino-1-methyl-6-phenylimidazo-[4,5-b]-pyridine (PhIP), 2-amino-3,8-dimethylimidazo[4,5-f]quinoxaline (MeIQ$_x$), and 2-amino-3-methylimidazo[4,5-f]quinoline (IQ).[3] Sugars may enhance this process when they are added to marinades or during the processing of beef jerky.[19] During the grilling of meat, higher temperature cooking to the same final internal temperature produces significantly higher levels of HCAs.[3] Pan residues used in the production of gravy and food flavor products tend to have higher levels of HCAs than the meat itself, especially if the residue dried under heat. This concentrates the reactants and causes large increases in cooking temperature.[20] The recovery of free HCAs from cooked meat samples is traditionally used to estimate the degree of formation of these carcinogens. However, it is now known that half or more of the total mutagenic capacity remains covalently bound within the protein structure, to be released during digestion.[21] This is likely due to the participation of amino acid side chains in HCA formation reactions without being released from the peptide structure, and it leads to significant underestimations of dietary HCA exposure if not corrected for.

The preservative nitrite forms reactive species that combine with secondary amines to form NA end products like dimethylnitrosamine (DMN). These reactions are encouraged by the acidic conditions of the stomach,[13,22] and by bacterial populations in other areas of the digestive tract or in cured, fermented foods.[10] N-nitrosamides are produced through the nitrosation of amides, and are unstable and short-lived.[23] They do, however, have an experimental carcinogenic profile that is more likely to cause leukemias and pediatric brain tumors, and future research should consider the role of endogenous nitrosamide formation following cured meat consumption.[23] Meats are cured using salt and nitrite to prevent bacterial growth and food poisoning, especially botulism. Cured, fermented fish are an excellent source of DMN, as high trimethylamine and dimethylamine levels and nitrite react with the aid of bacterial metabolism. These food products are associated with esophageal cancer in certain areas of the world.[10] Cured meats, like hot dogs and cold cuts, contain amino acids, which provide secondary amine substrates for nitrosamine formation.[23]

Figure 3.1 shows examples of the three major classes of secondary carcinogens. Both PAHs and HCAs are very lipophilic and planar molecules, and they are metabolized by similar P450 enzymes and have similar effects on gene expression through the aryl hydrocarbon receptor (AhR). NAs tend to be somewhat more water soluble and have different activation routes and induction patterns.

Tobacco smoke is a rich source of PAH, HCA, and NA carcinogens. Chewing tobacco is a more focused source of NAs, specifically the tobacco-specific nitrosamines, including N′-nitrosonornicotine (NNN) and 4-(methylnitrosamino)-1-(3-pyridyl)-1-butanone (NNK). These form in a reaction between nitrite (enhanced by fertilization practices) and nicotine during the curing of tobacco leaves.[24] Thus, tobacco products and cooked meats provide a similar spectrum of secondary carcinogens, albeit in different concentrations and via different routes of exposure. Importantly, the risks of contracting cancer from cooked meats and from cigarette smoke are both related to the balance of Phase I and II metabolic capacity of the individual, responding to diet, lifestyle and genetic factors.

Secondary carcinogens must be metabolized to prevent them from accumulating in the fashion of polychlorinated biphenyls (PCBs) or methyl mercury. The main enzyme system that accomplishes this is cytochrome P450, a family of broad spectrum enzymes that charge substrates with electrons until they oxidize (Phase I), creating functional groups that can be conjugated by Phase II reactions.[25] Essentially all dietary carcinogens require "bioactivation" by Phase I reactions to form the ultimate carcinogens that disrupt DNA structure, leading to mutations and cancer. Phase II reactions, especially glutathione and

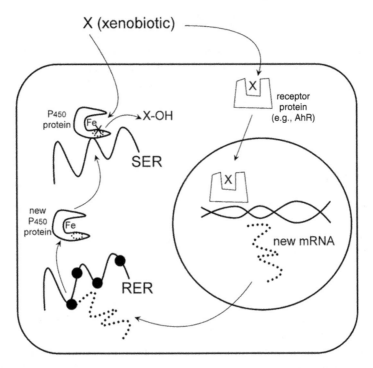

FIGURE 3.2 Secondary carcinogen bioactivation and conjugation. Stable secondary carcinogens require metabolism to prevent accumulation, leading to the formation of reactive intermediates that cause DNA damage and cancer. These can be safely metabolized to water-soluble conjugates, if the balance of Phase I and II enzymes and conjugating agents is favorable.

glucuronide conjugation, are usually protective in the detoxification of the reactive products of Phase I reactions. N-acetylation is a notable exception, in that it aids in the bioactivation of HCA.[25] These pathways are summarized in Figure 3.2.

While dietary carcinogens need to be metabolized by P450 routes to prevent them from accumulating, they do not need to be metabolized rapidly. We consume carcinogens in relatively small amounts, and they can be effectively cleared with low levels of P450 activity. Very high levels of P450 activity will generally increase cancer risk, as ultimate carcinogens are generated more rapidly than they can be cleared by Phase II conjugation reactions. This has been demonstrated in many animal model systems and is supported by human epidemiological findings. Higher levels of dietary protein enhance liver P450 activity and, in turn, increase the hepatocarcinogenicity of aflatoxin in rats.[26] Similarly, ethanol intake by rats induces specific forms of P450, increasing the bioactivation of NA compounds.[27] This reflects the synergism in human populations between alcohol abuse, cigarette smoking, and head and neck cancer incidence.[28]

As expected, a high capacity for Phase II conjugation reactions will generally decrease cancer risk. This can also be seen in the protective effect of dietary sulfur amino acids during the treatment of acetaminophen toxicity, where support of glutathione levels aids in the conjugation of the reactive acetaminophen metabolite created by P450 metabolism.[29] Thus, diet and lifestyle have a large impact on the susceptibility to a given dose of secondary carcinogens, through the expression of genes for P450 enzymes, conjugation enzymes, and the enzymes that generate conjugating agents.

3.3 ANIMAL-BASED RESEARCH ON COOKED MEAT CARCINOGENS

It is important to note that well done meat contains a wide variety of HCA and PAH carcinogens, with additional NAs associated with meat preservative use. Animal models have followed reductionist approaches in testing potential carcinogens individually and usually using high, single-dose models, many of which are not even based on oral exposure routes. Large numbers of PAHs, HCAs, and NAs have been shown to be potent multiple organ and transplacental carcinogens in mice and rats.[30] These data are too extensive to cover here. Very little work has been conducted on the consumption of cooked and preserved meat products in rodent models, or even chronic low-level dietary exposure to mixtures representing the different classes of secondary carcinogens. Feeding hot dogs to rats and mice was shown to cause a progressive increase in NA levels as the diet moved along the gastrointestinal tract (GIT).[31] Feeding a well-cooked beef diet enhanced 1,2-dimethylhydrazine-induced cancer in rats.[32] Conversely, diets containing fried chicken, beef, lamb, pork, and fish were not found to cause mutations in the Dlb-1 locus in mice,[33] and cooked beef was not found to cause PhIP adducts or genomic instability in the GI tissues of rats.[34] A standardized rodent model for exposure to cooked and preserved meats would allow important work to be conducted on cancer prevention strategies.

3.4 METABOLISM OF DIETARY SECONDARY CARCINOGENS

3.4.1 METABOLISM OF NAs

NAs are converted by P450 enzymes to reactive intermediates that break down to form diazonium ions, which in turn react with DNA bases, leading to adducts and mutations. DMN is bioactivated most actively by CYP2E1, the P450 enzyme that is induced by ethanol exposure. The association of head and neck (oral, nasal, esophageal, larynx, pharynx) cancer risk with ethanol use is likely due, in part, to the induction of P450 enzymes in these tissues, leading to more rapid bioactivation of dietary carcinogens. Ethanol exposure causes a rapid induction of CYP2E1 in gastrointestinal tissues and the liver, via protein stabilization. Ethanol also has a solvent effect in the transport of dietary carcinogens into epithelial tissues, and ethanol also causes cytotoxicity and cell division, which may also increase cancer risk. There is a dramatic synergism between ethanol consumption and smoking with respect to head and neck cancer risk.[28] The smoke-specific nitrosamine NNK is bioactivated by various P450 enzymes, including CYP2E1 and CYP2A family enzymes.[35]

NAs are metabolized by P450 to unstable intermediates that break down spontaneously to form alkyldiazonium ions, which are the ultimate carcinogen species.[36] These are short-lived and Phase II metabolism of these intermediates is not a popular research area, but they are electrophilic species and the majority of conjugation occurs with glutathione. Electrophiles are species with a net positive charge or a local area of positive charge that can react with other molecules. Glutathione contains a sulfhydryl group with a high electron density that allows it to react with electrophilic intermediates, preventing them from alkylating cellular proteins and DNA. This Phase II conjugation is enhanced by several forms of glutathione-S-transferase, an enzyme with high activity in tissues that have to metabolize xenobiotics, especially the liver. Oral support of glutathione via N-acetylcysteine supplementation decreased the induction of esophageal cancer in rats following diethylnitrosamine treatment.[37]

3.4.2 Metabolism of PAH and HCA Families

Conditions will tend to produce a mixture of PAHs and HCAs in most well-cooked meat products. High temperature cooking with flareups and noticeable black residue will indicate PAH formation. Any combustible substrate that burns incompletely will form small radicals, which polymerize to create PAHs.[25] These reactions are favored by a high fat content and high cooking temperatures. PAHs are also formed by the burning of woods chips in food smokers and in cigarette smoke. PAHs from smoke will diffuse into food products and lung tissue due to their lipophilic nature.

In contrast, HCAs are favored by slower cooking at lower temperatures, leading to drying, which concentrates the breakdown products of amino acids and creatinine, which polymerize to form HCA end products like PhIP and IQ.[3] PAH and HCA families are similar in several regards; the parent compounds are planar and lipophilic and are activated by CYP1A family enzymes. Activation may require more than one CYP1A oxidation (e.g., BaP) or the participation of Phase II conjugation (e.g., N-acetylation in the activation of HCAs). Both PAHs and HCAs interact with the AhR and induce CYP1A family enzymes.

3.4.3 Metabolism of PAHs

Most of the research on PAHs metabolism has been conducted on BaP, which is an excellent substrate for CYP1A family P450 enzymes (CYP1A1 in lung and the GIT, CYP1A2 in the liver). BaP is converted to a 7,8-epoxide by CYP1A enzymes, but this is quickly reduced to a 1,8-diol by epoxide hydratase. A second CYP1A epoxidation occurs at the 9,10 position, and further metabolism of this electrophilic residue is hindered by the presence of the bay-region ring structure. This impairs the activity of glutathione-*S*-transferase (GST) toward this intermediate, and UDP-glucuronyltransferase (UDPGT) is required to conjugate the 7,8-diols. In considering the whole family of PAHs metabolites, there will be a mixture of glutathione conjugation of electrophiles and glucuronic acid conjugation of nucleophiles[38]. Many dietary components that act as chemopreventative agents are found to induce the expression of GST and UDPGT enzymes (see Section 3.11).

3.4.4 METABOLISM OF HCAS

HCAs are also excellent substrates for CYP1A family enzymes and the resulting products are N-hydroxylated intermediates. These intermediates tend to be N-acetylated or sulfated in a Phase II reaction that creates the ultimate carcinogenic metabolites.[39] This is one of a small list of cases in which Phase II conjugations are procarcinogenic. HCAs metabolites are varied in structure and both glutathione and glucuronic acid conjugation appear to play a role in detoxification. PhIP is the most abundant HCAs in cooked meats, although others are more potent carcinogens. Reactive PhIP metabolites may be metabolized by conjugation with both glutathione and glucuronic acid,[40,41] while other HCA metabolites appear to be mainly conjugated via glucuronidation.[42] Individuals with low activity of the glutathione-*S*-transferase required for PhIP conjugation appear to be at higher risk for the development of colorectal cancer.[40] Conversely, high activity polymorphisms for N-acetyltransferase (fast acetylators) increase the risk for occurrence of colorectal cancer when combined with a high intake of red meat .[43]

3.5 AFLATOXIN AND FOOD SPOILAGE

Aflatoxin is an important hepatocarcinogen in developing countries. It represents a diversion from the previous examples in that it forms mainly on plant products, and it forms through spoilage rather than cooking. It is also a secondary carcinogen and its potency is also affected by changes in Phase I and II metabolism. Aflatoxin is activated to a hepatocarcinogenic epoxide by CYP3A4 and CYP1A2, and significant protection is provided by glutathione conjugation of this intermediate.[44] Human liver expression of the most protective form of glutathione-*S*-transferase is normally quite low and chemopreventative agents may function by inducing these enzymes.[44] Poorly stored grain products and peanuts are examples of foods that may be contaminated with aflatoxin.

3.6 EFFECTS OF CARCINOGEN EXPOSURE ON XENOBIOTIC METABOLISM

When xenobiotics enter a cell, they may interact with two main types of proteins, namely enzymes and receptors. The primary enzymes will be a variety of P450 gene products, with 57 individual members, with overlapping substrate recognition. This will usually lead to a catalytic reaction with the formation of oxidized products of the xenobiotics, possibly leading to the formation of reactive, ultimate carcinogens. Conversely, the xenobiotic may bind to a receptor protein, forming a complex that enters the nucleus and drives the expression of new mRNA from a specific group of genes. This is illustrated in Figure 3.2 and Figure 3.3.

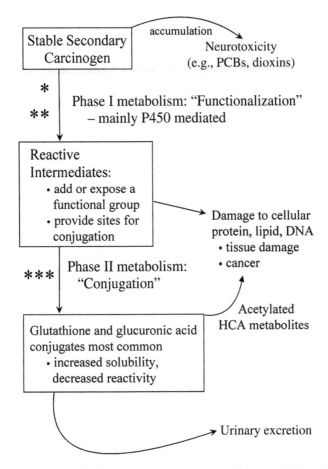

FIGURE 3.3 Cytochrome P450 activity and induction. Cytochrome P450 activity is limited to the catalytic cycle in the upper left of the diagram. Induction patterns, of both Phase I and II enzymes, play a critical role in the potency of dietary carcinogens. *Xenobiotics bind to specific receptors, which then act as transcription factors to induce the synthesis of new P450 enzymes, usually with a high capacity to metabolize that specific xenobiotic. **Phytochemicals tend to compete directly at the P450 active site to slow carcinogen bioactivation. Competition also takes place at the AhR, where phytochemicals can decrease the induction of P450 expression caused by secondary carcinogens. Large exposure to phytochemicals can activate the AhR, however, leading to procarcinogenic effects. ***Phytochemicals induce multiple forms of Phase II conjugation enzymes and agents.

As an example, benzo(a)pyrene (BaP) will enter a cell and be metabolized to reactive intermediates by CYP1A1/1A2 gene products. At the same time, BaP will also bind the aryl hydrocarbon receptor (AhR), forming a complex that induces the synthesis of a spectrum of new mRNA sequences, including that of CYP1A1/2 genes.[45] Therefore, with chronic exposure to BaP, there will be a progressive increase in CYP1A1/2 protein levels, which will enhance the rate of bioactivation and ultimate carcinogenicity of BaP. This has been shown in numerous animal models and even in human subjects consuming grilled meats.[46]

This system is logically designed to enhance the metabolic capacity for xenobiotics, which are present in tissues at a given time. It doesn't always favor long-term health, however. From an evolutionary perspective, it is more important to prevent the accumulation of lipophilic contaminants, which could disrupt fetal development, rather than prevent the long-term development of cancer. This is especially true in cultures where the average lifespan was shorter than that required to observe significant cancer incidence. This would have been true throughout the majority of evolutionary history, and the recent increase in human lifespan presents chronic disease conditions that were not a major issue in the distant past.

Some xenobiotics induce P450 genes that are not effective in metabolism of the inducing agent. Examples include dioxins and PCBs, which bind to and activate the AhR but are not metabolized by CYP1A1/2 with any efficiency. A broad spectrum of oncogenic genes are induced via dioxin-AhR activation, while other AhR ligands appear to decrease cancer risk.[45] These differences may be based on dose/potency and will be discussed later. Other receptors are present to control the expression levels of other P450 families, including the steroid and xenobiotic receptor (SXR) and the constitutive androstane receptor (CAR).[47] The SXR receptor controls the expression of some CYP3A family enzymes, which are the work horses of xenobiotic metabolism, comprising the majority of intestinal and liver P450 expression. The SXR is activated by binding with a wide variety of substrates, including endogenous and synthetic steroids, antibiotics, and various phytochemicals. One potent activator of the SXR is hyperforin, the active agent in St. John's wort, an antidepressive herbal product. There have been many cases of St. John's wort leading to failure of pharmaceutical regimens, including immunosuppressant medication and birth control, due to induction of CYP3A4 and decreased circulating drug concentration.[47] The CAR was found to mediate the classical induction of the CYP2B subfamily by phenobarbital, but the response is now known to be much more complex. CAR, SXR, and the retinoid X receptor (RXR) heterodimerize and generate complex patterns of P450 expression in response to xenobiotic and endobiotic exposure.[47] Other nuclear receptors that play a role in P450 expression include the peroxisome proliferator activated receptor (PPAR), the liver X receptor (LXR), and the farnesoid X receptor (FXR).[48]

Phase II conjugation enzymes, and the enzymes required to synthesize conjugating agents, are also regulated in response to environmental exposure to xenobiotics. The pattern of regulation is more complex than seen in Phase I genes. There are significant roles for the AhR, CAR, SXR/PXR, FXR, LXR, and PPAR receptors in the expression of Phase II enzymes like glutathione-S-transferases and UDP-glucuronyltransferases.[49] It is important to note that these receptors form a transcription factor after binding with a ligand, and the resulting complexes have unique actions. A dioxin-AhR complex is an excellent CYP1A inducer, while an indole-3-carbinol (a known AhR agonist) will induce both Phase I and II genes, but will antagonize the stronger dioxin-AhR induction of CYP1A genes.[50] There is an additional mechanism that detects oxidant stress through a complex of Keap1/Nrf2 proteins in the cytosol. Oxidant stress, induced by reactive oxygen species or electrophilic xenobiotic metabolites, causes the release of Nrf2, which travels to the nucleus and binds to antioxidant response elements (ARE) in numerous gene promoters.[51] This pathway is active in the induction of glutathione-S-transferase and UDP-glucuronyltransferase genes, and also induces gamma-glutamyl cysteine synthetase (rate limiting in GSH synthesis) and UDP-glucose dehydrogenase (last enzyme in UDP-glucuronic acid formation).[52]

These complex patterns of gene expression in Phase I and II enzymes play a central role in determining the potency of a given exposure to dietary secondary carcinogens and are central to the effects of chemopreventative agents. Human subjects who consumed a diet high in char-grilled meat for 7 days were found to have a significant induction of intestinal and liver CYP1A activity.[46] In a similar design with pan-fried meat consumption, HCAs alone were shown to induce hepatic CYP1A2 activity.[53] While these experiments did not determine the extent of DNA damage in target tissues, animal models suggest that the induced state following cooked meat consumption represents enhanced cancer risk, even if the exposure to secondary carcinogens was kept constant.

3.7 DIET AS A SOURCE OF CHEMOPREVENTATIVE AGENTS

Plant-based foods are a good source of almost all of the nutrients required by humans, but this is a relatively small number of chemicals (40 to 45, depending on interpretation). When we consume fruits and vegetables, we are exposed to thousands of additional compounds that may present health benefits or toxicological risks. The important concept is that these are xenobiotics (strange to life), not nutrients. Very few of these compounds are present for the purpose of being beneficial to human health, although long-term cultivation of certain plants has created some examples of this. Most represent chemical defenses (phytoalexins) designed to counter rodent, insect, or fungal attacks. When humans or experimental animals consume these compounds, the compounds are metabolized by typical xenobiotic enzymes and often have dramatic effects on Phase I and II enzyme activities and expression patterns.

In contrast to the effects of meat consumption, the incidence of various GI cancers[54] and lung cancers[55] decreases with increased vegetable consumption. Public attention, popular press, and the research community have focused attention on the antioxidant roles of nutrients and phytochemicals in fruits and vegetables. The antioxidant capacity of food extracts may be tested by methods that determine the ability of compounds to scavenge radicals in an *in vitro* system (e.g., FRAP, TEAC, and ORAC methods).[56] In these tests, both the phytochemicals and radicals are at high concentrations and placed in close proximity, which does not generally reflect the *in vivo* situation of tissue distribution and metabolism, and subcellular localization of these compounds. Interestingly, some whole animal and human intervention experiments show that biomarkers of oxidant stress are decreased and health end points, such as memory and brain function in aging rats, are improved.[57,58] These data are not as clear as it seems, however.

The main defense against reactive oxygen species in mammalian cells depends on glutathione (GSH) as a reducing agent, and the selenium-dependent enzyme glutathione peroxidase to detoxify hydrogen peroxide. During chronic oxidant stress, the pathway for glutathione synthesis is upregulated, namely the limiting enzyme, gamma-glutamylcysteine synthase.[59] If a diet actually protects against oxidant stress, this enzyme should be downregulated, but it is, in fact, upregulated with the consumption of a high berry diet,[60] and by flavonoids from onions and other vegetables.[61] The apparent explanation is that phytochemicals (which are xenobiotics) create a low level of oxidant stress that enhances oxidant defense, leading to improved health. There are many examples of small, manageable stresses working to strengthen a system and improve health. This is observed in the case of regular exercise, which increases the formation of reactive oxygen, but enhances defense systems,[59,62] in the end decreasing tissue biomarkers of oxidant stress[63] and delaying the development of chronic disease. This concept of low-level stress improving cellular function is an important and underappreciated concept in toxicology. The public, and many policy makers, view exposures to one group of compounds as good, and exposure to another group of compounds as dangerous, without proper consideration of dose response (further discussion in Section 3.13).

CARET and ATBC experience was an extension of the public and scientific obsession with oxidant stress and defense as a central theme in the fruit and vegetable cancer interaction. CARET and ATBC were two randomized human interventions in which human smokers were treated with large doses (about fivefold above normal dietary intake) of beta-carotene,[55,64–66] based on reasonably strong epidemiology associating high carotenoid intake with decreased lung cancer incidence. Assuming that oxidant stress was a central force in lung cancer development and that beta-carotene was an effective radical scavenger, it was hypothesized that supplementation would decrease lung cancer development. Both large studies found a significant increase in lung cancer incidence, cardiovascular events, and overall mortality with double-blinded beta-carotene supplementation, over the relatively short period of 5 to 8 years. One of the most interesting findings in both the CARET and ATBC studies was that people with higher baseline carotenoid status were still protected from lung cancer,[55,66] even in the beta-carotene supplemented group where the baseline carotenoids should have just been adding to the excessive carotenoid intake. It was clear from these studies that baseline carotenoids were acting as a proxy for the intake of other nutrients or phytochemicals, which were providing a significant protection against cigarette smoke-induced carcinogenesis.

One of the basic assumptions driving these clinical trials was that lung cancer is caused by oxidant stress. It has subsequently been shown that the mutations present in smoke-induced cancers are not similar to those caused by oxidant stress. Instead, they are similar to those caused by the two major classes of secondary carcinogens present in smoke, namely PAHs and smoke-specific nitrosamines, like NNK.[67] As described earlier in this chapter, PAHs and NAs are secondary carcinogens that require bioactivation by endogenous P450 enzymes, and the resulting reactive intermediates are not detoxified by enzymes involved in reactive oxygen metabolism. Animal models of lung cancer induced by these classes of chemicals have shown that various phytochemicals, and other agents that influence Phase I and II metabolism, have potent effects on lung cancer incidence.[68] Conversely, beta-carotene use in animal models has demonstrated pro-oxidant effects[69] and induction of P450 enzymes, which could enhance carcinogen bioactivation.[70]

Similar to the lung cancer situation, the incidence of GI cancers is associated with the exposure to secondary carcinogens (consumption of well-done and preserved meats) along with low vegetable and fruit consumption. Experiments on phytochemical fractions from sources such as vegetables (glucosinolates[68]), spices (curcumin[71]) and green tea (catechins like ECGC[72]) have shown that these are very active in the prevention of chemically-induced cancers.[73] Several types of cancers (e.g., GI, lung) are about 50% lower in the upper quartile of vegetable consumers.[74] This relationship is well explained by metabolic interactions between vegetable phytochemicals and dietary secondary carcinogens.[73] Changes in Phase I and II metabolism largely determine cancer risk from a given exposure to secondary carcinogens. Chronic exposure to carcinogens alone causes binding and activation of the aryl hydrocarbon receptor (AhR),[45] and other related receptors, which cause a dramatic upregualtion of specific P450 isozymes, like CYP1A1/2[46] (Figure 3.2). This increases the rate of formation of reactive intermediates and dramatically increases cancer risk from a given exposure to secondary carcinogens.[25,75] In contrast, the impact of phytochemical exposure on Phase I and II metabolism is complex, including the following effects:

1. Phytochemicals (alone) may activate AhR, causing a small induction of P450 activity.[76,78]
2. In combination with carcinogen exposure, phytochemicals compete with carcinogens for binding to the AhR, minimizing the large P450 induction seen with chronic exposure to carcinogens alone.[78,79]
3. Phytochemicals also compete for binding to the active site of P450 proteins, acting as direct competitive inhibitors and noncompetitive inactivators of CYP1A1/2 and CYP2E1 enzymes.[79–84]
4. Phytochemicals induce the major Phase II conjugation enzymes (glutathione-S-transferases and UDP-glucuronyltransferases),[48,77] and the enzymes that form the conjugating agents.[60,61,85,86]

The following sections will expand on these interactions between phytochemicals and xenobiotic metabolism.

3.8 PHYTOCHEMICAL ACTIVATION OF THE AHR

Many phytochemicals have been shown to bind to the AhR and/or induce CYP1A family P450 genes. Perhaps the most studied is indole-3-carbinol (I3C), which is an atypical breakdown product of a glucosinolate found in brassica plants like cabbage, Brussels sprouts, and broccoli. Most glucosinolates break down to form a mixture of thiocyanates and isothiocyanates, of which the thiocyanates impair iodine utilization (goitrogens) and the isothiocyanates interact with xenobiotic metabolism and have cancer preventative properties. I3C differs in that the parent indolylmethyl-glucosinolate breaks down to an isothiocyanate, but this rearranges and decomposes to release a simple thiocyanate ion and I3C, which is neither isothiocyanate nor thiocyanate in structure. I3C dimerizes to diindolylmethane (DIM) in the acid environment of the stomach. I3C and DIM are both capable of binding to and activating the AhR,[45,50,87] although they are considered weak agonists.[88] I3C and DIM will induce CYP1A family P450 genes in a variety of experimental models,[87] but tend to function in the low to mid micromolar range, compared to a low nanomolar range for the prototypical AhR agonist TCDD.[87,88]

Many other phytochemicals will bind to the AhR and induce CYP1A expression, including phenethyl isothiocyanate (PEITC) and sulforaphane (brassica), curcumin (turmeric), isoxanthohumol and 8-prenylnaringenin (flavonoids in beer hops), chrysin (various plant sources), phloretin (strawberries, apple skin), kaempferol (onions, grapes, apples, citrus family), galangin (tree bark, bee propolis), naringenin (citrus fruits and tomatoes), daidzein and genistein (soy), quercetin (onions, apples, tea, cranberries), myricetin (berries, grapes), luteolin (parsely, celery), baicalein (various herbals), apigenin (parsley, celery), and diosmin (citrus), cantharidin (beetle toxin), resveratrol (grapes, wine), green tea extracts, and emodin (aloe).[89–91]

It is interesting to consider the etiology of AhR activation by phytochemicals and the implications for cancer risk. It is a clear advantage to be able to induce forms of P450 capable of metabolizing dietary xenobiotics. Lipophilic xenobiotics will accumulate and tend to impair fetal brain development (like methyl-mercury, PCBs, dioxins), which would represent a selective disadvantage. Conversely, rapid bioactivation of xenobiotics may enhance cancer risk, but given the expected lifespan throughout the majority of our history and the fact that reproduction occurs at a younger age, avoiding cancer beyond the age of 30 or 40 years may not have created any selective pressure.

Of course, the epidemiological picture is that a high intake of fruit and vegetable phytochemicals is associated with cancer protection rather than enhanced risk. However, the induction of AhR by phytochemicals can be linked to increased cancer risk in animal models, most of which are unphysiological in nature. At high doses, I3C, an AhR agonist, is well recognized to promote carcinogenesis in several animal models. By inducing CYP1A genes, it increases the potency of PAHs and HCAs secondary carcinogens. Other genes induced by AhR activation are oncogenic in nature.[45] These levels of I3C are unphysiological with respect to a food-based diet, but may now be approached in human diets through the availability of potent supplements. In addition to excessively high exposures to I3C, some models divide the timing of exposure to I3C and carcinogen, where I3C exposure may induce P450 expression and then be removed from the diet before carcinogen exposure. Conversely, in other models, carcinogen exposure may be completed before I3C is introduced into the diet. In both of these cases, I3C may enhance carcinogenesis by activating the AhR, without the potential benefits that occur when I3C and secondary carcinogens are being metabolized simultaneously. Concurrent exposure is a more physiological model for human cancer risk, and the following sections describe further mechanisms that will function under these circumstances.

3.9   PHYTOCHEMICAL ANTAGONISM OF THE AHR

In real conditions that determine human health, people are usually exposed to small amounts of numerous chemicals for up to decades in time. Under these conditions, small changes in the balance of metabolism between Phase I and II pathways, or the routes of Phase I that handle certain xenobiotics, can lead to dramatic differences in life-long cancer risk. These conditions are poorly replicated by the high single-dose rodent models for carcinogen testing. Even when chemopreventative dietary components are introduced in high-dose rodent models, the routes of metabolism and role of DNA repair processes are responding to unphysiologically high metabolic burdens over a very short time frame, and the results may be a poor model of human diet–cancer relationships.

The induction of P450 genes, through activation of the AhR and other nuclear receptors, generally reflects a procarcinogenic effect, but this depends on the level of activation and whether it is accompanied by Phase II changes. While the previous section described unphysiological conditions under which dietary phytochemicals could be procarcinogenic, they tend to act differently when present for a long duration at low levels in the presence of other classes of xenobiotics. Under these conditions, phytochemicals and secondary carcinogens are both present inside the cell, with the ability to compete for binding and activation or inhibition of nuclear receptor function. This has been studied most extensively for the AhR. In general, when phytochemicals and planar carcinogens (PAHs and HCAs) are present concurrently, phytochemicals will antagonize the strong AhR activation of planar carcinogens. Some specific examples are provided below. The experimental models vary from *in vitro* transcription assays through cell culture work to *in vivo* animal data.

Several screening models have been developed based on AhR complex detection or the activity of reporter genes attached to CYP1A promoters in cultured cells.[91,92] These have been used to identify dietary components that agonize and antagonize the AhR. Allen et al. found that resveratrol, apigenin, curcumin, kaempferol, and green tea extract weakly enhanced the AhR function when used alone (two- to sixfold at 10 μM), and green tea extract, naringenin, and apigenin significantly antagonized the strong TCDD-induced activation of AhR (10-fold at 1 nM).[91] Curcumin and TCDD produced an additive effect on AhR activation. Amakura et al. found that green tea catechins and extracts of sage, spinach, and citrus fruits produced antagonism of TCDD-induced AhR activation.[92] In other studies, I3C and DIM, kaemferol, quercitin, myricetin, and luteolin antagonized TCDD-induce AhR activation.[50,89]

Green tea components are the best characterized phytochemicals with respect to AhR interactions. Individual catechins have shown lower antagonism than green tea extracts.[91] Williams et al. found that a mixture of the four major catechins displayed a strong antagonism similar to whole tea extract,[93] while Fukuda et al. showed that tea-derived lutein and chlorophyll a and b are also antagonists of AhR activation.[94] Inconsistent responses to epigallocatechin-3-gallate (EGCG), a major tea catechin, may be explained by the finding that this phytochemical does not compete at the binding site of the AhR, but appears to inhibit the conformation changes subsequent to binding, through interactions with accessory proteins.[95] Black tea theaflavins also suppress the transformation of TCDD-bound AhR to a transcriptionally active form.[96]

The importance of these observations is that, while many phytochemicals alone are weak agonists of the AhR, they are also antagonists of the strong activation of the AhR by compounds like TCDD and planar carcinogens. In a typical human diet, these compounds will be presented together and the effect of phytochemicals may be to modulate the AhR activation to a safer level, limiting the degree of P450 induction and encouraging a safe balance between Phase I and II metabolism. This has been verified by an elegant series of experiments in a physiologically relevant rat model by Thapliyal et al.[79,97,98] This model is based on the prevention of BaP and DMN-induced carcinogenesis by the root spice turmeric, in which the active ingredient is curcumin (diferuloylmethane). In this model, dietary turmeric provided dramatic protection against the formation of BaP adducts in liver, lung, and stomach tissues when consumed for 2 weeks preceding the dose of BaP, but not when the turmeric was introduced after the BaP dose.[98] DMN-induced cancer of the liver was also decreased by ongoing turmeric consumption, and not by turmeric following DMN treatment.[97] Thus, the effects in this model are mainly in the bioactivation and initiation period as has been discussed in this chapter. Further experiments showed that dietary turmeric alone had variable effects on P450 enzymes in the liver, lung, and GI tract, from small depressions to modest inductions,[79] as described in Section 3.8. When present in the diet during exposure to BaP, turmeric decreased the large induction of CYP1A1, 1A2, and 2B1 by 10 to 80%.[79] These studies also demonstrated direct inhibition of the catalytic activity of the P450 enzymes and the induction of Phase II enzymes, as will be discussed below.

3.10 PHYTOCHEMICAL INHIBITION OF THE CATALYTIC ACTIVITY OF P450

While various phytochemicals may cause some level of induction of P450 expression, many of the resulting enzymes will be rendered less active through different forms of inhibition if the phytochemicals continue to be present in the diet. Inhibition of the P450 catalytic cycle has been convincingly demonstrated for a long list of phytochemicals.

Thapliyal et al. have demonstrated this inhibition *in vitro*, showing that curcumins and isothiocyanates inhibit CYP1A1, 1A2, and 2B1 in rat microsomes, with IC_{50} values between 1 and 20 µM.[79] Diosmin, naringin, naringenin, rutin, and quercetin from citrus fruits inhibited CYP1A family enzymes and prevented the first step in the *in vitro* bioactivation of dietary HCAs and the tobacco nitrosamine NNK.[99,100] Phytochemicals from hops, used in the brewing of beer, including xanthohumol, isoxanthohumol, and 8-prenylnaringenin, largely eliminate CYP1A1/2 and 2B1 activity at 10 µM concentrations.[101] This prevented the *in vitro* bioactivation of aflatoxin, with very little impact on CYP2E1 or 3A4. Quercetin, ethoxyquin, tannic acid, theaflavins, and tea polyphenols inhibit the N-hydroxylation of HCAs by rat and human liver microsomes.[102] Benzyl and phenyl isothiocyanates and resveratrol, at levels below 1 µM, dramatically inhibited several forms of P450 in hamster liver microsomes.[103] Capsaicin (hot peppers) inhibited PhIP bioactivation by rat, hamster, and human liver S9 fractions.[104] PhIP mutagenicity (Salmonella reversion) was also inhibited by lycopene, caffeine, daidzein, and genistein.[105] Allyl sulfides (garlic) inhibit the bioactivation of nitrosamines by rat and human CYP2E1.[106]

Different flavanoid structures show selectivity for the inhibition CYP1A1 vs. 1A2,[107] which could change the route of metabolism of some secondary carcinogens or change the tissue in which metabolism takes place (CYP1A1 in the GIT and lung, CYP1A2 in the liver). Tea flavanols have demonstrated many protective effects *in vitro* and in animal models of carcinogenesis,[108,109] while the human epidemiology is favorable for the most part, but less clear.[109] Some of this uncertainty may be resolved by recent work showing that EGC and EGCG cause activation of EROD activity in rat liver microsomes at nM levels, while dramatically inhibiting the same activity at µM levels.[110] This assay measures CYP1A1 activity in rats and, if this effect also occurs in human CYP1A1 in extrahepatic tissues, it could explain some inconsistencies in the chemopreventative effects of green tea.

Soy, mushroom, and grape phytochemicals have been found to inhibit aromatase (CYP19), which plays a role in the formation of estrogens and may impact on hormonally sensitive cancers.[111]

Brassica isothiocyanates, such as PEITC and sulforaphane, have demonstrated a rather selective inhibition of rat CYP2E1 *in vitro*,[112] and have been shown to protect against CYP2E1-mediated *in vivo* endpoints like DMN-induced cancer,[113] and acetaminophen and ethanol-induced hepatotoxicity.[114] In a careful study of PEITC inhibition of human P450 enzymes, Nakajima et al. found competitive inhibition of CYP1A2 and 2A6, noncompetitive inhibition of CYP2B6, 2C9/19, 2D6, and 2E1, and mechanism-based inactivation of CYP2E1.[84] A similar inactivation process occurs between PEITC or BITC and CYP2B1, and it appears to involve a covalent modification of one amino acid on the enzyme protein by a reactive intermediate of the isothiocyanate molecule.[115] This type of inhibition can be potent and long-lived in an *in vivo* situation, as the protein is permanently inactivated by a short exposure to dietary phytochemicals, and activity will only recover as new protein is synthesized.

A number of studies have verified that phytochemicals can inhibit P450 activity *in vivo*, using both rodent[116] and human models. Human studies are usually limited to the use of probe drugs, which may not provide accurate data on the tissue site or species of P450 involved. The herbal products kava and goldenseal caused inhibition of CYP2E1 and CYP3A4/5, respectively.[117] Elderly patients experienced an induction of CYP3A4 with St. John's wort and an inhibition of CYP2E1 following garlic oil.[118] In these experiments, the treatment period was 4 weeks long, and changes may have been due to direct effects on the enzymes or through gene expression. In a more focused design, a single ingestion of watercress, a source of brassica isothiocyanates, decreased the clearance of a CYP2E1 probe.[119]

Direct inhibition or inactivation of P450 enzymes by acute exposure to phytochemicals has the potential to overcome any inducing effects that chronic exposure to phytochemicals or carcinogens may have caused. This effect may create a healthier balance between Phase I and II metabolism or force carcinogen metabolism through safer forms of P450.

3.11 PHYTOCHEMICAL INDUCTION OF PHASE II ENZYMES

As discussed earlier in this chapter, the induction of Phase II enzymes is responsive to the same nuclear receptors that control P450 gene expression, but is also controlled via cellular redox status, the Nrf2 transcription factor, and antioxidant response elements in gene promoters. Thus, the pattern of Phase II induction from a given xenobiotic exposure is generally different from the Phase I induction. Planar carcinogens, like PAHs and HCAs, are very active in the induction of CYP1A family enzymes, but are generally mild inducers of Phase II enzyme expression.

Many brassica isothiocyanates and metabolites are active in the induction of glutathione-*S*-transferase (GST), UDP-glucuronyltransferase (UDPGT), quinone reductase (QR), and gamma-glutamylcysteine synthase (GGCS) enzymes.[120] While PEITC, I3C, and DIM are "bifunctional inducers" that also enhance P450 expression, some brassica phytochemicals, like sulforaphane (4-methylsulfinylbutyl isothiocyanate), are very specific in the induction of Phase II enzymes. Sulforaphane is found at high levels in sprouting broccoli seeds, and extracts of these sprouts are effective chemopreventative agents.[121] The involvement of

Phase II enzymes is demonstrated by the enhanced sensitivity of Nrf2-null mice to BaP-induced cancers, and the fact that Nrf2-null mice are no longer protected by Phase II-inducing agents.[120]

Aliphatic sulfides from garlic and onions, including compounds, such as diallyl disulfide and trisulfide, are also well-known inducers of Phase II enzymes.[122] These have been associated with decreased risk of GIT cancers in humans and have proved effective in prevention of GIT and lung cancers in animal models.[123] Feeding of soy to rats also induces GST, UDPGT, and QR activities in various tissues.[124]

Phase II reactions are not always beneficial. The final step in the bioactivation of HCAs involves the acetylation or sulfation of an N-hydroxylated HCA metabolite. Fast acetylating phenotypes are associated with increased risk of certain cancers, and rapid sulfation could create similar risks. Garlic sulfides are inhibitors of N-acetyltransferase activity and may also decrease the risk of HCA-induced cancer by this mechanism.[125] Similar to the garlic sulfides, kahweol and cafestol palmitates from unfiltered coffee are inducers of GST and inhibitors of N-acetyltransferase activities, and feeding of these phytochemicals decreases the level of PhIP–DNA adducts in rat colon.[126] Compounds that inhibit N-acetyltransferase activity may be particularly useful for individuals with high activity polymorphisms for these genes, to avoid the enhanced cancer risk that may be associated with this genotype.[43] Interestingly, soy phytoestrogens are potent inhibitors of sulfotransferase activity, which could protect against HCA-induced cancers, but enhance the levels of active estrogens and increase breast cancer risk.[127]

The phytochemicals described above appear to have an ideal mixture of properties to act as chemopreventative agents. They appear to inhibit enzymes involved in carcinogen bioactivation (P450, N-acetyl transferase, sulfotransferase) and enhance the activities of those that are protective (GST, UDPGT, QR, etc.). While most of these chemicals appear to act as defenses against various stresses to the plant, some may have been selected over time in cultivated crops as beneficial to human health. It is important to remember that they are being handled by xenobiotic metabolism pathways and exerting many of their health benefits via interactions with potent carcinogens within these pathways. As we move towards more functional foods and nutraceutical products with enhanced levels of these products, we need to remember that they have toxic properties at higher levels of intake, perhaps to a greater extent than we now appreciate.

3.12 EXPERIMENTAL MODELS FOR FUTURE WORK AND OPPORTUNITIES FOR IMPROVING PUBLIC HEALTH

Because of the complex interactions between vegetable and meat consumption, meat doneness, preservative levels, and associated lifestyle variables, the role of cooked/preserved meats in carcinogenesis has remained controversial. Basic research has shown that most members of the PAH, HCA, and NA families are mutagenic *in vitro* and carcinogenic to rodents in large single dose models, but these lack physiological relevance to human exposures. The literature also lacks data on the effects of chronic exposure to low levels of complex mixtures of PAHs, HCAs, and NAs. Once a model for this is established, it may be used to examine cancer incidence, short-term biomarkers of exposure and injury, and the protective impact of plant products and phytochemical fractions.

In 2003, American consumers spent $1.8 billion on hot dogs in supermarkets alone[128] and much more at locations outside the home ($24.2 million in major league baseball parks[128]). Hot dogs are representative of a larger group of cured meats, including luncheon meats, bacon, and sausages. Norat et al. found that the 70th percentile of processed meat intake was around 40 g/d, while the 90th percentile was over 80 g/d,[5] representing 1 to 2 meals per day. While processed meats are often viewed as sources of NA exposure, these products are also smoked (causing PAH formation) and many are slow cooked to a low-moisture content (causing HCA formation). Children represent a high-risk group that consumes even greater levels of these products on a body weight basis, and at a young age are more susceptible to carcinogen exposure.

Consumers remain poorly informed about meat intake and cancer. Red and processed meat intake is not diminishing and barbequing appears to be increasing in popularity.[129] Interactions between phytochemicals and secondary carcinogens represent a potent approach to decrease the cancer risks associated with cooked meats. These phytochemicals can be introduced into processed meats, creating functional foods that play a role in disease prevention. Green tea is a promising source of active phytochemicals for this project. Green tea consumption is associated with a decreased risk of several human cancers,[130] and numerous animal-based experiments have shown that green tea phytochemical fractions and purified catechins inhibit high-dose PAH, HCA, and NA-induced cancers.[72] As mentioned earlier, PAHs, HCAs, and NAs are all secondary carcinogens, requiring bioactivation by P450 enzymes to cause DNA damage. There are about 60 different P450 gene products, with complex regulation in response to exposure to dietary carcinogens and phytochemicals.[16] This regulation occurs through receptors, like the AhR, which bind foreign compounds and become transcription factors that lead to increased expression of P450 proteins. The AhR is very active in the induction of CYP1A1/2 genes, which form P450 enzymes that bioactivate PAHs[25] and HCAs.[75] In human experiments, regular consumption of well-done meat increases intestinal CYP1A activity,[46] an effect that will increase cancer risk from a given carcinogen exposure. Basic research has demonstrated that green tea phytochemicals compete with carcinogens for binding to the AhR, and lessen the degree of P450 induction caused by carcinogens alone.[78] In addition, these phytochemicals compete directly at the active site of the P450 enzyme, decreasing the rate of production of reactive intermediates from carcinogens.[82] Lastly, green tea phytochemicals induce the expression of Phase II enzymes and conjugating agents.[48] The balance of these phytochemical effects is slower production and more rapid conjugation of reactive intermediates, decreasing the accumulation of harmful intermediates, DNA adducts, mutations, and cancer.

In addition, phytochemical fractions influence formation of PAHs, HCAs, and NAs in foods during storage and cooking. The formation of NAs has been shown to be inhibited by reducing agents, including green tea phytochemicals,[131] which encourage the conversion of nitrite to nitric oxide, preventing the formation of NAs.[22] Similarly, green tea phytochemicals have been shown to inhibit the formation of HCAs *in vitro* from purified components[131] and in cooked meats,[19] and appear to decrease nitrosamine formation in the GIT of humans consuming a nitrate-rich diet.[22]

3.13 PUBLIC PERCEPTION OF RISK AND RESULTING BEHAVIOR

The public has a very biased form of risk perception in relation to diet and health. Artificial "contaminants" of the food supply, including food additives and pesticide residues, are viewed as dangerous and carcinogenic, while natural products are seen as beneficial to health. Figure 3.4 shows several dose response curves, with increasing exposure on the horizontal axis, and health problems (cancer?) on the vertical axis. For the most part, these curves are theoretical extrapolations from very few actual data points. For example, pesticide X may be tested at very high doses in rats and found to cause or promote cancer. It is not possible to test X at lower doses, given the number of animals that would be required and the length of the experiment. Therefore, the low-dose area of the curve is modeled mathematically, which can be done using widely varying models. The simplest model is the linear response, which states that the incidence of disease will decrease in direct relationship with the exposure to X and will never completely disappear as long as X is present in the food supply. A second model assumes that there is a threshold level at which X may be safely metabolized and the risk of low exposures disappears at some point. The threshold point is very hard to determine and is obviously critical to regulation policy. There are two more dramatic curves to consider, the first of which states that low levels of X actually start to be beneficial, for example, leading to levels of cancer below that observed spontaneously (with an absence of X in the food supply). This response is called "hormesis" and it is thought to be very common, but difficult to study experimentally. Some dangerous exposures, like radiation, have been thought to present a linear form of risk because radiation produces DNA damage at very low levels of exposure. Surprisingly, radiation exposure produces one of the clearest and most studied forms of hormesis. Low levels of radiation extend lifespan and decrease cancer incidence in experimental animals. These effects are even reflected by non-thyroid cancer incidence data from Japan and Chernobyl that are well below predictive models.

Another established model of hormesis involves exposure to dioxin, which demonstrates health benefits in rodents at low doses. It seems likely that some of the pesticide residues that cause cancer at high doses in rodents may be harmless or "beneficial" at the levels found in the human diet. Calabrese and

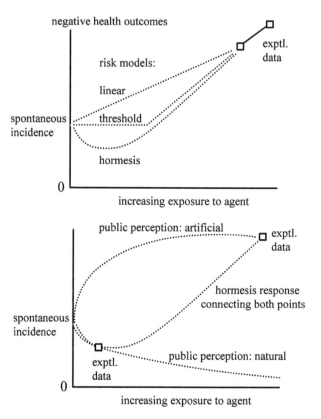

FIGURE 3.4 Risk models for extrapolation of cancer data. The top panel shows risk models used by toxicologists and public health policy makers. The bottom panel shows risk models perceived by the public, in which much higher risk is attached to artificial components in the food supply, while natural products are perceived as increasingly beneficial at high exposures, in the form of natural health products.

Baldwin have examined published data for evidence of hormesis in various areas of toxicology and found that close to 10% of toxicological studies demonstrate hormesis, although few are properly designed to do so. Among the different categories of compounds, metals are very likely to produce hormetic dose response curves, with herbicides, pesticides, insecticides, and hydrocarbons averaging around 5% of studies. Hormesis is poorly dealt with by health policy and basically incomprehensible in the forum of public risk perception.

The last curve to consider is the public perception curve, where a food additive or residue shown to cause cancer in rodents at high doses is considered to be as dangerous, or more so, in trace amounts in human populations. This is the top curve in the lower panel, and represents the illogical public perception of pesticide residues and additives like aspartame. To gain an accurate working knowledge of diet and cancer, the public has to stop considering natural products as healthy and artificial products as dangerous. They share common pathways of metabolism, and many of the benefits of phytochemicals are due to the fact that they are xenobiotics and they interact directly with more potent carcinogens in Phase I and II metabolism. Some of the problems resulting from public perception of risk are summarized below.

One of the strongest public fears is of pesticide residues in food, which is often focused on fruits and vegetables. This may lead to decreased intake through avoidance or due to the higher cost of organic products. Insufficient intake of fruits and vegetables is the major nutritional problem in developed countries. A low intake of fruits and vegetables may lead to increased meat intake, with associated exposure to carcinogens produced by cooking and preservation.

Producers of natural health products are taking advantage of the public desire to attain the benefits of fruit and vegetable consumption without incurring the risk of pesticide exposure or the basic lack of desire to eat these foods. This leads us to the final curve shown in Figure 3.4. Indole-3-carbinol is a breakdown product of brassica glucosinolates, known to be associated with decreased cancer risk in human populations (through consumption of brassica vegetables) and shown to prevent cancer, at low levels, in rodent models. An unbiased observer might place this data point in the lowest region of a hormetic response curve and expect that at high levels the health benefits would diminish and the compound would eventually become toxic. This follows the basic assumptions of toxicology that all substances become toxic if the dose is increased sufficiently (Paracelsus, 1493-1541). This has been established for indole-3-carbinol, which is shown to promote cancer development at high doses in rodent models. The public views this natural health product in a different light, however, and assumes that the benefits will increase with increasing intake, as shown in the bottom curve in the lower panel of Figure 3.4. Indole-3-carbinol is currently marketed in 200 mg capsules, with recommended intakes of 2 per day, equivalent to 30 pounds of cabbage per day. The justification for this extremely high intake by marketers of these compounds uses data from the regression of cervical dysplasia, which is actually an example of chemotherapy-like treatment of a dividing cell population, and in themselves could be interpreted as a toxic end point. This chemotherapy-like dose of I3C is being recommended and marketed to an unsuspecting public.

3.14 CONCLUSIONS

Current dietary patterns in developed countries favor exposure to carcinogens derived from meat processing and cooking techniques, and dietary habits have decreased the intake of chemopreventative phytochemicals. The growth of research, business, and public interest in functional foods and nutraceuticals provides opportunities to bring some of the beneficial metabolic effects back to the modern, highly processed diet. This movement also increases the risk of toxicity due to unnaturally high exposures to natural xenobiotics. Further research will help to maximize the benefits and minimize the risks associated with the novel use of natural products in cancer prevention.

REFERENCES

1. Ames BN, Gold LS. Environmental pollution, pesticides, and the prevention of cancer: misconceptions. *FASEB J.* 1997; 11: 1041–52.
2. Parkin DM. Global cancer statistics in the year 2000. *Lancet Oncol.* 2001; 2: 533–43.
3. Knize MG, Felton JS. Formation and human risk of carcinogenic heterocyclic amines formed from natural precursors in meat. *Nutr. Rev.* 2005; 63: 158–65.
4. Chao A, Thun MJ, Connell CJ, et al. Meat consumption and risk of colorectal cancer. *JAMA* 2005; 293: 172–82.
5. Norat T, Bingham S, Ferrari P, et al. Meat, fish, and colorectal cancer risk: the European Prospective Investigation into cancer and nutrition. *J. Natl. Cancer Inst.* 2005; 97: 906–16.
6. Sinha R, Chow WH, Kulldorff M, et al. Well-done, grilled red meat increases the risk of colorectal adenomas. *Cancer Res.* 1999; 59: 4320–4.
7. Peters JM, Preston-Martin S, London SJ, Bowman JD, Buckley JD, Thomas DC. Processed meats and risk of childhood leukemia (California). *Cancer Causes Control* 1994; 5: 195–202.
8. Levi F, Pasche C, Lucchini F, Bosetti C, La Vecchia C. Processed meat and the risk of selected digestive tract and laryngeal neoplasms in Switzerland. *Ann. Oncol.* 2004; 15: 346–9.
9. Armstrong RW, Imrey PB, Lye MS, Armstrong MJ, Yu MC, Sani S. Nasopharyngeal carcinoma in Malaysian Chinese: salted fish and other dietary exposures. *Int. J. Cancer* 1998; 77: 228–235.
10. Ke L, Yu P, Zhang ZX. Novel epidemiologic evidence for the association between fermented fish sauce and esophageal cancer in South China. *Int. J. Cancer* 2002; 99: 424–426.
11. Ngoan LT, Mizoue T, Fujino Y, Tokui N, Yoshimura T. Dietary factors and stomach cancer mortality. *Br. J. Cancer* 2002; 87: 37–42.
12. Jian L, Zhang DH, Lee AH, Binns CW. Do preserved foods increase prostate cancer risk? *Br. J. Cancer* 2004; 90: 1792–1795.
13. Dietrich M, Block G, Pogoda JM, Buffler P, Hecht S, Martin SP. A review: dietary and endogenously formed N-nitroso compounds and risk of childhood brain tumors. *Cancer Causes Control* 2005; 16: 619–635.
14. Sinha R. An epidemiologic approach to studying heterocyclic amines. *Mutat. Res.* 2002; 506-507: 197–204.
15. Sinha R, Cross A, Curtin J, et al. Development of a food frequency questionnaire module and databases for compounds in cooked and processed meats. *Mol. Nutr. Food Res.* 2005; 49: 648–655.
16. Jagerstad M, Skog K. Genotoxicity of heat-processed foods. *Mutat. Res.* 2005; 574: 156–172.
17. Lijinsky W. The formation and occurrence of polynuclear aromatic hydrocarbons associated with food. *Mutat. Res.* 1991; 259: 251–261.
18. Simko P. Factors affecting elimination of polycyclic aromatic hydrocarbons from smoked meat foods and liquid smoke flavorings. *Mol. Nutr. Food Res.* 2005; 49: 637–647.
19. Nerurkar PV, Le Marchand L, Cooney RV. Effects of marinating with Asian marinades or western barbecue sauce on PhIP and MeIQx formation in barbecued beef. *Nutr. Cancer* 1999; 34: 147–152.

20. Laser RA, Skog K, Jagerstad M. Effects of creatine and creatinine content on the mutagenic activity of meat extracts, bouillons and gravies from different sources. *Food Chem. Toxicol.* 1987; 25: 747–754.

21. Martin FL, Cole KJ, Phillips DH, Grover PL. The proteolytic release of genotoxins from cooked beef. *Biochem. Biophys. Res. Commun.* 2002; 293: 1497–1501.

22. Choi SY, Chung MJ, Sung NJ. Volatile N-nitrosamine inhibition after intake Korean green tea and Maesil (Prunus mume SIEB. et ZACC.) extracts with an amine-rich diet in subjects ingesting nitrate. *Food Chem. Toxicol.* 2002; 40: 949–957.

23. Dietrich M, Block G, Pogoda JM, Buffler P, Hecht S, Preston-Martin S. A review: dietary and endogenously formed N-nitroso compounds and risk of childhood brain tumors. *Cancer Causes Control* 2005; 16: 619–635.

24. Wogan GN, Hecht SS, Felton JS, Conney AH, Loeb LA. Environmental and chemical carcinogenesis. *Semin. Cancer Biol.* 2004; 14: 473–486.

25. Xue W, Warshawsky D. Metabolic activation of polycyclic and heterocyclic aromatic hydrocarbons and DNA damage: a review. *Toxicol. Appl. Pharmacol.* 2005; 206: 73–93.

26. Blanck A, Lindhe B, Porsch H, I, Lindeskog P, Gustafsson JA. Influence of different levels of dietary casein on initiation of male rat liver carcinogenesis with a single dose of aflatoxin B1. *Carcinogenesis* 1992; 13: 171–176.

27. Mori Y, Koide A, Kobayashi Y, Morimura K, Kaneko M, Fukushima S. Effect of ethanol treatment on metabolic activation and detoxification of esophagus carcinogenic N-nitrosamines in rat liver. *Mutagenesis* 2002; 17: 251–256.

28. Castellsague X, Quintana MJ, Martinez MC, et al. The role of type of tobacco and type of alcoholic beverage in oral carcinogenesis. *Int. J. Cancer* 2004; 108: 741–749.

29. Marzullo L. An update of N-acetylcysteine treatment for acute acetaminophen toxicity in children. *Curr. Opin. Pediatr.* 2005; 17: 239–245.

30. Cross AJ, Sinha R. Meat-related mutagens/carcinogens in the etiology of colorectal cancer. *Environ. Mol. Mutagen.* 2004; 44: 44–55.

31. Mirvish SS, Haorah J, Zhou L, Clapper ML, Harrison KL, Povey AC. Total N-nitroso compounds and their precursors in hot dogs and in the gastrointestinal tract and feces of rats and mice: possible etiologic agents for colon cancer. *J. Nutr.* 2002; 132: 3526S–3529S.

32. Pence BC, Landers M, Dunn DM, Shen CL, Miller MF. Feeding of a well-cooked beef diet containing a high heterocyclic amine content enhances colon and stomach carcinogenesis in 1,2-dimethylhydrazine-treated rats. *Nutr. Cancer* 1998; 30: 220–226.

33. Heddle JA, Knize MG, Dawod D, Zhang XB. A test of the mutagenicity of cooked meats *in vivo. Mutagenesis* 2001; 16: 103–107.

34. Shen CL, Purewal M, San Francisco S, Pence BC. Absence of PhIP adducts, p53 and Apc mutations, in rats fed a cooked beef diet containing a high level of heterocyclic amines. *Nutr. Cancer* 1998; 30: 227–231.

35. Smith GB, Bend JR, Bedard LL, Reid KR, Petsikas D, Massey TE. Biotransformation of 4-(methylnitrosamino)-1-(3-pyridyl)-1-butanone (NNK) in peripheral human lung microsomes. *Drug Metab. Dispos.* 2003; 31: 1134–1141.

36. Teiber JF, Mace K, Hollenberg PF. Metabolism of the beta-oxidized intermediates of N-nitrosodi-n-propylamine: N-nitroso-beta-hydroxypropylpropylamine and N-nitroso-beta-oxopropylpropylamine. *Carcinogenesis* 2001; 22: 499–506.

37. Balansky RM, Ganchev G, D'Agostini F, De Flora S. Effects of N-acetylcysteine in an esophageal carcinogenesis model in rats treated with diethylnitrosamine and diethyldithiocarbamate. *Int. J. Cancer* 2002; 98: 493–497.

38. Hsie AW, Recio L. Modulative effects of metabolic effectors on benzo(a)pyrene-induced cytotoxicity and mutagenicity in mammalian cells. *Toxicol. Ind. Health* 1994; 10: 181–189.

39. Di Paolo OA, Teitel CH, Nowell S, Coles BF, Kadlubar FF. Expression of cytochromes P450 and glutathione *S*-transferases in human prostate, and the potential for activation of heterocyclic amine carcinogens via acetyl-CoA. *Int. J. Cancer* 2005; 117: 8–13.

40. Coles B, Nowell SA, MacLeod SL, Sweeney C, Lang NP, Kadlubar FF. The role of human glutathione *S*-transferases (hGSTs) in the detoxification of the food-derived carcinogen metabolite N-acetoxy-PhIP, and the effect of a polymorphism in hGSTA1 on colorectal cancer risk. *Mutat. Res.* 2001; 482: 3–10.

41. Strickland PT, Qian Z, Friesen MD, Rothman N, Sinha R. Metabolites of 2-amino-1-methyl-6-phenylimidazo(4,5-b)pyridine (PhIP) in human urine after consumption of charbroiled or fried beef. *Mutat. Res.* 2002; 506-507: 163173.

42. Turesky RJ, Garner RC, Welti DH, et al. Metabolism of the food-borne mutagen 2-amino-3,8-dimethylimidazo[4,5-f]quinoxaline in humans. *Chem. Res. Toxicol.* 1998; 11: 217–225.

43. Chan AT, Tranah GJ, Giovannucci EL, Willett WC, Hunter DJ, Fuchs CS. Prospective study of N-acetyltransferase-2 genotypes, meat intake, smoking and risk of colorectal cancer. *Int. J. Cancer* 2005; 115: 648–652.

44. Eaton DL, Bammler TK, Kelly EJ. Interindividual differences in response to chemoprotection against aflatoxin-induced hepatocarcinogenesis: implications for human biotransformation enzyme polymorphisms. *Adv. Exp. Med. Biol.* 2001; 500: 559–576.

45. Safe S. Molecular biology of the Ah receptor and its role in carcinogenesis. *Toxicol. Lett.* 2001; 120: 1–7.

46. Fontana RJ, Lown KS, Paine MF, et al. Effects of a chargrilled meat diet on expression of CYP3A, CYP1A, and P-glycoprotein levels in healthy volunteers. *Gastroenterology* 1999; 117: 89–98.

47. Francis GA, Fayard E, Picard F, Auwerx J. Nuclear receptors and the control of metabolism. *Annu. Rev. Physiol.* 2003; 65: 261–311.

48. Xu C, Li CY, Kong AN. Induction of Phase I, II and III drug metabolism/transport by xenobiotics. *Arch. Pharm. Res.* 2005; 28:2 49–68.

49. Tirona RG, Kim RB. Nuclear receptors and drug disposition gene regulation. *J. Pharm. Sci.* 2005; 94: 1169–1186.

50. Chen I, Safe S, Bjeldanes L. Indole-3-carbinol and diindolylmethane as aryl hydrocarbon (Ah) receptor agonists and antagonists in T47D human breast cancer cells. *Biochem. Pharmacol.* 1996; 51: 1069–1076.

51. Kwak MK, Wakabayashi N, Kensler TW. Chemoprevention through the Keap1-Nrf2 signaling pathway by Phase 2 enzyme inducers. *Mutat. Res.* 2004; 555: 133–148.

52. Kwak MK, Wakabayashi N, Itoh K, Motohashi H, Yamamoto M, Kensler TW. Modulation of gene expression by cancer chemopreventive dithiolethiones through the Keap1-Nrf2 pathway. Identification of novel gene clusters for cell survival. *J. Biol. Chem.* 2003; 278: 8135–8145.

53. Sinha R, Rothman N, Brown ED, et al. Pan-fried meat containing high levels of heterocyclic aromatic amines but low levels of polycyclic aromatic hydrocarbons induces cytochrome P4501A2 activity in humans. *Cancer Res.* 1994; 54: 6154–6159.

54. McCullough ML, Robertson AS, Chao A, et al. A prospective study of whole grains, fruits, vegetables and colon cancer risk. *Cancer Causes Control* 2003; 14: 959–970.

55. Omenn GS, Goodman GE, Thornquist MD, et al. Risk factors for lung cancer and for intervention effects in CARET, the beta-carotene and retinol efficacy trial. *J. Natl. Cancer Inst.* 1996; 88: 1550–1559.

56. Decker EA, Warner K, Richards MP, Shahidi F. Measuring antioxidant effectiveness in food. *J. Agric. Food Chem.* 2005; 53: 4303–4310.

57. Aviram M, Dornfeld L, Kaplan M, et al. Pomegranate juice flavonoids inhibit low-density lipoprotein oxidation and cardiovascular diseases: studies in atherosclerotic mice and in humans. *Drugs Exp. Clin. Res.* 2002; 28: 49–62.

58. Natella F, Belelli F, Gentili V, Ursini F, Scaccini C. Grape seed proanthocyanidins prevent plasma postprandial oxidative stress in humans. *J. Agric. Food Chem.* 2002; 50: 7720–7725.

59. Marin E, Kretzschmar M, Arokoski J, Hanninen O, Klinger W. Enzymes of glutathione synthesis in dog skeletal muscles and their response to training. *Acta Physiol. Scand.* 1993; 147: 369–373.

60. Carlsen H, Myhrstad MC, Thoresen M, Moskaug JO, Blomhoff R. Berry intake increases the activity of the gamma-glutamylcysteine synthetase promoter in transgenic reporter mice. *J. Nutr.* 2003; 133: 2137–2140.

61. Myhrstad MC, Carlsen H, Nordstrom O, Blomhoff R, Moskaug JO. Flavonoids increase the intracellular glutathione level by transactivation of the gamma-glutamylcysteine synthetase catalytical subunit promoter. *Free Radic. Biol. Med.* 2002; 32: 386–393.

62. Gunduz F, Senturk UK, Kuru O, Aktekin B, Aktekin MR. The effect of one year's swimming exercise on oxidant stress and antioxidant capacity in aged rats. *Physiol. Res.* 2004; 53: 171–176.

63. Metin G, Gumustas MK, Uslu E, Belce A, Kayserilioglu A. Effect of regular training on plasma thiols, malondialdehyde and carnitine concentrations in young soccer players. *Chin. J. Physiol.* 2003; 46: 35–39.

64. Virtamo J, Pietinen P, Huttunen JK, et al. Incidence of cancer and mortality following alpha-tocopherol and beta-carotene supplementation: a postintervention follow-up. *JAMA* 2003; 290: 476–485.

65. Goodman GE, Thornquist MD, Balmes J, et al. The beta-carotene and retinol efficacy trial: incidence of lung cancer and cardiovascular disease mortality during 6-year follow-up after stopping beta-carotene and retinol supplements. *J. Natl. Cancer Inst.* 2004; 96: 1743–1750.

66. Albanes D, Heinonen OP, Huttunen JK, et al. Effects of alpha-tocopherol and beta-carotene supplements on cancer incidence in the Alpha-Tocopherol Beta-Carotene Cancer Prevention Study. *Am. J. Clin. Nutr.* 1995; 62: 1427S–1430S.

67. Pfeifer GP, Denissenko MF, Olivier M, Tretyakova N, Hecht SS, Hainaut P. Tobacco smoke carcinogens, DNA damage and p53 mutations in smoking-associated cancers. *Oncogene* 2002; 21: 7435–7451.

68. Stoner GD, Morse MA. Isothiocyanates and plant polyphenols as inhibitors of lung and esophageal cancer. *Cancer Lett.* 1997; 114: 113–119.

69. El Agamey A, Lowe GM, McGarvey DJ, et al. Carotenoid radical chemistry and antioxidant/pro-oxidant properties. *Arch. Biochem. Biophys.* 2004; 430: 37–48.
70. Paolini M, Antelli A, Pozzetti L, et al. Induction of cytochrome P450 enzymes and over-generation of oxygen radicals in beta-carotene supplemented rats. *Carcinogenesis* 2001; 22: 1483–1495.
71. Duvoix A, Blasius R, Delhalle S, et al. Chemopreventive and therapeutic effects of curcumin. *Cancer Lett.* 2005; 223: 181–190.
72. Crespy V, Williamson G. A review of the health effects of green tea catechins in *in vivo* animal models. *J. Nutr.* 2004; 134: 3431S–3440S.
73. van Iersel ML, Verhagen H, van Bladeren PJ. The role of biotransformation in dietary (anti)carcinogenesis. *Mutat. Res.* 1999; 443: 259–270.
74. Food, Nutrition and the Prevention of Cancer: a Global Perspective. Washington, DC: American Institute for Cancer Research (AICR), 1997.
75. Kim D, Guengerich FP. Cytochrome P450 activation of arylamines and heterocyclic amines. *Annu. Rev. Pharmacol. Toxicol.* 2005; 45: 27–49.
76. Kassie F, Uhl M, Rabot S, et al. Chemoprevention of 2-amino-3-methylimidazo[4,5-f]quinoline (IQ)-induced colonic and hepatic preneoplastic lesions in the F344 rat by cruciferous vegetables administered simultaneously with the carcinogen. *Carcinogenesis* 2003; 24: 255–261.
77. Steinkellner H, Rabot S, Freywald C, et al. Effects of cruciferous vegetables and their constituents on drug metabolizing enzymes involved in the bioactivation of DNA-reactive dietary carcinogens. *Mutat. Res.* 2001; 480–481: 285–97.
78. Williams SN, Shih H, Guenette DK, et al. Comparative studies on the effects of green tea extracts and individual tea catechins on human CYP1A gene expression. *Chem. Biol. Interact.* 2000; 128: 211–229.
79. Thapliyal R, Maru GB. Inhibition of cytochrome P450 isozymes by curcumins *in vitro* and *in vivo*. *Food Chem. Toxicol.* 2001; 39: 541–547.
80. Barcelo S, Gardiner JM, Gescher A, Chipman JK. CYP2E1-mediated mechanism of anti-genotoxicity of the broccoli constituent sulforaphane. *Carcinogenesis* 1996; 17: 277–282.
81. Smith TJ, Guo Z, Guengerich FP, Yang CS. Metabolism of 4-(methylnitrosamino)-1-(3-pyridyl)-1-butanone (NNK) by human cytochrome P450 1A2 and its inhibition by phenethyl isothiocyanate. *Carcinogenesis* 1996; 17: 809–813.
82. Muto S, Fujita K, Yamazaki Y, Kamataki T. Inhibition by green tea catechins of metabolic activation of procarcinogens by human cytochrome P450. *Mutat. Res.* 2001; 479: 197–206.
83. Thapliyal R, Deshpande SS, Maru GB. Effects of turmeric on the activities of benzo(a)pyrene-induced cytochrome P-450 isozymes. *J. Environ. Pathol. Toxicol. Oncol.* 2001; 20: 59–63.
84. Nakajima M, Yoshida R, Shimada N, Yamazaki H, Yokoi T. Inhibition and inactivation of human cytochrome P450 isoforms by phenethyl isothiocyanate. *Drug Metab. Dispos.* 2001; 29: 1110–1113.
85. Moskaug JO, Carlsen H, Myhrstad MC, Blomhoff R. Polyphenols and glutathione synthesis regulation. *Am. J. Clin. Nutr.* 2005;81:277S-83S.
86. Bishayee A, Chatterjee M. Anticarcinogenic biological response of *Mikania cordata*: reflections in hepatic biotransformation systems. *Cancer Lett.* 1994; 81: 193–200.

87. Jellinck PH, Forkert PG, Riddick DS, Okey AB, Michnovicz JJ, Bradlow HL. Ah receptor binding properties of indole carbinols and induction of hepatic estradiol hydroxylation. *Biochem. Pharmacol.* 1993; 45: 1129–1136.

88. Sanderson JT, Slobbe L, Lansbergen GW, Safe S, van den BM. 2,3,7,8-tetrachlorodibenzo-p-dioxin and diindolylmethanes differentially induce cytochrome P450 1A1, 1B1, and 19 in H295R human adrenocortical carcinoma cells. *Toxicol. Sci.* 2001; 61: 40–48.

89. Zhang S, Qin C, Safe SH. Flavonoids as aryl hydrocarbon receptor agonists/antagonists: effects of structure and cell context. *Environ. Health Perspect.* 2003; 111: 1877–1882.

90. Gross-Steinmeyer K, Stapleton PL, Liu F, et al. Phytochemical-induced changes in gene expression of carcinogen-metabolizing enzymes in cultured human primary hepatocytes. *Xenobiotica* 2004; 34: 619–632.

91. Allen SW, Mueller L, Williams SN, Quattrochi LC, Raucy J. The use of a high-volume screening procedure to assess the effects of dietary flavonoids on human cyp1a1 expression. *Drug Metab. Dispos.* 2001; 29: 1074–1079.

92. Amakura Y, Tsutsumi T, Nakamura M et al. Preliminary screening of the inhibitory effect of food extracts on activation of the aryl hydrocarbon receptor induced by 2,3,7,8-tetrachlorodibenzo-p-dioxin. *Biol. Pharm. Bull.* 2002; 25: 272–274.

93. Williams SN, Pickwell GV, Quattrochi LC. A combination of tea (*Camellia senensis*) catechins is required for optimal inhibition of induced CYP1A expression by green tea extract. *J. Agric. Food Chem.* 2003; 51: 6627–6634.

94. Fukuda I, Sakane I, Yabushita Y, et al. Pigments in green tea leaves (*Camellia sinensis*) suppress transformation of the aryl hydrocarbon receptor induced by dioxin. *J. Agric. Food Chem.* 2004; 52: 2499–2506.

95. Palermo CM, Westlake CA, Gasiewicz TA. Epigallocatechin gallate inhibits aryl hydrocarbon receptor gene transcription through an indirect mechanism involving binding to a 90 kDa heat shock protein. *Biochemistry* 2005; 44: 5041–5052.

96. Fukuda I, Sakane I, Yabushita Y, Sawamura S, Kanazawa K, Ashida H. Black tea theaflavins suppress dioxin-induced transformation of the aryl hydrocarbon receptor. *Biosci. Biotechnol. Biochem.* 2005; 69: 883–890.

97. Thapliyal R, Naresh KN, Rao KV, Maru GB. Inhibition of nitrosodiethylamine-induced hepatocarcinogenesis by dietary turmeric in rats. *Toxicol. Lett.* 2003; 139: 45–54.

98. Thapliyal R, Deshpande SS, Maru GB. Mechanism(s) of turmeric-mediated protective effects against benzo(a)pyrene-derived DNA adducts. *Cancer Lett.* 2002; 175: 79–88.

99. Bear WL, Teel RW. Effects of citrus flavonoids on the mutagenicity of heterocyclic amines and on cytochrome P450 1A2 activity. *Anticancer Res.* 2000; 20: 3609–3614.

100. Bear WL, Teel RW. Effects of citrus phytochemicals on liver and lung cytochrome P450 activity and on the *in vitro* metabolism of the tobacco-specific nitrosamine NNK. *Anticancer Res.* 2000; 20: 3323–3329.

101. Henderson MC, Miranda CL, Stevens JF, Deinzer ML, Buhler DR. *In vitro* inhibition of human P450 enzymes by prenylated flavonoids from hops, Humulus lupulus. *Xenobiotica* 2000; 30: 235–251.

102. Hammons GJ, Fletcher JV, Stepps KR, et al. Effects of chemoprotective agents on the metabolic activation of the carcinogenic arylamines PhIP and 4-aminobiphenyl in human and rat liver microsomes. *Nutr. Cancer* 1999; 33: 46–52.

103. Teel RW, Huynh H. Modulation by phytochemicals of cytochrome P450-linked enzyme activity. *Cancer Lett.* 1998; 133: 135–141.
104. Huynh HT, Teel RW. *In vitro* antimutagenicity of capsaicin toward heterocyclic amines in *Salmonella typhimurium* strain TA98. *Anticancer Res.* 2005; 25: 117–120.
105. Weisburger JH, Dolan L, Pittman B. Inhibition of PhIP mutagenicity by caffeine, lycopene, daidzein, and genistein. *Mutat. Res.* 1998; 416: 125–128.
106. Morris CR, Chen SC, Zhou L, Schopfer LM, Ding X, Mirvish SS. Inhibition by allyl sulfides and phenethyl isothiocyanate of methyl-n-pentylnitrosamine depentylation by rat esophageal microsomes, human and rat CYP2E1, and Rat CYP2A3. *Nutr. Cancer* 2004; 48: 54–63.
107. Zhai S, Dai R, Friedman FK, Vestal RE. Comparative inhibition of human cytochromes P450 1A1 and 1A2 by flavonoids. *Drug Metab. Dispos.* 1998; 26: 989–992.
108. Weisburger JH, Chung FL. Mechanisms of chronic disease causation by nutritional factors and tobacco products and their prevention by tea polyphenols. *Food Chem. Toxicol.* 2002; 40: 1145–1154.
109. Kim M, Masuda M. Cancer chemoprevention by green tea polyphenols. In Yamamoto T, Juneja LR, Chu DC, Kim M, Eds. *Chemistry and Applications of Green Tea.* Boca Raton, FL: CRC Press 1997: 61–73.
110. Anger DL, Petre MA, Crankshaw DJ. Heteroactivation of cytochrome P450 1A1 by teas and tea polyphenols. *Br. J. Pharmacol.* 2005; 145: 926–933.
111. Chen S, Zhou D, Okubo T, et al. Prevention and treatment of breast cancer by suppressing aromatase activity and expression. *Ann. NY Acad. Sci.* 2002; 963: 229–238.
112. Ishizaki H, Brady JF, Ning SM, Yang CS. Effect of phenethyl isothiocyanate on microsomal N-nitrosodimethylamine metabolism and other monooxygenase activities. *Xenobiotica* 1990; 20: 255–264.
113. Solt DB, Chang K, Helenowski I, Rademaker AW. Phenethyl isothiocyanate inhibits nitrosamine carcinogenesis in a model for study of oral cancer chemoprevention. *Cancer Lett.* 2003; 202: 147–152.
114. Li Y, Wang EJ, Chen L, Stein AP, Reuhl KR, Yang CS. Effects of phenethyl isothiocyanate on acetaminophen metabolism and hepatotoxicity in mice. *Toxicol. Appl. Pharmacol.* 1997; 144: 306–314.
115. Goosen TC, Kent UM, Brand L, Hollenberg PF. Inactivation of cytochrome P450 2B1 by benzyl isothiocyanate, a chemopreventative agent from cruciferous vegetables. *Chem. Res. Toxicol.* 2000; 13: 1349–1359.
116. Smith TJ, Guo Z, Li C, Ning SM, Thomas PE, Yang CS. Mechanisms of inhibition of 4-(methylnitrosamino)-1-(3-pyridyl)-1-butanone bioactivation in mice by dietary phenethyl isothiocyanate. *Cancer Res.* 1993; 53: 3276–3282.
117. Gurley BJ, Gardner SF, Hubbard MA, et al. *In vivo* effects of goldenseal, kava kava, black cohosh, and valerian on human cytochrome P450 1A2, 2D6, 2E1, and 3A4/5 phenotypes. *Clin. Pharmacol. Ther.* 2005; 77: 415–426.
118. Gurley BJ, Gardner SF, Hubbard MA, et al. Clinical assessment of effects of botanical supplementation on cytochrome P450 phenotypes in the elderly: St. John's wort, garlic oil, Panax ginseng and Ginkgo biloba. *Drugs Aging* 2005; 22: 525–539.

119. Leclercq I, Desager JP, Horsmans Y. Inhibition of chlorzoxazone metabolism, a clinical probe for CYP2E1, by a single ingestion of watercress. *Clin. Pharmacol. Ther.* 1998; 64: 144–149.
120. Talalay P, Fahey JW. Phytochemicals from cruciferous plants protect against cancer by modulating carcinogen metabolism. *J. Nutr.* 2001; 131: 3027S–3033S.
121. Fahey JW, Zhang Y, Talalay P. Broccoli sprouts: an exceptionally rich source of inducers of enzymes that protect against chemical carcinogens. *Proc. Natl. Acad. Sci. USA* 1997; 94: 10367–10372.
122. Munday R, Munday CM. Relative activities of organosulfur compounds derived from onions and garlic in increasing tissue activities of quinone reductase and glutathione transferase in rat tissues. *Nutr. Cancer* 2001; 40: 205–210.
123. Bianchini F, Vainio H. Allium vegetables and organosulfur compounds: do they help prevent cancer? *Environ. Health Perspect.* 2001; 109: 893–902.
124. Appelt LC, Reicks MM. Soy feeding induces Phase II enzymes in rat tissues. *Nutr. Cancer* 1997; 28: 270–275.
125. Chung JG, Lu HF, Yeh CC, Cheng KC, Lin SS, Lee JH. Inhibition of N-acetyltransferase activity and gene expression in human colon cancer cell lines by diallyl sulfide. *Food Chem. Toxicol.* 2004; 42: 195–202.
126. Huber WW, Teitel CH, Coles BF, et al. Potential chemoprotective effects of the coffee components kahweol and cafestol palmitates via modification of hepatic N-acetyltransferase and glutathione S-transferase activities. *Environ. Mol. Mutagen.* 2004; 44: 265–276.
127. Harris RM, Wood DM, Bottomley L, et al. Phytoestrogens are potent inhibitors of estrogen sulfation: implications for breast cancer risk and treatment. *J. Clin. Endocrinol. Metab.* 2004; 89: 1779–1787.
128. National Hot Dog and Sausage Council (www.hot-dog.org/facts/hd_vitalstats.htm). Accessed October 6, 2005.
129. Barbecue'n Statistics (www.barbecuen.com/bbqstats.htm). Accessed October 6, 2005.
130. Fujiki H, Suganuma M, Imai K, Nakachi K. Green tea: cancer preventive beverage and/or drug. *Cancer Lett.* 2002; 188: 9–13.
131. Weisburger JH, Nagao M, Wakabayashi K, Oguri A. Prevention of heterocyclic amine formation by tea and tea polyphenols. *Cancer Lett.* 1994; 83: 143–147.

4 Nutrient and Phytochemical Modulation of Cancer Treatment

Kelly Anne Meckling

CONTENTS

4.1 INTRODUCTION

Epidemiological data have consistently demonstrated that fruit and vegetable consumption are associated with decreased risk of cancer at a variety of tissue sites. A number of nutrients and phytochemical components of these foods have been identified as potential cancer chemopreventive agents acting through a variety of mechanisms (as described in Chapter 3). Many of these same compounds or additional ones may also have activity in the later stages of cancer development, including metastasis and the response of the patient to surgery, chemotherapy, and radiation therapy. In some cases, the effects may be opposite to those found in the early initiating events of carcinogenesis. Good examples here are the results from clinical intervention trials using β-carotene in smokers and finding an increased risk of lung tumor development, despite the fact that high carotenoid intake is frequently associated with decreased risk of developing lung cancer.[1,2]

Additional examples include phytochemicals that modify expression of P-glycoprotein that may be useful as chemopreventive agents since they can promote the efflux of certain carcinogens including 7,12-dimethylbenz(a)-anthracene. On the other hand, researchers are looking for ways to antagonize P-glycoprotein activity during chemotherapy since this activity in tumor cells can promote drug resistance and treatment failure. It is clear then that treatment of the cancer patient is a separate case from the prevention of cancer itself. Some strategies may be specifically useful in the treatment phase, and it can be appreciated that potential risks may be more acceptable at this point in the disease than they might be when considered for long-term use in otherwise healthy populations.

4.2 MAGNITUDE OF THE PROBLEM

Based on the best available current data, a comprehensive study estimated that in 2002 there were 10.9 million new cases of cancer worldwide, 6.7 million deaths, and 24.6 million people who had been diagnosed with cancer in the last 5 years.[3] The risk of developing cancer is highest in North American men and women, but the risk of dying from cancer is highest in Eastern European men and Northern European women.[4] Lung cancer has been the most common cancer in the world since 1985. However, because of differences in survival statistics, four times as many women are breast cancer survivors (5 years since diagnosis) as men and women who survive lung cancer. While the impression has been that cancer is largely a problem of the developed world, this is rapidly changing with cancer rates at many sites steadily rising in the developing world and only barely lagging behind rates in North America and Europe.

One estimate puts the number of new cancer cases in 2020 at 15 million, a 50% increase over the rate in the year 2000. The increase in the average age of the population as a whole is one contributor, but others include lifestyle factors, such as smoking, decreased physical activity, and increased consumption of "unhealthy diets," as well as communicable diseases. Given that we can expect an increase in the burden of cancer worldwide, at least for the next few decades, improved treatment strategies to effect cure and/or improve the quality of life for those suffering, are international objectives.

Given that a large number of cancer cases are likely to be attributed to dietary and lifestyle factors, it is perhaps not surprising that a significant proportion of the population is using supplements to "ward off disease" and may increase their use following a diagnosis of cancer.[5] Depending on the population studied, as many as 84% of patients may report using complementary and alternative medicine (CAM) and half of these report this use to their treating physician. One-third of Australian and Finnish women with breast cancer reported substantial changes to their dietary and lifestyle habits in the months following diagnosis.[6] These included smoking cessation, changes in macronutrient composition, increasing physical activity, and the use of vitamin and herbal supplements as well as visits to CAM practitioners, including naturopaths. The highest users of CAM appear to be pediatric oncology patients (84%)[7] followed by breast cancer survivors with more than 66% of Canadian women, living in Ontario, reporting use of CAM.[5] Sixty-one percent of U.S. armed forces veterans diagnosed with cancer admitted using dietary supplements[8] and about 30% of Canadian men with prostate cancer report using some form of alternative medicine, although only one-third of these were seeing a CAM practitioner.[9]

While the move toward informing clinicians about the use of CAM therapies may be increasing, there are still 30% or more of certain patient groups that fail to report. In order to provide useful resources for patients and clinicians on specific therapies, prevalence data and outcome measures need to be available. Both positive and negative interactions of CAMs with other therapies, including chemotherapy, need to be identified and reported by both traditional and alternative healthcare practitioners. If properly applied, diet, nutritional, and herbal supplements could increase drug efficacy in cancer treatment and potentially lessen drug toxicity, leading to increased cure and better quality of life for those suffering from cancer.

4.3 EFFECTS OF OVERALL NUTRITIONAL STATUS ON TREATMENT OUTCOMES

There is marked individual variation in drug pharmacokinetics based on genetic polymorphisms, gene-environment interactions, presence or absence of disease, the type and pattern of nutrient intake, and the scheduling/dosage of drug administration. In the area of food–drug interactions the main focus has been on the effects of food on drug absorption in the small intestine. Some adverse reactions to particular treatment protocols have been attributed to food–drug interactions without ever identifying the mechanisms or factors involved. Even when the complicating food/nutrient is identified, the typical response by treating physicians and pharmacists is to put the "food" on the "do not consume" list. While this may seem like a reasonable approach, the possible nutritional deficits that may result from eliminating large numbers of foods from one's diet, combined with the possible benefits that a mechanistic understanding of the nature of the interaction may have on drug efficacy, side effects, and normal tissue toxicity, speaks to the need for more rational treatment design (see Table 4.1).

4.3.1 Changes in Nutritional Status of the Cancer Patient

Substantial weight loss is often observed in cancer patients, particularly those with advanced disease. This may come about as a result of the disease process

TABLE 4.1
Nutritional Components with Potential Activity in Adjuvant Cancer Therapy

Nutrient/ Phytochemical	Molecular Target(s) or Activity	Confounding Factors
Green tea polyphenols	Multidrug resistance proteins NFB signaling AP-1 transcription factor Cell cycle inhibitory proteins p21, p27, cyclins D1, E IGF-II EGFR Increase ovarian cancer survival	
Sulforaphane	NFκB signaling	
Resveratrol	NFκB signaling	
Soy isoflavones (genistein)	Decrease breast cancer risk Decrease prostate cancer in TRAMP model	May stimulate growth of ER+ breast tumors Antagonizes benefit of Tamoxifen
Curcumin	Antiangiogenic Cardioprotectant Lung protection from bleomycin	Possible activation of multidrug resistance proteins Inhibition of camptothecin and doxorubicin killing of breast cancer cells
Ellagic acid	VEGFR-2 PDGFR Antiangiogenic	
Lutein	Bax:Bcl-2 ratio Angiogenesis Induce apoptosis	May increase ACF formation at high concentrations
Grape seed extract (procyanidins)	Angiogenesis (VEGF) IGFBP-3 Apoptosis induction	
Mushroom polysaccharides (Krestin)	Immune enhancement Th1/Th2 balance Dendritic cell differentiation	
Flaxseed lignans	HER-2/neu Apoptosis cascade Estrogen and progesterone receptors	

TABLE 4.1 (CONTINUED)
Nutritional Components with Potential Activity in Adjuvant Cancer Therapy

Nutrient/ Phytochemical	Molecular Target(s) or Activity	Confounding Factors
Omega-3 fatty acids EPA/DHA	Cachexia reversal agent 20 S proteosome Lipoxygenase Cyclooxygenase NFB signaling Improve cytokine profile Decrease iNOS Decrease metastatic spread Improved liver and pancreatic function	Low levels inhibit breast carcinogenesis, but high levels increase risk if exposed during prepubescent period
Antioxidant vitamins (E, C, β-carotene)	Enhance chemotherapy in some adult populations Low dose -carotene inhibits formation of colonic aberrant crypts High carotenoid levels associated with recurrence-free survival in breast cancer patients	Interfere with chemotherapy in some adult and childhood cancers May promote tumor progression in smokers High dose β-carotene stimulates ACF formation

itself or from therapies that affect tissue metabolism or the patient's ability to assimilate nutrients.[10] As well as there being different incidence between cancer types, there are also differences in the presentation and pattern of body composition changes between men and women.[11] Regardless of treatment modality, the incidence of deficiency signs and symptoms frequently increases as treatment progresses.[12] These can include the appearance of stomatitis, edema, and changes in body composition. The anorexia-cachexia syndrome is typical of patients suffering from many solid tumors and occurs in greater than 50% of all cancer patients and more than 85% of pancreatic and lung cancer patients.[13] Presence of cachexia is associated with increased morbidity and mortality, and research efforts are focused on improving quality of life and functional capacity for those suffering.[14] Both fat stores (predominantly triglyceride) and skeletal muscle protein are targets of the hypermetabolic state resulting from a number of inflammatory mediator and cytokine changes, including release of lipid mobilizing factor (LIF) and proteolysis inducing factor (PIF) from tumor cells and other tissues.

Recent studies using oral nutritional supplements containing eicosapentaenoic acid (EPA, 20:5n-3) in cachectic patients have demonstrated improvements in weight or decreases in the rate of weight loss, improvements in body composition, functional status, and quality of life.[15–18] Many of the early studies focused on untreated pancreatic patients where effective therapy and survival are limited. However, a recent pilot study demonstrated improved outcomes in lung cancer and pancreatic cancer patients with cachexia undergoing gemcitabine chemotherapy.[19] These studies have demonstrated that an energy- and protein-rich supplemental drink, providing at least 1 g of EPA per day, can improve weight gain, physical activity, and quality of life.[18,19]

EPA has been shown to inhibit the muscle catabolism induced by PIF through antagonism of the ubiquitin proteosomal pathway.[20] EPA attenuates the release of arachidonic acid (AA, 20:4n-6) from membrane phospholipids and its subsequent metabolism to various eicosanoid products, including 15-hydroxyeicosatetraenoic acid (15-HETE).[21] Both PIF and 15-HETE can directly modify the proteosomal pathway by promoting NFB translocation to the nucleus. β-hydroxy-β-methybutyrate (HMB), a metabolite of the amino acid leucine, has similar antagonistic activity to EPA; however, it appears to act at a step downstream from AA release by inhibiting phosphorylation of the p42/44 mitogen-activated protein kinase, key to the upregulation of the 20 S proteosome.[22]

Even when patients with advanced cancer are in seemingly good medical condition, there is considerable interindividual response to therapy. The ability to identify those factors that predict a patient's ability to tolerate a specific therapeutic regimen is highly desirable. Severe clinical hematopoietic toxicity is a frequent and often life-threatening complication of chemotherapy. Although the incidence does correlate with dose, complications can follow or copresent with any cytotoxic therapy. It is conceivable that chemotherapy-induced DNA and cellular damage may be more toxic to normal tissues, promoting hematopoietic toxicity, in the presence of inflammatory cytokines and metabolic factors associated with the anorexia-cachexia syndrome. Alexandre and coworkers recently reported on the frequency of neutropenic fever or severe thrombocytopenia in patients undergoing chemotherapy for advanced breast, gynecological, or gastrointestinal neoplasias.[23] Drugs that were included in the various regimens included anthracyclines, topoisomerase I or II inhibitors, platinum compounds, and alkylating agents. Using an NIS index, calculated as the ratio (C-reative protein X alpha-1 glycoprotein)/(albumin X prealbumin),[24] the authors were able to predict severe hematopoietic toxicity with a sensitivity of 89% and specificity of 66%. Combined with the WHO measure of performance status, these two measurements together should be able to identify those most likely to experience severe chemotherapeutic toxicity. It remains to be seen whether nutritional supplementation or antiinflammatory drug treatment can reverse this sensitivity in such patients.

In addition to hematopoietic toxicity, a number of drug and radiation regimens produce substantial dose-limiting gastrointestinal toxicity, including mucositis.[25] This cannot only impair the patient's desire to eat, but can also make them vulnerable to infection at the site of injury. In a model of intestinal injury repair, we showed that long-chain omega-3 fatty acids, docosahexaenoic acid (DHA, 22:6n-3) and eicosapentaenoic acid (EPA, 20:5n-3) promoted faster wound healing than short-chain fatty acids or omega-6 fatty acids [26] and decreased mucosal damage in the small intestine of drug-treated rats.[27] Compared to other areas of nutrition and cancer research, there have been relatively few studies examining effective therapies for mucositis. Most efforts have been on palliation and pain control (for review, see Reference 25). One clinical trial demonstrated that supplementation of parenteral nutrition formula with glutamine reduced the severity of mucositis in patients undergoing high dose chemotherapy followed by autologous bone marrow transplantation.[28] Another found that treatment with human recombinant keratinocyte growth factor substantially improved oral mucositis symptoms in patients about to undergo myeloablation and autologous stem cell transplantation for hematologic malignancies.[29] Though not specifically tested in cancer patients, a traditional herbal medicine, Throat Coat®, containing elm bark, licorice root, and marshmallow root, substantially improved symptoms of pharyngitis in clinical patients.[30]

4.3.2 THE ANTIOXIDANT CONUNDRUM

The association between consumption of foods rich in antioxidants and reduced risk of several types of cancer has often been interpreted as indicating that high antioxidant intake will inevitably reduce cancer risk and improve cancer therapy. As noted in Chapter 3, antioxidants can also act as prooxidants depending on dose and interaction with other biologicals, including other antioxidant vitamins, minerals, and phytochemicals. While some trials have demonstrated that dietary supplementation with antioxidants may enhance the response to chemotherapy, improve the quality of life of patients by reducing toxic side effects, or recovery of normal tissues to therapeutic insult,[31–34] others have shown that supplementation of antioxidants during chemotherapy may actually interfere with the activity of the drug.[35–38] This is particularly the case when oxidant stress and generation of free radical damage are part of the mechanism by which the drugs kill tumor cells. For example, the enhanced therapeutic effect of anthracyclines in the background of an omega-3 fatty acid supplementation on mammary cancer treatment is suppressed in the presence of α-tocopherol (vitamin E).[38]

Saintot and coworkers also found a negative correlation between α-tocopherol levels and subsequent survival in women with breast cancer.[39] In other models, however, vitamin E has been shown to reduce cardiotoxicity of doxorubicin,[40] healing of chemotherapy-induced stomatitis[41] and increase efficacy of 5-fluorouracil treatment of colon cancer.[42] Similar inconsistencies exist for other antioxidant vitamins including vitamin C and beta-carotene (reviewed in Reference 42). In a recent trial, patients with low vitamin C plasma concentrations had shorter survival times than those with higher levels.[44] While vitamin C levels did correlate with high C-reactive protein levels, none of these patients were undergoing chemotherapy, as treatment was strictly palliative.

In contrast to the results in adult cancer patients, children suffering from acute lymphoblastic leukemia (the most common cancer in children) seem particularly vulnerable to low antioxidant vitamin status. In this population, higher intake of vitamins A, C, and E were associated with fewer therapy delays, less chemotherapeutic drug toxicity, fewer days spent in hospital, and decreased incidence of infection.[45] The authors of this work suggested that the additional burden of chemotherapy combined with the disease process itself would lead to an increased free radical load and, therefore, tax the antioxidant defenses even in the presence of apparent dietary adequacy. Given the inconsistencies between reports and the large variation between specific patient populations, generalizations about the benefits and/or risks of antioxidant supplementation during chemotherapy cannot be made. Rather, recommendations for their use must be based on the specific drug regimen and tumor type being treated and a molecular understanding of the relevant targets (see Table 4.1).

4.4 SPECIFIC MOLECULAR TARGETS

4.4.1 P-Glycoprotein and Other Drug Efflux Pumps

P-glycoprotein (Pgp) is a 170 kDa phosphorylated glycoprotein encoded by the human MDR1 gene. It belongs to a family of adenosine triphosphate (ATP)-dependent membrane ABC cassette transporters normally responsible for transport of structurally unrelated chemicals, including xenobiotics, lipophilic, and amphipathic natural compounds, hormones, and pharmacological agents. Other members include ABCG2 (breast cancer resistance protein) and MRPs 1 to 8 (multidrug resistance proteins, reviewed by Choi,[46]). MRP1 is a 190 kDa protein with several conserved regions common to ABC members, but with a distinct transport mechanism and substrate specificity from Pgp. Substrates for MRP include leukotriene C4 and glucuronide conjugates of 17-β-estradiol,[47] and for drug transport, it is frequently dependent on the presence of reduced glutathione.[48] Pgps, along with several other members of this family, are ubiquitously expressed, but tend to be concentrated on the apical surfaces of epithelial cells, particularly those in the gastrointestinal tract tissues,[49] the blood–brain barrier,[50] and in bone marrow progenitors.[51]

One of the major reasons for treatment failure in chemotherapy is the development of drug resistance. This can occur as a result of over-expression of one or more of the drug resistance transporters (MDR) listed above, in tumor targets. Drug therapy becomes ineffective, even at high dose levels, because the activity of these transporters to extrude drug from tumor cells becomes incredibly efficient. A variety of strategies including the development of chemosensitizers has been attempted to overcome the resistant phenotype. Some chemosensitizers are active against more than one MDR product while others are highly selective. Verapamil, a calcium channel blocker, was shown to be an effective sensitizer in both models and in a recent clinical trial of metastatic breast cancer;[52] however, at effective doses that bring about sensitization, verapamil causes cardiotoxicity. Cyclosporin A and related derivatives have also shown some promise clinically, but again the side effects, in this case immunosuppression, are major clinical issues. A variety of second-generation chemosensitizing agents are currently under development by a number of companies with the emphasis being on reducing toxicity while maximizing drug reversal in tumor cells (reviewed by Choi[46]). It is interesting to note that a variety of flavonoid compounds are being examined as potential chemosensitizers, as it has been proposed that these would have fewer side effects than pharmacologic agents. Whether this is the case remains to be determined.

As are the cases with many of the P450 enzymes, Pgp and MRP1 expression and activity can be regulated by nutrients and phytochemicals, including many herbal constituents. Identifying the chemical components and target specificity are keys to developing these "natural" therapeutic agents that may be active alone or in combination with conventional pharmacologic agents. Dr. Susan Cole's group was the first to report that a wide range of flavonoids found in commonly consumed foodstuffs were inhibitors of conjugated organic anion transport via MRP1.[53] Apigenin, naringenin, genistein, and quercetin were all shown to inhibit the transport of LTC4 and 17-β-estradiol 17-(β-D-glucoronide), while at the same time promoting GSH transport by MRP1 without acting as substrates themselves.[53,54]

An important consideration for their utility as cancer therapeutic agents is their bioavailability *in vivo*. While many polyphenols have been shown to be active *in vitro*, the real question is whether they are effective, particularly when given orally to patients. For example, curcumin, a polyphenol found in *Curcuma longa* (the spice tumeric), has been shown to have antioxidant, antiinflammatory, hypolipidemic, antimutagenic, anticancer, and antimetastatic properties, presumably through regulation of key signaling cascades involving NFB, c-myc, p21, and bcl-X_L.[55] Even though curcumin has been shown to be nontoxic at doses up to 10 g/d in humans, serum metabolites are virtually undetectable (or at most in the nM range) at this level largely because liver and intestinal conjugation are so efficient.[56] Curcumin at doses of 50 to 150 μM is cytotoxic to freshly isolated hepatocytes, but if added to progressively older cultures is nontoxic as a result of upregulation of Pgp.[57] In cervical carcinoma cells, curcumin down regulates MDR1 activity and increases sensitivity to vinblastine, possibly by directly binding Pgp and antagonizing its activity.[58] However, once again these results were only achieved at μM concentrations of curcumin. Thus, although curcumin appears to be a good drug reversal agent *in vitro*, the key to its clinical utility will be in improving its bioavailability.

Similarly, various ginseng components including ginsenosides have been shown to have activity in reversing drug resistant in several tumor cell lines by inhibiting Pgp.[59] Several were active *in vivo* in prolonging the life of leukemia P388 transplanted mice treated with doxorubicin[60] and in reversing drug resistance *in vitro* in several daunorubicin and doxorubicin acute myelogenous leukemia cell lines with activity greater than observed with verapamil.[61] While there are, as yet, no clinical reports of specific drug interactions with Pgp substrates, one could predict that Panax ginseng could be used as a complementary therapy in human cancer chemotherapy.

A variety of catechins in green tea have been associated with decreased cancer risk at various sites. While some of these same components (EGCG, epicatechin gallate, and catechin gallate) have been shown to be active Pgp inhibitors and, therefore, may be useful in adjuvant chemotherapy settings, others (i.e, epicatechin) have shown the opposite activity.[62,63] Whether these heterologous activities have importance clinically for drug interactions in cancer or any other disease, remains to be determined. Similarly, while St. John's wort has been shown to modify drug activity modulated by CYP3A4 and has a particularly critical effect when used in combination with psychiatric drugs (see Chapter 6, Nutrients and Herbals in the Pharmacotherapy of Unipolar/Major Depression), it has also been shown to stimulate Pgp expression in a number of cell lines and peripheral blood lymphocytes.[64–66] The potential impact of hyperforin and other St. John's wort constituents on cancer chemotherapeutics have not been examined clinically and, thus, the potential for significant worsening of the drug-resistant phenotype during therapy is entirely possible.

4.4.2 NFκB, AP-1, AND COX-2

NFκB (nuclear transcription factor κB) describes a family of dimeric transcription factors involved in cell cycle control, cell differentiation, apoptosis, cell adhesion and migration, and angiogenesis. NFκB is maintained in the cytoplasm in an inactive form by binding to one of the inhibitory κIBs (inhibitory kappa binding protein). Phosphorylation of κIB by an Iκkinase (IKK) promotes its ubiquitination and proteosomal degradation, thereby releasing NFκB for translocation to the nucleus to target specific genes. While controlled expression of NFκB is critical to normal cell fate determination, abnormal expression has been associated with the transformed phenotype (reviewed by Dorai and Aggarwal[67] and Nakanishi and Toi[68]).

Activated protein-1 (AP-1) is also a hetero- or homodimeric transcription factor composed of various combinations of fos and jun proteins. Targets of AP-1 activity include genes such as urokinase-type plasminogen activator (uPA) and matrix metalloproteinases (MMPs), two types of proteins critical to acquisition of the metastatic phenotype and the androgen receptor in prostate cancer.[69] Several phytochemicals, including green tea catechins, curcumin, resveratrol, and capsaicin, have been shown to suppress AP-1 activation (possibly NFκB as well[70]) and may specifically down-regulate Bcl-2 and Bcl-X$_L$, two antiapoptotic proteins. In addition, some of these same compounds and additional ones from grape seed extract (procyanidins) have been shown to inhibit growth factor receptors including those for insulin-like growth factor (IGF-1), epidermal growth factor (EGF), fibroblast growth factor-2 (FGF2), and vascular endothelial growth factor (VEGF), which have roles in promoting tumor growth and angiogenesis.[71–78] The activity and expression of HER-2/neu, a receptor that is over-expressed in many breast cancers and associated with poor prognosis, is inhibited by curcumin[79] and flaxseed lignans.[80]

Curcumin has additional targets, such as the Src-homology domain tyrosine phosphatase (SHP-2), where it activates the protein's activity, thereby interfering with the JAK-STAT signaling pathway and suppressing proliferation in tumors, such as multiple myeloma.[81] The tetracyclic phenolic, ellagic acid, has similar molecular targets to its cousin curcumin. Ellagic acid is richly produced in raspberries, strawberries, cranberries, walnuts, and pecans, where it is concentrated in the seeds/nuts. As well as inhibiting VEGFR-2 in endothelial cells, ellagic acid also inhibits PDGFR activity in smooth muscle cells.[82] These dual effects result in profound inhibition of angiogenesis and point to ellagic acid's potential as a useful adjuvant in human cancer therapy.

In addition to their activities on NFκB and growth factor signaling, directly or indirectly, a number of food components also modulate the levels of eicosanoids. Depending on the initial polyunsaturated fatty acid substrate, and relative levels of the various cyclooxygenase and lipoxygenase activities, a wide variety of pro- and antiinflammatory eicosanoid metabolites can be produced. Typical substrates, such as arachidonic acid (AA), can be metabolized to the proinflammatory hormone-like compound, prostaglandin E_2, via cyclooxygenase enzymes (COX-1 or COX-2) (Figure 4.2). COX-1 is ubiquitously expressed and tends to be constitutively expressed in most cells, suggesting a generalized housekeeping role for this form of the enzyme. On the other hand, COX-2, the inducible form of the enzyme, tends to be stimulated in response to inflammatory signals. A large body of literature now exists demonstrating an important role for COX-2 products in tumorigenesis (for review, see Wallace[83]).

Chemoprevention studies using nonsteroidal, antiinflammatory agents (NSAIDS), such as celecoxib and aspirin, showed that colon carcinogenesis could be profoundly inhibited in Min mice and in controlled trials of patients with familial adenomatous polyposis (FAP). There are a whole host of side effects of long-term NSAID treatment and, thus, this approach is of limited utility in populations other than those with FAP. However, given that COX-2 over expression is an extremely common occurrence in malignancy and interferes with tumor cell killing and promotes angiogenesis, targeting this enzyme in adjuvant cancer therapy may be a realistic option. In this respect, it is interesting that certain phytochemicals, such as curcumin, can act similarly to NSAIDs in that they inhibit COX-2 activity.

COX-2 is overexpressed in more than 80% of human colorectal adenomas and carcinomas, and is associated with constitutively higher levels of PGE_2 than normal surrounding mucosa.[84,85] Colon cells expressing high levels of COX-2 are also resistant to the differentiation effects of the bacterial fiber fermentation metabolite, butyrate. In general, high level COX-2 expression is associated with more advanced tumor grade, increased frequency of metastasis, and shorter survival times in colon cancer patients[86,87] Glioblastoma multiforme also seems to be a cancer where COX-2 over expression is predictive of poor survival, and there is some suggestion that inhibitors may be helpful as adjuvant therapy for brain tumors. In breast cancer, an association has been made between overactive HER-2/neu and elevated COX-2 expression. Activation of HER-2/neu in cultured cells leads to upregulation of COX-2 and increased production of PGE_2 in the medium. Conversely, treatment with the antibody Herceptin® reduced COX-2 and PGE_2 expression. Additionally important in the breast, COX-2-derived prostaglandins stimulate aromatase activity in the breast providing local production of active estrogens for breast cancer promotion.[88,89] Other cancers where a role for

COX-2 in tumor progression have been suggested include cervical carcinoma, endometrial carcinoma, squamous cell carcinoma of the head and neck, adeno-carcinoma of the lung, pancreatic cancer, prostate cancer, and bladder cancer (reviewed by Wallace[83]).

COX-2 products including PGE_2, PGI_2, and thromboxane A_2 (TXA_2) reduce endothelial apoptosis and directly stimulate endothelial migration[90,91] by stimu-lating production of basic fibroblast growth factor (BFGF), platelet-derived growth factor (PDGF), and VEGF. VEGF, in particular, seems to be critical in establishing the vasculature necessary for tumor angiogenesis and progression. Furthermore, these products also stimulate tumor production of MMPs facilitating extravasation and metastatic spread.[92] In addition, COX-2 products have been reported to upset the balance of interleukins and cytokines necessary for normal immunocompetence (see below), thereby impairing host attempts at tumor cell killing. There are a wide variety of natural inhibitors of COX-2 that have been described, many of which have been tested *in vitro*. Many of these are flavonoids or related in structure to these. *Scutellaria baicalensis* and several other Chinese medicinal herbs demonstrate breast and prostate anticancer activity through sup-pression of PGE_2 via COX-2.[93]

In addition to being active antitumor agents on their own, curcumin and resveratrol may also be important in adjuvant therapy settings. They can make cells more sensitive to radiation and chemotherapy by inducing p21[Cip1/waf-1], which promotes cell cycle arrest, decreasing drug resistance through depressed glu-tathione levels through GST-Pi inhibition, and down-regulation of the survival protein surviving (reviewed by Dorai and Aggarwal[67]). As well, several chemo-therapy agents may inadvertently transactivate NFκB signaling as they simulta-neously trigger apoptotic cascades through activation of p53 (reviewed by Nakan-ishi and Toi[68]). Taxanes, Vinca alkaloids, and topoisomerase I and II inhibitors are all examples of drugs that appear to simultaneously induce NFκB nuclear translocation. This, in itself, could contribute to drug resistance and may be overcome by simultaneous administration of NFκB targeting phytochemicals. The exploitation of green tea polyphenols, resveratrol, curcumin, and related phy-tochemicals in adjuvant therapy needs to be examined in clinical trials of human cancer patients. Furthermore, combining some of these compounds into "nutri-tional cocktails" may be particularly useful. A mixture of lysine, proline, arginine, vitamin C, and epigallocatechin gallate was recently shown to inhibit osteosar-coma cell production of MMPs, and VEGF.[94] Given that osteosarcoma is associ-ated with poor prognosis and increased frequency of second site tumors as a result of chemotherapy, new therapies like this need to be tested in clinical trials.

4.4.3 THE MEVALONATE PATHWAY

Statins are probably the most safe and effective hypolipidemic medicines cur-rently available. Specifically, they are competitive inhibitors of the rate-limiting enzyme in cholesterol biosynthesis, 3-hydroxy-3-methylglutaryl-coenzyme A reductase (HMG-CoAR). Mevalonate, in addition to being a precursor of cholesterol, is also a key intermediate in the formation of isoprenoid groups that localize and maintain the activity of small GTP-binding proteins, including ras, rac, and rho. Activating ras mutations or defects in ras signaling are typical of many cancers. A number of studies have now shown that treatment with statins has antitumor activity both *in vitro* and *in vivo* (reviewed by Katz[95]). Recently, Duncan and coworkers showed that EPA and DHA attenuated the up-regulation of HMG-CoAR in MCF-7 breast cancer cells in response to mevastatin and suggested that these may be useful in adjuvant breast cancer therapy.[96]

4.4.4 IMMUNOMODULATORS

Patients undergoing surgery, radiation, or chemotherapy have a high risk of complications, including wound infections and septicemia. Alterations in host defense associated with disease or treatment may make the cancer patient particularly vulnerable. Although there is no single contributor to immune dysfunction, there are indicators that specific nutritional substrates may be effective in rebalancing the immune system in cancer patients. As already mentioned, the n-3 fatty acid, EPA, has anticachectic properties that lead to decreased weight loss in treated patients. Recent studies have shown that EPA and the amino acids, arginine or glutamine, when supplemented orally, improved postoperative infectious and wound complications in head and neck cancer[97,98] pancreatic cancer,[99] colon cancer[100] patients, and during bone marrow transplantation.[101]

Recently, green tea polyphenols were also shown to promote cytotoxic CD8+ T cell invasion of UV-induced tumors and promoted apoptosis via activation of caspase-3 in animals.[102,103] As well, mistletoe lectins (ML-1) have considerable immunomodulatory activity in human beings. Healthy human subjects administered mistletoe lectins responded with an initial proliferation of peripheral blood mononuclear cells, accompanied by increased production of TNFα and IL-6 and less pronounced elevation of INF-γ and IL-4 (reviewed by Pryme et al.[104]). Expansion in the CD8+ cytotoxic T cell population and NK activity have also been reported in response to ML-1.[105]

Additional compounds that have interesting immunomodulatory activity include a variety of polysaccharides from herbs used in traditional Chinese medicine (TCM). There are important structure–function relationships that have not been completely delineated but that seem critical to their activity (reviewed by Chang[106]). The most important bioactives appear to have a β1,3 1,4 or 1,6 branching pattern, and the more highly branched and higher molecular weight species seem to be the most potent.[107] More than 200 species have been identified, mostly fungal or botanicals. One representative example is the polysaccharide, Lentinan, from Shiitake mushrooms, *Lentinus edodes*; it inhibits the growth of transplanted tumors in rodents[108] and, in a controlled clinical trial, it increased survival in recurrent and metastatic gastric and colorectal cancer patients when given in combination with chemotherapy.[109] This latter study was carried out in Japan, published in Japanese, and, as far as one can tell, has not been reproduced in larger clinical trials. Thus, the utility of this agent remains to be examined.

However, another agent, Krestin, has been shown to extend survival in several clinical trials, including patients with gastrointestinal tumors at various tissue sites, nonsmall-cell lung carcinoma, and some breast cancers.[110-115] This protein-bound polysaccharide has recently shown great promise as an adjuvant with 5-fluorouracil in colon cancer patients after surgical resection.[111,116,117] In an animal model of bone metastatic breast cancer, Krestin also substantially affected the rates of metastases and long-term survival when combined with Tamoxifen[118,119] and, in one clinical trial, improved response in combination chemotherapy for operable breast cancer.[120] It has also been shown to restore the cytotoxic T-cell profile toward Th1 dominance, critical to successful vaccine therapy, and promoted the differentiation of dendritic cells in similar patient populations.[121] Jimenez et al. also suggested that this compound may have important NK stimulatory activity as it was potent in NK-derived cell lines *in vitro*.[122] Polysaccharide preparations from the mushroom *Coriolus versicolor* have antileukemic activity by lowering IL-8 and increasing IL-1β and IL-6 production.[123] IL-8 excess is thought to be important in cancer progression by promoting mitotic, angiogenic, and migrational activity of tumor cells. Interestingly, glutamine restriction or deprivation promotes the expression of IL-8 and several other genes in breast cancer and other cell types[124] through NFκB. An oral supplement mixture containing arginine, n-3 fatty acids, and RNA as a source of nucleosides improved the IL-8 and cytokine profile, markers of inflammation (including prostaglandins and leukotrienes) in preoperative patients about to undergo major surgery for cancer.[125]

4.5 POLYUNSATURATED FATTY ACIDS AS THERAPEUTIC AND ADJUVANT CHEMOTHERAPY AGENTS

Long-chain polyunsaturated fatty acids (PUFA) found in the human body are derived either from foods and/or metabolism of shorter versions consumed in the diet. Omega-3 (ω-3 or n-3) and omega-6 (ω-6 or n-6) represent two families of fatty acids required for normal human growth and development. Human beings do not have the ability to desaturate fatty acids at the 3 or 6 positions from the methyl end and, thus, these must be provided in the diet as essential fatty acids. Two examples of essential fatty acids are linoleic acid (LA, 18:2n-6) and alpha-linolenic acid (LNA, 18:3n-3), both of which can be elongated and desaturated to form longer versions, such as arachidonic acid (20:4n-6), eicosapentaenoic acid (EPA, 20:5n-3), and docosahexaenoic acid (DHA, 22:6n-3) (Figure 4.1). Rich natural sources of LA include sunflower and corn oil, LNA includes flaxseed and canola oils, and EPA and DHA are found in some algae and cold water fishes. These fatty acids can in turn be esterified into mono-, di- and triglycerides and into various membrane phospholipids. Following their release through the action of phopholipases (including phospholipase A$_2$ [PLA$_2$], which releases fatty acids from the *sn*-2 position), 20-carbon (and possibly 22 carbon) fatty acids can either

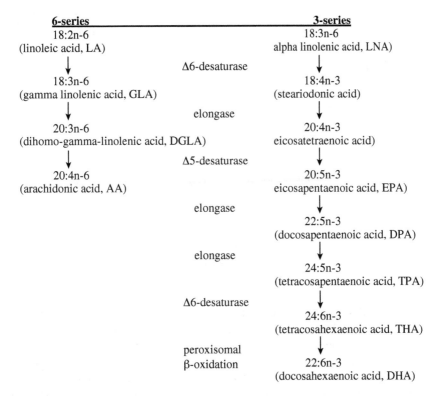

6-series

18:2n-6
(linoleic acid, LA)

↓   Δ6-desaturase

18:3n-6
(gamma linolenic acid, GLA)

↓   elongase

20:3n-6
(dihomo-gamma-linolenic acid, DGLA)

↓   Δ5-desaturase

20:4n-6
(arachidonic acid, AA)

elongase

elongase

Δ6-desaturase

peroxisomal
β-oxidation

3-series

18:3n-6
alpha linolenic acid, LNA)

↓

18:4n-3
(steariodonic acid)

↓

20:4n-3
eicosatetraenoic acid)

↓

20:5n-3
eicosapentaenoic acid, EPA)

↓

22:5n-3
(docosapentaenoic acid, DPA)

↓

24:5n-3
(tetracosapentaenoic acid, TPA)

↓

24:6n-3
(tetracosahexaenoic acid, THA)

↓

22:6n-3
(docosahexaenoic acid, DHA)

FIGURE 4.1 Metabolism of essential fatty acids in man

be reesterified or metabolized into one of several eicosanoid products including prostaglandins, leukotrienes, and thromboxanes (Figure 4.2).

The balance of eicosanoid products is dependent on the relative concentrations of n-6 and n-3 PUFAs in membrane phospholipids (which is largely dependent on dietary intake), the activity of PLA_2 (and related enzymes), and the activity of the various isoforms of COX, LOX, and cytochrome P_{450} enzymes. In addition to enzymatic catalysis, AA is particularly vulnerable to free radical attack promoting the formation of longer-lived isoprostanes, which are potent inflammatory molecules. Compared to AA metabolites, DGLA and EPA eicosanoids tend to be less inflammatory or may even be antiinflammatory depending on the specific series created. Many of the benefits of fish consumption on cardiovascular disease risk are related to the antiinflammatory properties of EPA metabolites and their roles in inhibiting platelet aggregation, promoting vasodilation, and lowering arterial blood pressure.

Most eicosanoid products are relatively short-lived, surviving only seconds or minutes after release and only able to act locally. In contrast, some LOX byproducts, such as 5-HETE and 12-HETE, may survive up to hours in the circulation, giving them ample time to act and reach more targets. As well, several eicosanoid products have the ability to bind to fatty acid binding proteins in blood,

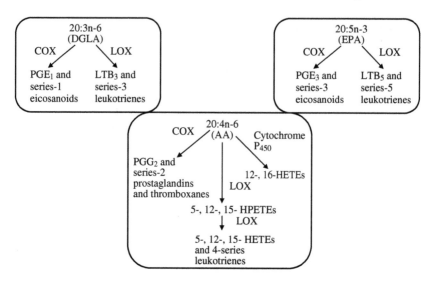

FIGURE 4.2 Eicosanoid metabolism of n-6 and n-3 fatty acids.

which can substantially stabilize them and extend their half-lives further.[126] 5-HETE and 12-HETE tend to be associated with increased cancer cell growth and may act through specific receptors or receptor-independent pathways.[127,128] Some tumor types, including gliomas, breast cancer, and leukemia cells, both produce and respond to HETEs in an autocrine fashion; LOX inhibitors have been demonstrated to have antitumor activity in these cell lines *in vitro.*[129] 5-HETE is a particularly important survival factor for prostate cancer cells. When its synthesis is blocked, both hormone responsive and nonresponsive tumor cells undergo rapid apoptosis.[130,131] 12-HETE promotes proliferation and the metastatic phenotype of colon, pancreatic, breast, melanoma, and prostate tumor cell lines.[83,131] Elevated 12-LOX activity is typical of high-grade tumors, which release 12-HETE promoting angiogenesis in neighboring endothelial cells, changes in extracellular matrix proteins, and invasive properties in the primary tumor.[132,133] Molecular targets of 12-HETE include protein kinase C, activation of Erk1/2, src, and activation of NFκB.[134] Often times, both COX and LOX products have cancer promoting and antiapoptotic activity in the same tumor. MCF-7, ER+ breast cancer cells are stimulated by both LOX and COX products of AA; inhibition of only one or the other produces much less growth inhibition than inhibiting both routes simultaneously.[135]

From a therapeutic view, it seems reasonable to use COX and LOX inhibitors in chemopreventive or in adjuvant cancer therapies. Despite the evidence from epidemiological data demonstrating clear chemopreventive effects of NSAIDs, the long-term use of such pharmacologic agents is associated with substantial side-effects including gastric ulceration, perforation, and obstruction and have been linked to thousands of deaths per year.[136] This is where dietary modification and nutritional supplementation come into play. The goal here is to reset the balance of eicosanoids so as to inhibit tumorigenesis while leaving normal cells and developmental programs intact. The key here is to use inherent differences in metabolism of lipids and fatty acids between tumor and normal cells to achieve selective targeting.

With the exception of Inuit or Japanese following traditional diet and lifestyles patterns, most populations around the world consume ratios of n-6:n-3 fatty acids on the order of 10 to 20:1. While there is no definitive proof of the ideal ratio, the suggested ratio for optimal health is about 2 to 4:1. This is the ratio that would be consumed in a traditional Japanese diet (where total fat is low and total carbohydrate high) or Greenland Inuit diet (high in total fat, low in carbohydrate). Thus, most North Americans and many other populations around the world consume diets rich in n-6 fatty acids that will inevitably lead to higher membrane and tissue levels of LA, DGLA, and AA, relative to the levels of LNA, EPA, and DHA. In order to achieve this "ideal ratio," one would need to consume at least 2 to 3 fatty fish (herring, mackerel, salmon, trout, tuna) meals per week. While plant sources, such as canola and flax, do provide short-chain n-3 fatty acids, predominantly LNA, these are only very poorly converted to the longer chain PUFAs, EPA, and DHA in humans. The efficiency of conversion has been estimated to be between 1 and 5% in healthy tissues, and cancer cells are notoriously deficient in $\Delta 6$-desaturase compared to normal cells from the same tissue.[137–140] As a result, fish oil supplements appear to be the most effective way of getting additional long-chain PUFAs into the human diet. A variety of studies both *in vitro* and *in vivo* using fish oil supplements and purified EPA and DHA have demonstrated selective antitumor action. Supplementation with n-3 fatty acids has been shown to inhibit proliferation and invasion of various tumor cell lines, induce cell cycle arrest and/or apoptosis, and enhance response to cell differentiation agents.[141–147]

EPA and DHA compete with AA and DGLA for incorporation into membrane phospholipids (PLs). As one might expect, providing additional EPA and DHA in culture medium through dietary supplementation increases the relative concentrations of these fatty acids in specific PL classes. This occurs via direct competition for esterification, particularly at the *sn-2* position of PLs, where highly unsaturated fatty acids are the preferred substrates. As well, because EPA and DHA are more highly unsaturated than AA precursors, they bind with higher affinity to desaturase enzymes, thereby inhibiting *de novo* AA synthesis. Thus, upon appropriate stimulation of PLA_2, relative levels of EPA will be higher than AA and, thus, fewer AA fatty acids will be available for eicosanoid production. Not only are PGE_2, 5-HETE, and LTB_4 produced in lower amounts, but higher levels of EPA metabolites, which do not have cancer promoting activity, are created through LOX and COX activity. Interestingly, EPA and DHA seem to selectively inhibit COX-2 with little or no effect on COX-1.[148]

In addition to providing a reduction in inflammatory AA eicosanoids, supplementation with EPA and DHA also affect a number of other activities in cells in which they are incorporated. Human trials have shown that TNF-α and IL-1 synthesis are inhibited.[149] Activity of membrane receptors including those for insulin,[150] RANKL,[151] HER-2/neu,[152] nuclear PPARs, and mitochondrial activity[153] have all been shown to be influenced by EPA and/or DHA. As well, DHA appears to down-regulate the expression of inducible nitric oxide synthase in colon cancer cells, which indirectly leads to decreased COX-2 production and associated decreases in NFκB, interferons, cyclic GMP, and up-regulation of a number of cyclin-dependent kinase inhibitors, including p21 and p27.[154] All of these activities have been associated with reduced tumorigenesis, tumor cell arrest or apoptosis, and decreased tumor progression. As well, recent studies have suggested that liver and pancreatic function in postoperative cancer patients can be improved with n-3 supplementation.[155] The benefits of n-3 supplementation alone seem to be relatively limited, though. No "cures" have been demonstrated with this approach by itself and the levels of fatty acid needed to achieve many of the effects *in vitro* were in the high μM range, which is difficult to achieve through oral supplementation of patients. Where the n-3s are showing the greatest promise is in combination or adjuvant therapy settings, with surgery, radiation, and chemotherapy.

More than a decade ago, it was shown that supplementation of fibrosarcoma and murine leukemia cells with EPA and DHA increased the toxicity of nucleoside drugs and doxorubicin selectively in the tumor cells while leaving the normal cells unaffected or even protected.[141,142] This resulted in a substantial theoretical improvement in therapeutic index for arabinosylcytosine (araC) and doxorubicin. Later, we demonstrated that *in vivo* supplementation of rat or mouse diets with purified DHA decreased tumor burden (fibrosarcoma and leukemia) and enhanced the therapeutic activity of araC in these animals while simultaneously protecting bone marrow progenitors and gastrointestinal mucosa, two key sites of potential dose-limiting injury.[27,156,157] While we have been able to demonstrate altered nucleoside transport activity in a variety of cell types incubated with DHA and EPA,[158,159] we showed that at least part of the chemopotentiation by DHA was due to altered activity of enzymes involved in araC activation and degradation that was tumor-specific.[160] In our models, both *in vitro* and *in vivo*, adding vitamin E did not attenuate the beneficial effects of DHA on drug toxicity, suggesting that oxidant-stress *per se* was not critical; however, a study by Colas and coworkers[38] showed that α-tocopherol did suppress mammary tumor sensitivity to anthracyclines, so this possibility remains open.

In experimental breast cancer, long-chain n-3 PUFAs themselves have anti-angiogenic and antmetastatic activity, but tumor kill can synergistically be improved with several drugs, including mitomycin C, doxorubicin, and cyclo-phosphamide.[161,162] Importantly Colas showed that the effectiveness of the n-3 supplementation with doxorubicin in a breast cancer model was attenuated with α-tocopherol, suggesting that oxidant stress was part of the killing synergism.[38] Their studies had previously indicated that women with higher n-3 levels in breast adipose tissue fared better following chemotherapy to a variety of regimens than those with low n-3 status in breast adipose.[163] It is not clear from the human studies to date whether the antioxidant status of the patient is important during the adjuvant treatment with omega-3 supplements and any of the other drugs.

Colon cancer, despite its prevalence and the availability of tools that have generally aided in early detection and removal of preneoplastic polyps resulting in increased cure, remains one of the most difficult cancers to treat. Less than 25% of colon cancer patients treated with chemotherapy are responsive. The most efficacious therapy utilizes a combination of 5-fluorouracil with leucovorin rescue. Some recent successes have also been demonstrated with new therapeutic regimens utilizing two other classes of drugs, irinotecan/camptothecin, and oxaliplatin.[164,165] While not typically used in colon cancer therapy (Grem et al., 1995), araC and gemcitabine have recently been explored as antitumor agents in colon cancer cells.[166] We showed that the therapeutic index of araC could be improved 40-fold with supplementation of rat colon tumor cells while protecting normal colonic cells from toxicity.[167] Jordan and Stein demonstrated that a fish oil-based lipid emulsion, combined with 5-fluorouracil, promoted apoptosis and cell cycle arrest in Caco-2 human colon cancer cells as well.[168] Wynter et al. showed increased sensitivity of the MAC16 colon tumor in mice when EPA/DHA were given in combination with epothiline, gemcitabine, 5-fluorouracil, and cyclophosphamide.[169] As well as sarcomas, breast cancers, colon cancers, and some leukemias, DHA and EPA have also been tested and found effective as adjuvant agents in prostate cancer with celecoxib[170,171] and in cervical carcinoma.[172] A recent study using more than 30 different colon tumor cell lines identified a series of genes that identified tumor cells that were, or were not, responsive to 5-fluorouracil and/or camptothecin.[165] Signatures such as these may be useful in the future to predict which adjuvant therapy setting may provide the best outcome in specific clinical patients (see Chapters 2, 8, and 9).

4.6 OTHER FOODS, PHYTOCHEMICALS, AND SUPPLEMENTS USEFUL IN ADJUVANT CHEMOTHERAPY

Flaxseed, in addition to being a great source of LNA, is also one of the richest sources of the phytoestrogen secoisolariciresinol diglycoside (SDG), a plant lignan that can be metabolized by colonic bacteria to the mammalian lignans enterodiol and enterolactone. A related lignan to the one identified in flaxseed, 7-hydroxymatairesinol, is richly expressed in Norway spruce (*Picea abies*) and can also be metabolically converted to the mammalian lignan enterolactone. SDG itself antagonizes mammary tumor growth in nude mice, both for ER+ and ER- tumor types.[173] 7-hydroxymatairesinol also has activity against breast tumors in animal models, but has additional activity against prostate cancer as well.[174] When used in combination with Tamoxifen, even in the presence of high circulating 17-β-estradiol levels, flaxseed enhanced the antitumorigenic response by inhibiting tumor cell growth and promoting apoptosis.[175] This could have important implications for human breast cancer therapy where Tamoxifen is being used in treatment or chemoprevention. A recent placebo-controlled trial using 25 g/d flaxseed in patients with newly diagnosed breast cancer demonstrated that 4 weeks of treatment with the flaxseed muffin (between the confirmation biopsy and surgical resection of the tumor) significantly reduced Ki-67 labeling index, HER-2/neu expression, progesterone, and estrogen receptor levels, and increased apoptosis in tumor tissue.[80] It will be interesting to see if this approach results in long-term successful treatment outcomes and/or benefits those who go on for radiation or chemotherapy treatments.

Indole-3-carbinol has been shown to inhibit the hepatotoxicity of the tetrahydroisoquinoline alkyloid, trabectidin, without compromising the drug's mammary carcinoma killing ability in rats.[176] Maitake mushroom β-glucan was recently shown to enhance the *in vitro* activity of carmustine in drug-resistant prostate cancer cells;[177] human clinical trials using this preparation in hormone refractory prostate cancer are needed. Several studies have suggested utility of other natural medicines, including Rasayanas, which is a complex group of herbals used in Ayurveda traditional Indian medicine.[178] This complex formulation showed reduced leukopenia and enhanced bone marrow cellularity in cyclophosphamide-treated mice and enhanced NK activity following radiation therapy[179] and inhibited tumor growth and metastasis in melanoma and prostate cancer models.[180,181] There is a single report of reduced myelosuppression in a pilot study using human cancer patients receiving radiation or chemotherapy.[182]

In addition to certain supplementation conditions, there is evidence that dietary deficiency of some specific nutrients may actually improve therapy outcome. While this is generally not the case, a specific example where limiting nutrient availability may be helpful for cancer treatment is methionine restriction. A number of studies suggest that tumor cells are dependent on methionine, while normal cells can use homocysteine instead if provided (reviewed by Cellarier et al.[183]). Many tumor types including gliomas and melanomas appear to have low methionine synthase activity compared to normal surrounding tissue. This could result from enzymatic mutations or defects in the generation of cofactors B_{12} and folate for activity. Alternatively, methionine salvage for polyamine biosynthesis may be limiting because of deficiencies in methylthioadenosine phosphorylase, which seems typical of nonsmall-cell lung cancer, leukemia, glioma, rectal adenocarcinoma, and melanoma. Additionally, there is evidence that the requirement for methionine in tumor cells may simply be much higher than in normal cells because of increased rates of transmethylation. Capitalizing on these metabolic differences, some success has occurred in animal models combining methionine-deficient diets with methionine analogs, such as ethionine in prostate, glioma, and sarcoma.[183] Furthermore, because of the link between folate metabolism and methionine, deficiency combined with 5-fluorouracil treatment has synergistic antitumor activity in these same models. Benefits have also been observed with methionine deficiency in combination with doxorubicin, antimitotics (such as vincristine), with the alkylating agent carmustine and with cisplatin in human colon and breast cancer models.[184–188] Large-scale clinical trials are still lacking for these approaches, but are certainly worthy of additional study.

4.7 CONCLUSIONS

As the population continues to age and the numbers of individuals afflicted with cancer continues to climb over the next few decades, substantial new treatments will need to be available. While there have been considerable strides in the detection and treatment of some cancers, there continues to be a substantial problem of drug resistance and failure of therapies for a large portion of those with disease. Furthermore, incidence of secondary or recurrent malignancies continues to be a problem for those who survive their first diagnosis and go on to surgery, radiation, and/or chemotherapy. A large number of children and adults are currently using nutritional strategies to either decrease their risk of developing cancer or to improve their likelihood of cure. While there are still numerous unanswered questions regarding mechanisms, interactions with conventional drugs, and very few human clinical intervention trials, this "adjuvant" strategy is likely to be adopted and expanded over the next several years. Understanding the molecular targets of drugs and nutrients/phytochemicals should lead to improvements in cancer therapies, increased cure rates, and much more immediately, improved quality of life for cancer patients. The findings presented here are encouraging and give hope that together conventional practitioners and those that practice complementary and alternative medicine can cooperate to provide the best possible treatment options for their patients.

REFERENCES

1. Goodman GE, Thornquist MD, Balmes J, Cullen MR, Meyskens FL, Jr., Omenn GS, Valanis B, Williams JH Jr. The Beta-Carotene and Retinol Efficacy Trial: incidence of lung cancer and cardiovascular disease mortality during 6-year follow-up after stopping beta-carotene and retinol supplements. *J Natl Cancer Inst* 2004; 96(23): 1743–1750.
2. Albanes D, Heinonen OP, Huttunen JK, Taylor PR, Virtamo J, Edwards BK, Haapakoski J, Rautalahti M, Hartman AM, Palmgren J. Effects of alpha-tocopherol and beta-carotene supplements on cancer incidence in the Alpha-Tocopherol Beta-Carotene Cancer Prevention Study. *Am J Clin Nutr* 1995; 62(6 Suppl): 1427S–1430S.
3. Pisani P, Bray F, Parkin DM. Estimates of the world-wide prevalence of cancer for 25 sites in the adult population. *Int J Cancer* 2002; 97(1): 72–81.
4. Bray F, Sankila R, Ferlay J, Parkin DM. Estimates of cancer incidence and mortality in Europe in 1995. *Eur J Cancer* 2002; 38(1): 99–166.
5. Boon H, Stewart M, Kennard MA, Gray R, Sawka C, Brown JB, McWilliam C, Gavin A, Baron RA, Aaron D, Haines-Kamka T. Use of complementary/alternative medicine by breast cancer survivors in Ontario: prevalence and perceptions. *J Clin Oncol* 2000; 18(13): 2515–2521.
6. Salminen E, Bishop M, Poussa T, Drummond R, Salminen S. Dietary attitudes and changes as well as use of supplements and complementary therapies by Australian and Finnish women following the diagnosis of breast cancer. *Eur J Clin Nutr* 2004; 58(1): 137–144.

7. Kelly KM, Jacobson JS, Kennedy DD, Braudt SM, Mallick M, Weiner MA. Use of unconventional therapies by children with cancer at an urban medical center. *J Pediatr Hematol Oncol* 2000; 22(5): 412–416.

8. Jazieh AR, Kopp M, Foraida M, Ghouse M, Khalil M, Savidge M, Sethuraman G. The use of dietary supplements by veterans with cancer. *J Altern Complement Med* 2004; 10(3): 560–564.

9. Boon H, Westlake K, Stewart M, Gray R, Fleshner N, Gavin A, Brown JB, Goel V. Use of complementary/alternative medicine by men diagnosed with prostate cancer: prevalence and characteristics. *Urology* 2003; 62(5): 849–853.

10. Ockenga J, Valentini L. Review article: anorexia and cachexia in gastrointestinal cancer. *Aliment Pharmacol Ther* 2005; 22(7): 583–594.

11. Harvie MN, Campbell IT, Thatcher N, Baildam A. Changes in body composition in men and women with advanced nonsmall cell lung cancer (NSCLC) undergoing chemotherapy. *J Hum Nutr Diet* 2003; 16(5): 323–326.

12. Usharani K, Roy RK, Vijayalakshmi, Prakash J. Nutritional status of cancer patients given different treatment modalities. *Int J Food Sci Nutr* 2004; 55(5): 363–369.

13. Tisdale MJ. Molecular pathways leading to cancer cachexia. *Physiology* (Bethesda) 2005; 20: 340–348.

14. Yeh SS, Hafner A, Chang CK, Levine DM, Parker TS, Schuster MW. Risk factors relating blood markers of inflammation and nutritional status to survival in cachectic geriatric patients in a randomized clinical trial. *J Am Geriatr Soc* 2004; 52(10): 1708–1712.

15. Barber MD, Ross JA, Fearon KC. Cancer cachexia. *Surg Oncol* 1999; 8(3): 133–141.

16. Fearon KC, Von Meyenfeldt MF, Moses AG, Van Geenen R, Roy A, Gouma DJ, Giacosa A, Van Gossum A, Bauer J, Barber MD, Aaronson NK, Voss AC, Tisdale MJ. Effect of a protein and energy dense N-3 fatty acid enriched oral supplement on loss of weight and lean tissue in cancer cachexia: a randomised double blind trial. *Gut* 2003; 52(10): 1479–1486.

17. Isenring E, Capra S, Bauer J, Davies PS. The impact of nutrition support on body composition in cancer outpatients receiving radiotherapy. *Acta Diabetol* 2003; 40 Suppl 1: S162–S164.

18. Moses AW, Slater C, Preston T, Barber MD, Fearon KC. Reduced total energy expenditure and physical activity in cachectic patients with pancreatic cancer can be modulated by an energy and protein dense oral supplement enriched with n-3 fatty acids. *Br J Cancer* 2004; 90(5): 996–1002.

19. Bauer JD, Capra S. Nutrition intervention improves outcomes in patients with cancer cachexia receiving chemotherapy — a pilot study. *Support Care Cancer* 2005; 13(4): 270–274.

20. Lorite MJ, Cariuk P, Tisdale MJ. Induction of muscle protein degradation by a tumour factor. *Br J Cancer* 1997; 76(8): 1035–1040.

21. Smith HJ, Lorite MJ, Tisdale MJ. Effect of a cancer cachectic factor on protein synthesis/degradation in murine C2C12 myoblasts: modulation by eicosapentaenoic acid. *Cancer Res* 1999; 59(21): 5507–5513.

22. Smith HJ, Wyke SM, Tisdale MJ. Mechanism of the attenuation of proteolysis-inducing factor stimulated protein degradation in muscle by beta-hydroxy-beta-methylbutyrate. *Cancer Res* 2004; 64(23): 8731–8735.

23. Alexandre J, Gross-Goupil M, Falissard B, Nguyen ML, Gornet JM, Misset JL, Goldwasser F. Evaluation of the nutritional and inflammatory status in cancer patients for the risk assessment of severe haematological toxicity following chemotherapy. *Ann Oncol* 2003; 14(1): 36–41.

24. Ingenbleek Y, Carpentier YA. A prognostic inflammatory and nutritional index scoring critically ill patients *Int J Vitam Nutr Res* 1985; 55(1): 91–101.

25. Scully C, Epstein J, Sonis S. Oral mucositis: a challenging complication of radiotherapy, chemotherapy, and radiochemotherapy. Part 2: diagnosis and management of mucositis. *Head Neck* 2004; 26(1): 77–84.

26. Ruthig DJ, Meckling-Gill KA. Both (n-3) and (n-6) fatty acids stimulate wound healing in the rat intestinal epithelial cell line, IEC-6. *J Nutr* 1999; 129(10): 1791–1798.

27. Atkinson TG, Murray L, Berry DM, Ruthig DJ, Meckling-Gill KA. DHA feeding provides host protection and prevents fibrosarcoma-induced hyperlipidemia while maintaining the tumor response to araC in Fischer 344 rats. *Nutr Cancer* 1997; 28(3): 225–235.

28. Piccirillo N, De Matteis S, Laurenti L, Chiusolo P, Sora F, Pittiruti M, Rutella S, Cicconi S, Fiorini A, D'Onofrio G, Leone G, Sica S. Glutamine-enriched parenteral nutrition after autologous peripheral blood stem cell transplantation: effects on immune reconstitution and mucositis. *Haematologica* 2003; 88(2): 192–200.

29. Spielberger R, Stiff P, Bensinger W, Gentile T, Weisdorf D, Kewalramani T, Shea T, Yanovich S, Hansen K, Noga S, McCarty J, LeMaistre CF, Sung EC, Blazar BR, Elhardt D, Chen MG, Emmanouilides C. Palifermin for oral mucositis after intensive therapy for hematologic cancers. *N Engl J Med* 2004; 351(25): 2590–2598.

30. Brinckmann J, Sigwart H, van Houten TL. Safety and efficacy of a traditional herbal medicine (Throat Coat) in symptomatic temporary relief of pain in patients with acute pharyngitis: a multicenter, prospective, randomized, double-blinded, placebo-controlled study. *J Altern Complement Med* 2003; 9(2): 285–298.

31. Prasad KN, Kumar A, Kochupillai V, Cole WC. High doses of multiple antioxidant vitamins: essential ingredients in improving the efficacy of standard cancer therapy. *J Am Coll Nutr* 1999; 18(1): 13–25.

32. Lamson DW, Brignall MS. Antioxidants in cancer therapy; their actions and interactions with oncologic therapies. *Altern Med Rev* 1999; 4(5): 304–329.

33. Conklin KA. Dietary antioxidants during cancer chemotherapy: impact on chemotherapeutic effectiveness and development of side effects. *Nutr Cancer* 2000; 37(1): 1–18.

34. Kumar A, Qiblawi S, Khan AK, Banerjee S, Rao AR. Chemomodulatory action of Brassica compestris (var sarason) on hepatic carcinogen metabolizing enzymes, antioxidant profiles and lipid peroxidation. *Asian Pac J Cancer Prev* 2004; 5(2): 190–195.

35. Labriola D, Livingston R. Possible interactions between dietary antioxidants and chemotherapy. *Oncology* (Williston Park) 1999; 13(7): 1003–1008.

36. Kong Q, Lillehei KO. Antioxidant inhibitors for cancer therapy. *Med Hypotheses* 1998; 51(5): 405–409.

37. Salganik RI, Albright CD, Rodgers J, Kim J, Zeisel SH, Sivashinskiy MS, Van Dyke TA. Dietary antioxidant depletion: enhancement of tumor apoptosis and inhibition of brain tumor growth in transgenic mice. *Carcinogenesis* 2000; 21(5): 909–914.

38. Colas S, Germain E, Arab K, Maheo K, Goupille C, Bougnoux P. Alpha-tocopherol suppresses mammary tumor sensitivity to anthracyclines in fish oil-fed rats. *Nutr Cancer* 2005; 51(2): 178–183.

39. Saintot M, Mathieu-Daude H, Astre C, Grenier J, Simony-Lafontaine J, Gerber M. Oxidant-antioxidant status in relation to survival among breast cancer patients. *Int J Cancer* 2002; 97(5): 574–579.

40. Wagdi P, Fluri M, Aeschbacher B, Fikrle A, Meier B. Cardioprotection in patients undergoing chemo- and/or radiotherapy for neoplastic disease. A pilot study. *Jpn Heart J* 1996; 37(3): 353–359.

41. Wadleigh RG, Redman RS, Graham ML, Krasnow SH, Anderson A, Cohen MH. Vitamin E in the treatment of chemotherapy-induced mucositis. *Am J Med* 1992; 92(5): 481–484.

42. Chinery R, Brockman JA, Peeler MO, Shyr Y, Beauchamp RD, Coffey RJ. Antioxidants enhance the cytotoxicity of chemotherapeutic agents in colorectal cancer: a p53-independent induction of p21WAF1/CIP1 via C/EBPbeta. *Nat Med* 1997; 3(11): 1233–1241.

43. Norman HA, Butrum RR, Feldman E, Heber D, Nixon D, Picciano MF, Rivlin R, Simopoulos A, Wargovich MJ, Weisburger EK, Zeisel SH. The role of dietary supplements during cancer therapy. *J Nutr* 2003; 133(11 Suppl 1): 3794S–3799S.

44. Mayland CR, Bennett MI, Allan K. Vitamin C deficiency in cancer patients. *Palliat Med* 2005; 19(1): 17–20.

45. Kennedy DD, Tucker KL, Ladas ED, Rheingold SR, Blumberg J, Kelly KM. Low antioxidant vitamin intakes are associated with increases in adverse effects of chemotherapy in children with acute lymphoblastic leukemia. *Am J Clin Nutr* 2004; 79(6): 1029–1036.

46. Choi CH. ABC transporters as multidrug resistance mechanisms and the development of chemosensitizers for their reversal. *Cancer Cell Int* 2005; 5: 30.

47. Lautier D, Canitrot Y, Deeley RG, Cole SP. Multidrug resistance mediated by the multidrug resistance protein (MRP) gene. *Biochem Pharmacol* 1996; 52(7): 967–977.

48. Ballatori N, Hammond CL, Cunningham JB, Krance SM, Marchan R. Molecular mechanisms of reduced glutathione transport: role of the MRP/CFTR/ABCC and OATP/SLC21A families of membrane proteins. *Toxicol Appl Pharmacol* 2005; 204(3): 238–255.

49. Stride BD, Valdimarsson G, Gerlach JH, Wilson GM, Cole SP, Deeley RG. Structure and expression of the messenger RNA encoding the murine multidrug resistance protein, an ATP-binding cassette transporter. *Mol Pharmacol* 1996; 49(6): 962–971.

50. Mizutani T, Hattori A. New horizon of MDR1 (P-glycoprotein) study. *Drug Metab Rev* 2005; 37(3): 489–510.

51. Raaijmakers HG, Van Den BG, Boezeman J, De Witte T, Raymakers RA. Single-cell image analysis to assess ABC-transporter-mediated efflux in highly purified hematopoietic progenitors. *Cytometry* 2002; 49(4): 135–142.

52. Belpomme D, Gauthier S, Pujade-Lauraine E, Facchini T, Goudier MJ, Krakowski I, Netter-Pinon G, Frenay M, Gousset C, Marie FN, Benmiloud M, Sturtz F. Verapamil increases the survival of patients with anthracycline-resistant metastatic breast carcinoma. *Ann Oncol* 2000; 11(11): 1471–1476.

53. Leslie EM, Deeley RG, Cole SP. Bioflavonoid stimulation of glutathione transport by the 190-kDa multidrug resistance protein 1 (MRP1). *Drug Metab Dispos* 2003; 31(1): 11–15.

54. Leslie EM, Mao Q, Oleschuk CJ, Deeley RG, Cole SP. Modulation of multidrug resistance protein 1 (MRP1/ABCC1) transport and atpase activities by interaction with dietary flavonoids. *Mol Pharmacol* 2001; 59(5): 1171–1180.

55. Aggarwal BB, Kumar A, Bharti AC. Anticancer potential of curcumin: preclinical and clinical studies. *Anticancer Res* 2003; 23(1A): 363–398.

56. Garcea G, Jones DJ, Singh R, Dennison AR, Farmer PB, Sharma RA, Steward WP, Gescher AJ, Berry DP. Detection of curcumin and its metabolites in hepatic tissue and portal blood of patients following oral administration. *Br J Cancer* 2004; 90(5): 1011–1015.

57. Romiti N, Tongiani R, Cervelli F, Chieli E. Effects of curcumin on P-glycoprotein in primary cultures of rat hepatocytes. *Life Sci* 1998; 62(25): 2349–2358.

58. Anuchapreeda S, Leechanachai P, Smith MM, Ambudkar SV, Limtrakul PN. Modulation of P-glycoprotein expression and function by curcumin in multidrug-resistant human KB cells. *Biochem Pharmacol* 2002; 64(4): 573–582.

59. Jia WW, Bu X, Philips D, Yan H, Liu G, Chen X, Bush JA, Li G. Rh2, a compound extracted from ginseng, hypersensitizes multidrug-resistant tumor cells to chemotherapy. *Can J Physiol Pharmacol* 2004; 82(7): 431–437.

60. Kim SW, Kwon HY, Chi DW, Shim JH, Park JD, Lee YH, Pyo S, Rhee DK. Reversal of P-glycoprotein-mediated multidrug resistance by ginsenoside Rg(3). *Biochem Pharmacol* 2003; 65(1): 75–82.

61. Choi CH, Kang G, Min YD. Reversal of P-glycoprotein-mediated multidrug resistance by protopanaxatriol ginsenosides from Korean red ginseng. *Planta Med* 2003; 69(3): 235–240.

62. Sadzuka Y, Sugiyama T, Sonobe T. Efficacies of tea components on doxorubicin induced antitumor activity and reversal of multidrug resistance. *Toxicol Lett* 2000; 114(1-3): 155–162.

63. Jodoin J, Demeule M, Beliveau R. Inhibition of the multidrug resistance P-glycoprotein activity by green tea polyphenols. *Biochim Biophys Acta* 2002; 1542(1-3): 149–159.

64. Durr D, Stieger B, Kullak-Ublick GA, Rentsch KM, Steinert HC, Meier PJ, Fattinger K. St. John's wort induces intestinal P-glycoprotein/MDR1 and intestinal and hepatic CYP3A4. *Clin Pharmacol Ther* 2000; 68(6): 598–604.

65. Hennessy M, Kelleher D, Spiers JP, Barry M, Kavanagh P, Back D, Mulcahy F, Feely J. St. John's wort increases expression of P-glycoprotein: implications for drug interactions. *Br J Clin Pharmacol* 2002; 53(1): 75–82.

66. Perloff MD, von Moltke LL, Stormer E, Shader RI, Greenblatt DJ. St. John's wort: an *in vitro* analysis of P-glycoprotein induction due to extended exposure. *Br J Pharmacol* 2001; 134(8): 1601–1608.

67. Dorai T, Aggarwal BB. Role of chemopreventive agents in cancer therapy. *Cancer Lett* 2004; 215(2): 129–140.

68. Nakanishi C, Toi M. Nuclear factor-κB inhibitors as sensitizers to anticancer drugs. *Nat Rev Cancer* 2005; 5(4): 297–309.

69. Yuan H, Pan Y, Young CY. Overexpression of c-Jun induced by quercetin and resverol inhibits the expression and function of the androgen receptor in human prostate cancer cells. *Cancer Lett* 2004; 213(2): 155–163.
70. Kundu JK, Surh YJ. Molecular basis of chemoprevention by resveratrol: NF-κB and AP-1 as potential targets. *Mutat Res* 2004; 555(1-2): 65–80.
71. Min JK, Han KY, Kim EC, Kim YM, Lee SW, Kim OH, Kim KW, Gho YS, Kwon YG. Capsaicin inhibits *in vitro* and *in vivo* angiogenesis. *Cancer Res* 2004; 64(2): 644–651.
72. Oak MH, El Bedoui J, Schini-Kerth VB. Antiangiogenic properties of natural polyphenols from red wine and green tea. *J Nutr Biochem* 2005; 16(1): 18.
73. Korutla L, Cheung JY, Mendelsohn J, Kumar R. Inhibition of ligand-induced activation of epidermal growth factor receptor tyrosine phosphorylation by curcumin. *Carcinogenesis* 1995; 16(8): 1741–1745.
74. Aggarwal S, Ichikawa H, Takada Y, Sandur SK, Shishodia S, Aggarwal BB. Curcumin (diferuloylmethane) downregulates expression of cell proliferation, antiapoptotic and metastatic gene products through suppression of I{kappa}B{alpha} kinase and AKT activation. *Mol Pharmacol* Epub, October 11, 2005.
75. Vyas S, Asmerom Y, De Leon DD. Resveratrol regulates insulin-like growth factor-II in breast cancer cells. *Endocrinology* 2005; 146(10): 4224–4233.
76. Mousa AS, Mousa SA. Anti-angiogenesis efficacy of the garlic ingredient alliin and antioxidants: role of nitric oxide and p53. *Nutr Cancer* 2005; 53(1): 104–110.
77. Mousa SS, Mousa SS, Mousa SA. Effect of resveratrol on angiogenesis and platelet/fibrin-accelerated tumor growth in the chick chorioallantoic membrane model. *Nutr Cancer* 2005; 52(1): 59–65.
78. Singh RP, Tyagi AK, Dhanalakshmi S, Agarwal R, Agarwal C. Grape seed extract inhibits advanced human prostate tumor growth and angiogenesis and upregulates insulin-like growth factor binding protein-3. *Int J Cancer* 2004; 108(5): 733–740.
79. Hong RL, Spohn WH, Hung MC. Curcumin inhibits tyrosine kinase activity of p185neu and also depletes p185neu. *Clin Cancer Res* 1999; 5(7): 1884–1891.
80. Thompson LU, Chen JM, Li T, Strasser-Weippl K, Goss PE. Dietary flaxseed alters tumor biological markers in postmenopausal breast cancer. *Clin Cancer Res* 2005; 11(10): 3828–3835.
81. Kim HY, Park EJ, Joe EH, Jou I. Curcumin suppresses Janus kinase-STAT inflammatory signaling through activation of Src homology 2 domain-containing tyrosine phosphatase 2 in brain microglia. *J Immunol* 2003; 171(11): 6072–6079.
82. Labrecque L, Lamy S, Chapus A, Mihoubi S, Durocher Y, Cass B, Bojanowski MW, Gingras D, Beliveau R. Combined inhibition of PDGF and VEGF receptors by ellagic acid, a dietary-derived phenolic compound. *Carcinogenesis* 2005; 26(4): 821–826.
83. Wallace JM. Nutritional and botanical modulation of the inflammatory cascade — eicosanoids, cyclooxygenases, and lipoxygenases — as an adjunct in cancer therapy. *Integr Cancer Ther* 2002; 1(1): 737.
84. Dimberg J, Samuelsson A, Hugander A, Soderkvist P. Differential expression of cyclooxygenase 2 in human colorectal cancer. *Gut* 1999; 45(5): 730–732.
85. Sheng H, Shao J, Kirkland SC, Isakson P, Coffey RJ, Morrow J, Beauchamp RD, DuBois RN. Inhibition of human colon cancer cell growth by selective inhibition of cyclooxygenase-2. *J Clin Invest* 1997; 99(9): 2254–2259.

86. Masunaga R, Kohno H, Dhar DK, Ohno S, Shibakita M, Kinugasa S, Yoshimura H, Tachibana M, Kubota H, Nagasue N. Cyclooxygenase-2 expression correlates with tumor neovascularization and prognosis in human colorectal carcinoma patients. *Clin Cancer Res* 2000; 6(10): 4064–4068.
87. Sheehan KM, Sheahan K, O'Donoghue DP, MacSweeney F, Conroy RM, Fitzgerald DJ, Murray FE. The relationship between cyclooxygenase-2 expression and colorectal cancer. *JAMA* 1999; 282(13): 1254–1257.
88. Subbaramaiah K, Dannenberg AJ. Cyclooxygenase 2: a molecular target for cancer prevention and treatment. *Trends Pharmacol Sci* 2003; 24(2): 96–102.
89. Iniguez MA, Rodriguez A, Volpert OV, Fresno M, Redondo JM. Cyclooxygenase-2: a therapeutic target in angiogenesis. *Trends Mol Med* 2003; 9(2): 73–78.
90. Gately S. The contributions of cyclooxygenase-2 to tumor angiogenesis. *Cancer Metastasis Rev* 2000; 19(1-2): 19–27.
91. Leahy KM, Koki AT, Masferrer JL. Role of cyclooxygenases in angiogenesis. *Curr Med Chem* 2000; 7(11): 1163–1170.
92. Attiga FA, Fernandez PM, Weeraratna AT, Manyak MJ, Patierno SR. Inhibitors of prostaglandin synthesis inhibit human prostate tumor cell invasiveness and reduce the release of matrix metalloproteinases. *Cancer Res* 2000; 60(16): 4629–4637.
93. Ye F, Xui L, Yi J, Zhang W, Zhang DY. Anticancer activity of *Scutellaria baicalensis* and its potential mechanism. *J Altern Complement Med* 2002; 8(5): 567–572.
94. Roomi MW, Ivanov V, Kalinovsky T, Niedzwiecki A, Rath M. Antitumor effect of nutrient synergy on human osteosarcoma cells U-2OS, MNNG-HOS and Ewing's sarcoma SK-ES.1. *Oncol Rep* 2005; 13(2): 253–257.
95. Katz MS. Therapy insight: potential of statins for cancer chemoprevention and therapy. *Nat Clin Pract Oncol* 2005; 2(2): 82–89.
96. Duncan RE, el Sohemy A, Archer MC. Regulation of HMG-CoA reductase in MCF-7 cells by genistein, EPA, and DHA, alone and in combination with mevastatin. *Cancer Lett* 2005; 224(2): 221–228.
97. Riso S, Aluffi P, Brugnani M, Farinetti F, Pia F, D'Andrea F. Postoperative enteral immunonutrition in head and neck cancer patients. *Clin Nutr* 2000; 19(6): 407–412.
98. De Luis DA, Izaola O, Aller R, Cuellar L, Terroba MC. A randomized clinical trial with oral immunonutrition (omega3-enhanced formula vs. arginine-enhanced formula) in ambulatory head and neck cancer patients. *Ann Nutr Metab* 2005; 49(2): 95–99.
99 Di C, V, Gianotti L, Balzano G, Zerbi A, Braga M. Complications of pancreatic surgery and the role of perioperative nutrition. *Dig Surg* 1999; 16(4): 320–326.
100. Gianotti L, Braga M, Fortis C, Soldini L, Vignali A, Colombo S, Radaelli G, Di C, V. A prospective, randomized clinical trial on perioperative feeding with an arginine-, omega-3 fatty acid-, and RNA-enriched enteral diet: effect on host response and nutritional status. *JPEN J Parenter Enteral Nutr* 1999; 23(6): 314–320.
101. Coghlin Dickson TM, Wong RM, offrin RS, Shizuru JA, Johnston LJ, Hu WW, Blume KG, Stockerl-Goldstein KE. Effect of oral glutamine supplementation during bone marrow transplantation. *JPEN J Parenter Enteral Nutr* 2000; 24(2): 61–66.

102. Mantena SK, Meeran SM, Elmets CA, Katiyar SK. Orally administered green tea polyphenols prevent ultraviolet radiation-induced skin cancer in mice through activation of cytotoxic T cells and inhibition of angiogenesis in tumors. *J Nutr* 2005; 135(12): 2871–2877.

103. Mantena SK, Roy AM, Katiyar SK. Epigallocatechin-3-gallate inhibits photocarcinogenesis through inhibition of angiogenic factors and activation of CD8(+) T cells in tumors. *Photochem Photobiol* 2005; 81(5): 1174–1179.

104. Pryme IF, Bardocz S, Pusztai A, Ewen SW, Pfuller U. A mistletoe lectin (ML-1)-containing diet reduces the viability of a murine non-Hodgkin lymphoma tumor. *Cancer Detect Prev* 2004; 28(1): 52–56.

105. Baxevanis CN, Voutsas IF, Soler MH, Gritzapis AD, Tsitsilonis OE, Stoeva S, Voelter W, Arsenis P, Papamichail M. Mistletoe lectin I-induced effects on human cytotoxic lymphocytes. I. Synergism with IL-2 in the induction of enhanced LAK cytotoxicity. *Immunopharmacol Immunotoxicol* 1998; 20(3): 355–372.

106. Chang R. Bioactive polysaccharides from traditional Chinese medicine herbs as anticancer adjuvants. *J Altern Complement Med* 2002; 8(5): 559–565.

107. Cleary JA, Kelly GE, Husband AJ. The effect of molecular weight and beta-1,6-linkages on priming of macrophage function in mice by (1,3)-beta-D-glucan. *Immunol Cell Biol* 1999; 77(5): 395–403.

108. Ng ML, Yap AT. Inhibition of human colon carcinoma development by lentinan from shiitake mushrooms (*Lentinus edodes*). *J Altern Complement Med* 2002; 8(5): 581–589.

109. Wakui A, Kasai M, Konno K, Abe R, Kanamaru R, Takahashi K, Nakai Y, Yoshida Y, Koie H, Masuda H. Randomized study of lentinan on patients with advanced gastric and colorectal cancer. Tohoku Lentinan Study Group. *Gan To Kagaku Ryoho* 1986; 13(4 Pt 1): 1050–1059.

110. Nakazato H, Koike A, Saji S, Ogawa N, Sakamoto J. Efficacy of immunochemotherapy as adjuvant treatment after curative resection of gastric cancer. Study Group of Immunochemotherapy with PSK for Gastric Cancer. *Lancet* 1994; 343(8906): 1122–1126.

111. Ito K, Nakazato H, Koike A, Takagi H, Saji S, Baba S, Mai M, Sakamoto J, Ohashi Y. Long-term effect of 5-fluorouracil enhanced by intermittent administration of polysaccharide K after curative resection of colon cancer. A randomized controlled trial for 7-year follow-up. *Int J Colorectal Dis* 2004; 19(2): 157–164.

112. Mitomi T, Tsuchiya S, Iijima N, Aso K, Suzuki K, Nishiyama K, Amano T, Takahashi T, Murayama N, Oka H. Randomized, controlled study on adjuvant immunochemotherapy with PSK in curatively resected colorectal cancer. The Cooperative Study Group of Surgical Adjuvant Immunochemotherapy for Cancer of Colon and Rectum (Kanagawa). *Dis Colon Rectum* 1992; 35(2): 123–130.

113. Ogoshi K, Satou H, Isono K, Mitomi T, Endoh M, Sugita M. Immunotherapy for esophageal cancer. A randomized trial in combination with radiotherapy and radiochemotherapy. Cooperative Study Group for Esophageal Cancer in Japan. *Am J Clin Oncol* 1995; 18(3): 216–222.

114. Go P, Chung CH. Adjuvant PSK immunotherapy in patients with carcinoma of the nasopharynx. *J Int Med Res* 1989; 17(2): 141–149.

115. Hayakawa K, Mitsuhashi N, Saito Y, Takahashi M, Katano S, Shiojima K, Furuta M, Niibe H. Effect of krestin (PSK) as adjuvant treatment on the prognosis after radical radiotherapy in patients with non-small cell lung cancer. *Anticancer Res* 1993; 13(5C): 1815–1820.

116. Ohwada S, Ikeya T, Yokomori T, Kusaba T, Roppongi T, Takahashi T, Nakamura S, Kakinuma S, Iwazaki S, Ishikawa H, Kawate S, Nakajima T, Morishita Y. Adjuvant immunochemotherapy with oral Tegafur/Uracil plus PSK in patients with stage II or III colorectal cancer: a randomised controlled study. *Br J Cancer* 2004; 90(5): 1003–1010.

117. Takahashi Y, Mai M, Nakazato H. Preoperative CEA and PPD values as prognostic factors for immunochemotherapy using PSK and 5-FU. *Anticancer Res* 2005; 25(2B): 1377–1384.

118. Iino Y, Yokoe T, Maemura M, Takei H, Horiguchi J, Morishita Y. A new endocrine therapy strategy for bone metastasis of breast cancer: the effect of biological response modifiers and 22-oxacarcitriol on animal models. *Breast Cancer* 1997; 4(4): 311–313.

119. Aoyagi H, Iino Y, Takeo T, Horii Y, Morishita Y, Horiuchi R. Effects of OK-432 (picibanil) on the estrogen receptors of MCF-7 cells and potentiation of antiproliferative effects of tamoxifen in combination with OK-432. *Oncology* 1997; 54(5): 414–423.

120. Yokoe T, Iino Y, Takei H, Horiguchi J, Koibuchi Y, Maemura M, Ohwada S, Morishita Y. HLA antigen as predictive index for the outcome of breast cancer patients with adjuvant immunochemotherapy with PSK. *Anticancer Res* 1997; 17(4A): 2815–2818.

121. Kanazawa M, Yoshihara K, Abe H, Iwadate M, Watanabe K, Suzuki S, Endoh Y, Takita K, Sekikawa K, Takenoshita S, Ogata T, Ohto H. Effects of PSK on T and dendritic cells differentiation in gastric or colorectal cancer patients. *Anticancer Res* 2005; 25(1B): 443–449.

122. Jimenez E, Garcia-Lora A. Martinez M, Garrido F. Identification of the protein components of protein-bound polysaccharide (PSK) that interact with NKL cells. *Cancer Immunol Immunother* 2005; 54(4): 395–399.

123. Hsieh TC, Kunicki J, Darzynkiewicz Z, Wu JM. Effects of extracts of Coriolus versicolor (I'm-Yunity) on cell-cycle progression and expression of interleukins-1 beta,-6, and -8 in promyelocytic HL-60 leukemic cells and mitogenically stimulated and nonstimulated human lymphocytes. *J Altern Complement Med* 2002; 8(5): 591–602.

124. Bobrovnikova-Marjon EV, Marjon PL, Barbash O, Vander Jagt DL, Abcouwer SF. Expression of angiogenic factors vascular endothelial growth factor and interleukin-8/CXCL8 is highly responsive to ambient glutamine availability: role of nuclear factor-kappaB and activating protein-1. *Cancer Res* 2004; 64(14): 4858–4869.

125. Nakamura K, Kariyazono H, Komokata T, Hamada N, Sakata R, Yamada K. Influence of preoperative administration of omega-3 fatty acid-enriched supplement on inflammatory and immune responses in patients undergoing major surgery for cancer. *Nutrition* 2005; 21(6): 639–649.

126. Zimmer JS, Dyckes DF, Bernlohr DA, Murphy RC. Fatty acid binding proteins stabilize leukotriene A4: competition with arachidonic acid but not other lipoxygenase products. *J Lipid Res* 2004; 45(11): 2138–2144.

127. Kim JH, Hubbard NE, Ziboh V, Erickson KL. Attenuation of breast tumor cell growth by conjugated linoleic acid via inhibition of 5-lipoxygenase activating protein. *Biochim Biophys Acta* 2005; 1736(3): 244–250.

128. O'Flaherty JT, Rogers LC, Paumi CM, Hantgan RR, Thomas LR, Clay CE, High K, Chen YQ, Willingham MC, Smitherman PK, Kute TE, Rao A, Cramer SD, Morrow CS. 5-Oxo-ETE analogs and the proliferation of cancer cells. *Biochim Biophys Acta* 2005; 1736(3): 228–236.

129. Blomgren H, Kling-Andersson G. Growth inhibition of human malignant glioma cells *in vitro* by agents which interfere with biosynthesis of eicosanoids. *Anticancer Res* 1992; 12(3): 981–986.

130. Ghosh J, Myers CE. Central role of arachidonate 5-lipoxygenase in the regulation of cell growth and apoptosis in human prostate cancer cells. *Adv Exp Med Biol* 1999; 469: 577–582.

131. Gao X, Honn KV. Biological properties of 12(S)-HETE in cancer metastasis. Adv Prostaglandin Thromboxane. *Leukot Res* 1995; 23: 439–444.

132. Pidgeon GP, Tang K, Rice RL, Zacharek A, Li L, Taylor JD, Honn KV. Overexpression of leukocyte-type 12-lipoxygenase promotes W256 tumor cell survival by enhancing alphavbeta5 expression. *Int J Cancer* 2003; 105(4): 459–471.

133. Kandouz M, Nie D, Pidgeon GP, Krishnamoorthy S, Maddipati KR, Honn KV. Platelet-type 12-lipoxygenase activates NF-kappaB in prostate cancer cells. *Prostaglandins Other Lipid Mediat* 2003; 71(3-4): 189–204.

134. Szekeres CK, Trikha M, Honn KV. 12(S)-HETE, pleiotropic functions, multiple signaling pathways. *Adv Exp Med Biol* 2002; 507: 509–515.

135. Steele VE, Holmes CA, Hawk ET, Kopelovich L, Lubet RA, Crowell JA, Sigman CC, Kelloff GJ. Lipoxygenase inhibitors as potential cancer chemopreventives. *Cancer Epidemiol Biomarkers Prev* 1999; 8(5): 467–483.

136. Miller JL. Decisions loom on selective COX-2 inhibitors. *Am J Health Syst Pharm* 1999; 56(2): 106–107.

137. Young G, Conquer J. Omega-3 fatty acids and neuropsychiatric disorders. *Reprod Nutr Dev* 2005; 45(1): 1–28.

138. Marzo I, Pineiro A, Naval J. Loss of delta6-desaturase activity leads to impaired docosahexaenoic acid synthesis in Y-79 retinoblastoma cells. *Prostaglandins Leukot Essent Fatty Acids* 1998; 59(5): 293–297.

139. Marzo I, Martinez-Lorenzo MJ, Anel A, Desportes P, Alava MA, Naval J, Pineiro A. Biosynthesis of unsaturated fatty acids in the main cell lineages of human leukemia and lymphoma. *Biochim Biophys Acta* 1995; 1257(2): 140–148.

140. Lane J, Mansel RE, Jiang WG. Expression of human delta-6-desaturase is associated with aggressiveness of human breast cancer. *Int J Mol Med* 2003; 12(2): 253–257.

141. Atkinson TG, Meckling-Gill K.A. Regulation of nucleoside drug toxicity by transport inhibitors and omega-3 polyunsaturated fatty acids in mormal and transformed rat-2 fibroblasts. *Cell Pharmacol* 1995; 2: 259–264.

142. de Salis H, Meckling-Gill KA. EPA and DHA alter nucleoside drug and adriamycin toxicity in L1210 leukemia cells but not in normal bone marrow derived S1 macrophages. *Cell Pharmacol* 1995; 2: 69–74.

143. Rose DP, Connolly JM, Rayburn J, Coleman M. Influence of diets containing eicosapentaenoic or docosahexaenoic acid on growth and metastasis of breast cancer cells in nude mice. *J Natl Cancer Inst* 1995; 87(8): 587–592.

144. Brand A, Yavin E. Translocation of ethanolamine phosphoglyceride is required for initiation of apoptotic death in OLN-93 oligodendroglial cells. *Neurochem Res* 2005; 30(10): 1257–1267.

145. Kimura Y. New anticancer agents: *in vitro* and *in vivo* evaluation of the antitumor and antimetastatic actions of various compounds isolated from medicinal plants. *In Vivo* 2005; 19(1): 37–60.

146. Kimura Y, Sumiyoshi M. Antitumor and antimetastatic actions of eicosapentaenoic acid ethylester and its by-products formed during accelerated stability testing. *Cancer Sci* 2005; 96(7): 441–450.

147. Jia Y, Turek JJ. Inducible nitric oxide synthase links NF-kappaB to PGE2 in polyunsaturated fatty acid altered fibroblast *in vitro* wound healing. *Lipids Health Dis* 2005; 4: 14.

148. Singh J, Hamid R, Reddy BS. Dietary fat and colon cancer: modulation of cyclooxygenase-2 by types and amount of dietary fat during the post-initiation stage of colon carcinogenesis. *Cancer Res* 1997; 57(16): 3465–3470.

149. Endres S, von Schacky C. n-3 polyunsaturated fatty acids and human cytokine synthesis. *Curr Opin Lipidol* 1996; 7(1): 48–52.

150. Lardinois CK. The role of omega 3 fatty acids on insulin secretion and insulin sensitivity. *Med Hypotheses* 1987; 24(3): 243–248.

151. Bhattacharya A, Rahman M, Banu J, Lawrence RA, McGuff HS, Garrett IR, Fischbach M, Fernandes G. Inhibition of osteoporosis in autoimmune disease prone MRL/Mpj-Fas(lpr) mice by N-3 fatty acids. *J Am Coll Nutr* 2005; 24(3) 200–209.

152. Menendez JA, Lupu R, Colomer R. Exogenous supplementation with omega-3 polyunsaturated fatty acid docosahexaenoic acid (DHA; 22:6n-3) synergistically enhances taxane cytotoxicity and downregulates Her-2/neu (c-erbB-2) oncogene expression in human breast cancer cells. *Eur J Cancer Prev* 2005; 14(3): 263–270.

153. Guo W, Xie W, Lei T, Hamilton JA. Eicosapentaenoic acid, but not oleic acid, stimulates beta-oxidation in adipocytes. *Lipids* 2005; 40(8): 815–821.

154. Narayanan BA, Narayanan NK, Reddy BS. Docosahexaenoic acid regulated genes and transcription factors inducing apoptosis in human colon cancer cells. *Int J Oncol* 2001; 19(6): 1255–1262.

155. Heller AR, Rossel T, Gottschlich B, Tiebel O, Menschikowski M, Litz RJ, Zimmermann T, Koch T. Omega-3 fatty acids improve liver and pancreas function in postoperative cancer patients. *Int J Cancer* 2004; 111(4): 611–616.

156. Atkinson TG, Barker HJ, Meckling-Gill KA. Incorporation of long-chain n-3 fatty acids in tissues and enhanced bone marrow cellularity with docosahexaenoic acid feeding in post-weanling Fischer 344 rats. *Lipids* 1997; 32(3): 293–302.

157. Cha MC, Meckling KA, Stewart C. Dietary docosahexaenoic acid levels influence the outcome of arabinosylcytosine chemotherapy in l1210 leukemic mice. *Nutr Cancer* 2002; 44(2): 176–181.

158. Blackmore VL, Meckling-Gill KA. Fish oil and oleic acid-rich oil feeding alter nucleoside uptake in human erythrocytes. *Nutritional Biochemistry* 1995; 6: 438–444.

159. Martin D, Meckling-Gill KA. Omega-3 polyunsaturated fatty acids increase purine but not pyrimidine transport in L1210 leukaemia cells. *Biochem J* 1996; 315 (Pt 1): 329–333.

160. Cha MC, Meckling-Gill KA. Modifications of deoxycytidine kinase and deaminase activities by docosahexaenoic acid in normal and transformed rat fibroblasts. *Biochem Pharmacol* 2002; 63(4): 717–723.

161. Rose DP, Connolly JM. Regulation of tumor angiogenesis by dietary fatty acids and eicosanoids. *Nutr Cancer* 2000; 37(2): 119–127.

162. Hardman WE. (n-3) fatty acids and cancer therapy. *J Nutr* 2004; 134(12 Suppl): 3427S–3430S.

163. Bougnoux P, Germain E, Chajes V, Hubert B, Lhuillery C, Le Floch O, Body G, Calais G. Cytotoxic drugs efficacy correlates with adipose tissue docosahexaenoic acid level in locally advanced breast carcinoma. *Br J Cancer* 1999; 79(11-12): 1765–1769.

164. Martin MJ. Current stage-specific chemotherapeutic options in colon cancer. *Expert Rev Anticancer Ther* 2005; 5(4): 695–704.

165. Mariadason JM, Arango D, Shi Q, Wilson AJ, Corner GA, Nicholas C, Aranes MJ, Lesser M, Schwartz EL, Augenlicht LH. Gene expression profiling-based prediction of response of colon carcinoma cells to 5-fluorouracil and camptothecin. *Cancer Res* 2003; 63(24): 8791–8812.

166. Grem JL, Geoffroy F, Politi PM, Cuddy DP, Ross DD, Nguyen D, Steinberg SM, Allegra CJ. Determinants of sensitivity to 1-beta-D-arabinofuranosylcytosine in HCT 116 and NCI-H630 human colon carcinoma cells. *Mol Pharmacol* 1995; 48(2): 305–315.

167. Cha MC, Lin A, Meckling KA. Low dose docosahexaenoic acid protects normal colonic epithelial cells from araC toxicity. *BMC Pharmacol* 2005; 5(1): 7.

168. Jordan A, Stein J. Effect of an omega-3 fatty acid containing lipid emulsion alone and in combination with 5-fluorouracil (5-FU) on growth of the colon cancer cell line Caco-2. *Eur J Nutr* 2003; 42(6): 324–331.

169. Wynter MP, Russell ST, Tisdale MJ. Effect of n-3 fatty acids on the antitumour effects of cytotoxic drugs. *In Vivo* 2004; 18(5): 543–547.

170. Narayanan BA, Narayanan NK, Pttman B, Reddy BS. Adenocarcina of the mouse prostate growth inhibition by celecoxib: downregulation of transcription factors involved in COX-2 inhibition. *Prostate* 2006; 66: 257–265.

171. Narayanan NK, Narayanan BA, Reddy BS. A combination of docosahexaenoic acid and celecoxib prevents prostate cancer cell growth *in vitro* and is associated with modulation of nuclear factor-kappaB, and steroid hormone receptors. *Int J Oncol* 2005; 26(3): 785–792.

172. Madhavi N, Das UN, Prabha PS, Kumar GS, Koratkar R, Sagar PS. Suppression of human T-cell growth *in vitro* by cis-unsaturated fatty acids: relationship to free radicals and lipid peroxidation. *Prostaglandins Leukot Essent Fatty Acids* 1994; 51(1): 33–40.

173. Dabrosin C, Chen J, Wang L, Thompson LU. Flaxseed inhibits metastasis and decreases extracellular vascular endothelial growth factor in human breast cancer xenografts. *Cancer Lett* 2002; 185(1): 31–37.

174. Bylund A, Saarinen N, Zhang JX, Bergh A, Widmark A, Johansson A, Lundin E, Adlercreutz H, Hallmans G, Stattin P, Makela S. Anticancer effects of a plant lignan 7-hydroxymatairesinol on a prostate cancer model *in vivo*. *Exp Biol Med* (Maywood) 2005; 230(3): 217–223.

175. Chen J, Hui E, Ip T, Thompson LU. Dietary flaxseed enhances the inhibitory effect of tamoxifen on the growth of estrogen-dependent human breast cancer (mcf-7) in nude mice. *Clin Cancer Res* 2004; 10(22): 7703–7711.

176. Donald S, Verschoyle RD, Greaves P, Colombo T, Zucchetti M, Falcioni C, Zaffaroni M, D'Incalci M, Manson MM, Jimeno J, Steward WP, Gescher AJ. Dietary agent indole-3-carbinol protects female rats against the hepatotoxicity of the antitumor drug ET-743 (trabectidin) without compromising efficacy in a rat mammary carcinoma. *Int J Cancer* 2004; 111(6): 961–967.

177. Finkelstein MP, Aynehchi S, Samadi AA, Drinis S, Choudhury MS, Tazaki H, Konno S. Chemosensitization of carmustine with maitake beta-glucan on androgen-independent prostatic cancer cells: involvement of glyoxalase I. *J Altern Complement Med* 2002; 8(5): 573–580.

178. Vayalil PK, Kuttan G, Kuttan R. Protective effects of Rasayanas on cyclophosphamide- and radiation-induced damage. *J Altern Complement Med* 2002; 8(6): 787–796.

179. Kumar P, Kuttan R, Kuttan G. Radioprotective effects of Rasayanas. *Indian J Exp Biol* 1996; 34(9): 848–850.

180. Menon LG, Kuttan R, Kuttan G. Effect of rasayanas in the inhibition of lung metastasis induced by B16F-10 melanoma cells. *J Exp Clin Cancer Res* 1997; 16(4): 365–368.

181. Gaddipati JP, Rajeshkumar NV, Thangapazham RL, Sharma A, Warren J, Mog SR, Singh AK, Maheshwari RK. Protective effect of a polyherbal preparation, Brahma rasayana against tumor growth and lung metastasis in rat prostate model system. *J Exp Ther Oncol* 2004; 4(3): 203–212.

182. Joseph CD, Praveenkumar V, Kuttan G, Kuttan R. Myeloprotective effect of a non-toxic indigenous preparation Rasayana in cancer patients receiving chemotherapy and radiation therapy. A pilot study. *J Exp Clin Cancer Res* 1999; 18(3): 325–329.

183. Cellarier E, Durando X, Vasson MP, Farges MC, Demiden A, Maurizis JC, Madelmont JC, Chollet P. Methionine dependency and cancer treatment. *Cancer Treat Rev* 2003; 29(6): 489–499.

184. Stern PH, Hoffman RM. Enhanced *in vitro* selective toxicity of chemotherapeutic agents for human cancer cells based on a metabolic defect. *J Natl Cancer Inst* 1986; 76(4): 629–639.

185. Poirson-Bichat F, Goncalves RA, Miccoli L, Dutrillaux B, Poupon MF. Methionine depletion enhances the antitumoral efficacy of cytotoxic agents in drug-resistant human tumor xenografts. *Clin Cancer Res* 2000; 6(2): 643–653.

186. Kokkinakis DM, Hoffman RM, Frenkel EP, Wick JB, Han Q, Xu M, Tan Y, Schold SC. Synergy between methionine stress and chemotherapy in the treatment of brain tumor xenografts in athymic mice. *Cancer Res* 2001; 61(10): 4017–4023.

187. Tan Y, Sun X, Xu M, Tan X, Sasson A, Rashidi B, Han Q, Tan X, Wang X, An Z, Sun FX, Hoffman RM. Efficacy of recombinant methioninase in combination with cisplatin on human colon tumors in nude mice. *Clin Cancer Res* 1999; 5(8): 2157–2163.

188. Hoshiya Y, Kubota T, Matsuzaki SW, Kitajima M, Hoffman RM. Methionine starvation modulates the efficacy of cisplatin on human breast cancer in nude mice. *Anticancer Res* 1996; 16(6B): 3515–3517.

5 Role of Nutritional Antioxidants in the Prevention and Treatment of Neurodegenerative Disorders

Ennio Esposito

CONTENTS

Keywords: Neurodegeneration, Alzheimer's disease, Parkinson's disease, amyotrophic lateral sclerosis, oxidative stress, nuclear factor κB, antioxidants, polyphenols, neuroprotection, nutritional.

5.1 INTRODUCTION

There is an increasing attention toward the role played by certain nutritional components found in foods, including dietary flavonoids, in fruit, vegetables and beverages in the prevention of age-related decreases in cognitive, memory and learning tasks. Thus, aging is a major risk factor for neurodegenerative diseases including Alzheimer's disease (AD), Parkinson's disease (PD), and amyotrophic lateral sclerosis (ALS). An unbalanced overproduction of reactive oxygen species (ROS) may give rise to oxidative stress, which can induce neuronal damage, ultimately leading to neuronal death by apoptosis or necrosis. A large body of evidence indicates that oxidative stress is involved in the pathogenesis of AD, PD and ALS. An increasing number of studies show that nutritional antioxidants (especially vitamin E and polyphenols) can block neuronal death *in vitro*, and may have therapeutic properties in animal models of neurodegenerative diseases including AD, PD and ALS. Moreover, clinical data suggest that nutritional antioxidants might exert some protective effect against AD, PD and ALS. In this chapter, the biochemical mechanisms by which nutritional antioxidants can reduce or block neuronal death occurring in neurodegenerative disorders are reviewed. Particular emphasis will be given to the role played by the nuclear transcription factor-κB (NFκB) in apoptosis, and in the pathogenesis of neurodegenerative disorders, such as AD, PD and ALS. The effects of ROS and antioxidants on NFκB function and their relevance in the pathophysiology of neurodegenerative diseases will also be examined.

5.1.1 MAJOR NEURODEGENERATIVE DISORDERS

Neurodegenerative disorders, such as AD, PD and ALS, are among the most common neurological diseases. As the population of elderly increases, the prevalence of these age-related diseases is likely to increase. Thus, of the few risk factors that have been identified for these diseases, increasing age is the only one that is common to AD, PD and ALS. For AD, the incidence and prevalence of the disease increase dramatically after age 60; one study showed a 47% prevalence for patients over age 85.[1] Alzheimer's disease currently affects almost 2% of the population in industrialized countries,[2] and it is predicted that the incidence of AD will increase three-fold within the next 5 decades.[2] The causes of AD, PD and ALS are not known and, with the possible exception of PD, there is no treatment that alters significantly the progression of any of these disorders. Although the vast majority of these neurodegenerative disorders are sporadic, genetic and environmental factors can determine the individual risk for them.[2] For example, a low calorie diet decreases the risk of major neurodegenerative disorders including AD and PD,[3] and there is evidence that suppression of oxidative stress is one mechanism by which dietary restriction protects neurons.[4] However, aging appears to be the single most important factor in the occurrence of AD, PD and ALS.[1] In addition to their possible involvement in aging, mitochondrial dysfunction and oxidative damage may play important roles in the slowly progressive neuronal death that is characteristic of several different neurodegenerative disorders including AD, PD and ALS.[5–9]

5.1.2 OXIDATIVE STRESS AND ANTIOXIDANTS

There is substantial evidence that the brain, which consumes large amounts of oxygen, is particularly vulnerable to oxidative damage. Free radicals are normal products of cellular metabolism.[10] The predominant cellular free radicals are the superoxide (O_2^-) and hydroxyl ($OH\cdot$) species.[6,11] Other molecules, such as hydrogen peroxide (H_2O_2) and peroxynitrite ($ONOO^-$), although not themselves free radicals, can lead to the generation of free radicals through various chemical reactions. Thus, H_2O_2, in the presence of reduced metal, forms the highly reactive $OH\cdot$ via the Fenton reaction.[11] Peroxynitrite ($ONOO^-$), formed by the reaction of nitric oxide ($NO\cdot$) with O_2^-, is a highly reactive molecule that also breaks down to form $OH\cdot$. Together, these molecules are referred to as reactive oxygen species (ROS) to signify their ability to lead to oxidative changes within the cell.[11,12] Problems occur when the production of ROS exceeds the ability of cells to defend themselves against these substances. This imbalance between cellular production of ROS and the ability of cells to defend themselves against ROS is referred to as oxidative stress.[11] Oxidative stress can cause cellular damage and ROS oxidize critical cellular components such as membrane lipids, proteins and DNA, thereby inducing apoptosis or necrosis.[13–17] Necrosis is characterized by a loss of plasma membrane integrity, the formation of large vacuoles and cell swelling, whereas typical features of apoptotic cells are nuclear changes that include chromatin margination and condensation, DNA fragmentation, membrane blebbing and cell shrinkage.[18] There is large scientific literature regarding the relation between ROS production, the induction of apoptosis (or necrosis) and the pathogenesis of neurodegenerative disorders.[12,18–26] Although this subject is still a matter of debate, increasing evidence supports the hypothesis that neuronal death may occur primarily by apoptotic mechanisms in AD, PD and ALS.[27–31] Therefore, clinical evidence shows signs of apoptosis in patients with AD, PD and ALS.[30–33]

Cells normally have a number of mechanisms to resist against damage induced by free radicals.[10] The major antioxidant defenses consist of antioxidant scavengers, such as glutathione (GSH), vitamin C (ascorbic acid), vitamin E (α-tocopherol), carotenoids, polyphenols, flavonoids and antioxidant enzymes. Severe depletion of GSH in mice by administration of buthionine sulphoximine, which inhibits GSH synthesis, causes neuronal damage and mitochondrial degeneration.[13] There is a high concentration of ascorbic acid in the gray and white matter of the central nervous system in all species that have been examined.[34] Indeed, the brain, spinal cord and adrenal glands have the highest ascorbate concentrations of all the tissues in the body.[34] Ascorbate is a broad-spectrum radical scavenger that is effective against peroxyl and hydroxyl radicals, super-oxide, singlet oxygen and peroxynitrite.[34] Also, the lipid-soluble, chain-breaking antioxidant vitamin E exerts a very important protective function against oxidative stress in the brain[10] and interacts with ascorbate enhancing its antioxidant activity.[35] Little information is available on the levels of carotenoids and flavonoids in the human brain. The antioxidant enzymes in the brain include Cu/Zn super-oxide dismutase (SOD-1) and Mn superoxide dismutase (SOD-2), which catalyze the conversion of O_2^- to H_2O_2.[36] H_2O_2 is then converted to H_2O by either catalase or glutathione peroxidase (GSH-Px). Antioxidant defense mechanisms can be upregulated in response to increased ROS or peroxide production.[37] Although upregulating antioxidant defense systems may confer protection against ROS, they are not completely effective in preventing oxidative damage. Moreover, the efficiency of gene expression may decline with age or become defective as oxidative damage to the genome increases.

As already mentioned, the brain is especially vulnerable to ROS damage because of its high oxygen consumption rate, abundant lipid content and relative paucity of antioxidant enzymes compared with other organs.[38] If the increased demand on the cell's capacity to detoxify ROS is not met, alterations, such as aldehydes or isoprostanes from lipid peroxidation, protein carbonyls from protein oxidation, and oxidized base adducts from DNA oxidation may accumulate.[10] Oxidation of polyunsaturated fatty acids (PUFA) results in the production of multiple aldehydes with different carbon chain lengths including propanal, buta-nal, pentanal, hexanal and 4-hydroxy-2-*trans*-nonenal (4-HNE). There is evidence that 4-HNE is capable of inducing apoptosis in PC12 cells and cultured rat hippocampal neurons, suggesting that it is a mediator of oxidative stress-induced apoptosis.[39] These findings suggest that in addition to direct ROS damage to phospholipid membranes, there is an indirect mechanism involving 4-HNE, which may also be involved in neuronal death. In this regard, it noteworthy that 4-HNE has been suggested to be involved in the pathogenesis of PD.[40,41] Oxidative damage to proteins can be revealed by measuring protein carbonyl content,[42] which was found to be elevated in AD and ALS patients.[43] Another indication of protein oxidation is the formation of nitrotyrosine by peroxynitrite. This might represent a useful clinical parameter of the occurrence of oxidative stress in neurodegenerative diseases, inasmuch as increased levels of nitrotyrosine have been found in AD, PD and ALS.[21,44–49] The most useful marker of DNA oxidation is 8-hydroxy-2'-deoxyguanosine (8-OHdG), which is elevated in patients with AD, PD and ALS.[50–54]

Another index of oxidative is the activation of the transcription factor NFκB (nuclear factor kappa B). Thus, a large body of evidence indicates that ROS can act as second messengers mediating intracellular responses, including NFκB activation.[55–59] In turn, activated NFκB can influence the expression of a large number of genes, including SOD-2.[55,58,60] Hence, NFκB activation can be con-sidered as the executive branch of a feed-back mechanism that operates to regulate the intracellular concentration of ROS, trying to dampen an excessive accumu-lation of ROS, which can be dangerous for the cell. Moreover, NFκB induces the expression of the so-called IAPs (inhibitor of apoptosis proteins), Bcl-2, and calbindins.[60,61] All these biochemical actions of NFκB indicate that this transcription factor can exert an antiapoptotic effect, thereby protecting neurons against degeneration.[58,60] As we will discuss below, these data are consistent with clinical findings showing increased levels of NFκB in vulnerable regions of the central nervous system of AD, PD and ALS.[62-64]

5.1.3 EPIDEMIOLOGICAL STUDIES

Although the available data are still limited, epidemiological studies indicate that dietary habits can influence the incidence of neurodegenerative disorders, such as dementia (including AD) and PD.[65-69] For example, incidence data from the so-called PAQUID (Personnes Agees Quid) study showed that people drinking three to four glasses of wine per day had an 80% decreased incidence of dementia and AD 3 years later, compared to those who drank less or did not drink at all.[67,68,70] This protective effect was still highly significant after adjusting the data for potential confounding factors such as age, sex, education, occupation and baseline MMSE (Mini-Mental State Examination). However, in another study, moderate wine consumption was found to be associated with a fourfold reduction of the risk for AD, but this effect disappeared when institutionalization was taken into account.[71] These protective effects are most likely due to the presence of antioxidants in food and beverages,[65,68] inasmuch as it has been found that wine drinking and the consumption of other foods and drinks, which are rich in polyphenols, can increase the antioxidant activity in serum.[72-74] More recently, investigators in the Rotterdam Study[75] reported that any form of moderate alcohol would have the same beneficial effects. The risk reduction associated with alcohol is possibly related to its antioxidant properties or its effects on lipid metabolism.

Some observational studies have found a beneficial effect on the risk of dementia associated with vitamin supplements intake, although this effect has been observed with vitamin C alone in two studies[76,77] and only with combination of vitamin E and C in another.[78] Subsequently, other researchers failed to find such an association between vitamin supplement intake and incident AD, but they have demonstrated a decreased risk of incident AD among subjects with high dietary intake of vitamins, particularly vitamin E.[79,80] However, Varner[81] suggested a different interpretation for the inverse relationship between intake of vitamin E from food (not supplements) with the risk of AD; the predominant form of vitamin E, γ-tocopherol, but not the form found in supplements, α-tocopherol, has been shown to inhibit cyclooxygenase 2 (COX-2) production of prostaglandin E_2 in macrophage and epithelial cells.[82] Indeed, long-term use of nonsteroidal antiinflammatory drugs and COX-2 inhibition may protect against AD.[83] Moreover, commenting on a paper of Engelhart et al.,[79] Brenner[84] proposed that silicon might be the dietary element responsible for the positive effect of vitamin E-rich foods on the risk for AD. Thus, plant-based foods (e.g., grains and cereal products, which have high levels of vitamin E) are also the major dietary sources of silicon,[85] which could be associated with reduction in development of AD. Asian Indians have much higher silicon intakes than do Western populations because of higher intakes of plant-based foods[86] and it may be significant that Indians have among the lowest rates of AD.[87] More recently, it was found that subjects with low plasma vitamin E concentrations are at higher risk of developing a dementia in subsequent years.[88] However, this is a very controversial issue in that data obtained from the Honolulu–Asia Aging Study, a prospective community-based study of Japanese-American men who were age 45 to 68 in 1965 to1968, show that midlife dietary intake of antioxidants does not modify the risk of late-life dementia or its most prevalent subtypes.[89] Thus, intake of β-carotene, vitamin C and flavonoids was not associated with the risk of dementia and its subtypes either at 6 years or at 26 years of follow-up.[89,90]

Epidemiological studies have also found an inverse association between high intake of dietary vitamin E (but not flavonoids or vitamin C) and the occurrence of PD.[69,91] However, these data were not confirmed by other studies,[66,92] although Hellenbrand et al.[66] reported a significant statistical trend toward a protective effect of vitamin C in PD. Individuals over the age of 65 that had higher levels of β-carotene performed better on learning and memory tests compared with individuals with low β-carotene levels.[93] Lycopene is a carotenoid that has been suggested to protect against heart disease, stroke and certain cancers.[94,95] Lycopene can protect cultured hippocampal neurons against amyloid-beta (Aβ) and glutamate toxicity.[3] Uric acid is markedly effective in protecting cultured neurons against insults relevant to AD and PD, including exposure to Aβ and iron.[96,97] The clinical findings indicating a protective effect of dietary flavonoids against neurodegenerative disease are supported by data obtained in laboratory animals showing that a diet supplemented with fruits and vegetables rich in antioxidants (blueberries, strawberries and spinach) can have beneficial effects on age-related decline of neuronal and cognitive function in old rats.[98]

This chapter will focus on the actions of *in vitro* application of natural nutritional antioxidants in experimental models of neurodegenerative disorders. The capability of these compounds to counteract the damaging effects of ROS, and the relevance of this biochemical effect in their putative neuroprotective action will be examined. Among the numerous biochemical effects of ROS and antioxidants, particular emphasis will be given to their interference with NFκB function, whose role in the pathophysiology of neurodegenerative disorders is gaining increasing attention. Moreover, the effects of the administration of "pharmacological" doses of nutritional antioxidants in animal models and in patients with AD, PD and ALS will be reviewed. Finally, a detailed analysis on the role of dietary intake of polyphenols and other antioxidant vitamins in the prevention of AD and PD will be carried out.

5.2 NATURAL DIETARY ANTIOXIDANTS

Natural dietary antioxidants include vitamins A, C and E, carotenoids, polyphenols and flavonoids.· Vitamin C (ascorbate) and vitamin E (α-tocopherol) are absorbed from the gut. Ascorbate is rapidly distributed to all tissues, whereas α-tocopherol is incorporated into lipoproteins in the liver and is then secreted together into plasma.[13] Ascorbate can scavenge many reactive species including $O_2^{-\cdot}$, OH· and lipid hydroperoxides,[34] and may stabilize catecholamines from forming ROS. α-tocopherol is a powerful chain-breaking antioxidant that inhibits lipid peroxidation.[35] Carotenoids can scavenge singlet oxygen and a range of other ROS *in vitro*, but there is still little evidence that they contribute significantly to the antioxidant defense system in the central nervous system.[13] Several thousand molecules having a polyphenolic structure (i.e., several hydroxyl groups on aromatic rings) have been identified in higher plants and are generally involved in defense against ultraviolet radiation or aggression by pathogens.[99] These compounds may be classified into different groups as a function of the number of phenolic rings that they contain and of the structural elements that bind these rings to one another (Figure 5.1). Distinctions, thus, are made between the phenolic acids, flavonoids, stilbenes and lignans (Figure 5.1). The flavonoids, which share a common structure consisting of two aromatic rings (A and B), are bound together by three carbon atoms that form an oxygenated heterocycle (ring C) (Figure 5.2). Thus, the flavonoids belong to a group of natural substances with variable phenolic structures and are found in fruit, vegetables, grains, flowers, tea and wine.[100] More than 4000 varieties of flavonoids have been identified, many of which are responsible for the attractive colors of flowers, fruits and leaves.[70] Flavonoids represent the single most widely occurring group of phenolic phytochemicals.[101] They can be divided into various classes on the basis of their molecular structure. The six main groups of flavonoids are:

1. Flavones
2. Flavanones
3. Isoflavones
4. Flavonols
5. Catechins
6. Anthocyanins

The flavones are characterized by a planar structure because of a double bond in the central ring. One of the best described flavonoids, quercetin, is a member of this group. Quercetin is found in abundance in onions, apples, broccoli and berries. The second group is the flavanones, mainly found in citrus fruit. Flavonoids belonging to the catechins are mainly found in green and black tea and in red wine, whereas anthocyanins are found in strawberries and other berries, grapes, wine and tea.[70] Another phenolic antioxidant is curcumin, a yellow curry spice derived from turmeric, which is used as a food preservative and herbal medicine in India. Most flavonoids are glycosylated in their natural dietary forms with the exception of the catechins.[101] Generally, flavonoids may undergo three forms of intracellular metabolism: (1) conjugation with thiols, particularly GSH; (2) oxidative metabolism; and (3) P450-related metabolism.[102] Metabolic modifications of flavonoids will alter their "classical" antioxidant nature, which is defined mainly by the presence of a B-ring catechol group (dihydroxylated B-ring)

Hydroxybenzoic acid   Hydroxycinnamic acids

$R_1 = R_2 = OH, R_3 = H : Protocatechuic\ acid$
$R_1 = R_2 = R_3 = OH : Gallic\ acid$

$R_1 = OH : Coumaric\ acid$
$R_1 = R_2 = OH : Caffeic\ acid$
$R_1 = OCH_3 = OH : Ferulic\ acid$

Chlorogenic acid

Flavonoids

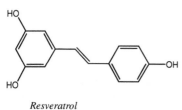

Stilbenes   Lignans

Resveratrol   *Secoisolariciresinol*

FIGURE 5.1 Chemical structure of polyphenols.

capable of readily donating hydrogen (electron) to stabilize a radical species.[102] Other structural features for antioxidant nature include the presence of 2,3 unsaturation in conjunction with 4-oxo- function in the C-ring and the presence of functional groups capable of binding transition metal ions, such as iron and copper. Circulating metabolites of flavonoids, such as glucuronides and O-methylated forms, and intracellular metabolites (e.g., flavonoid–GSH adducts) have reduced ability to donate hydrogen and are less effective scavengers of ROS and nitrogen species relative to their parent aglycone forms.[102]

Flavonols

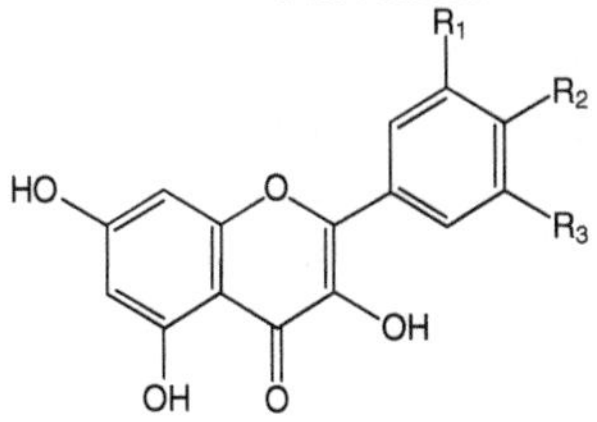

$R_2 = OH; R_1 = R_2 = H : Kaempferol$
$R_1 = R_2 = OH ; R_3 = H : Quercetin$
$R_1 = R_2 = R_3 = OH : Myricetin$

Flavones

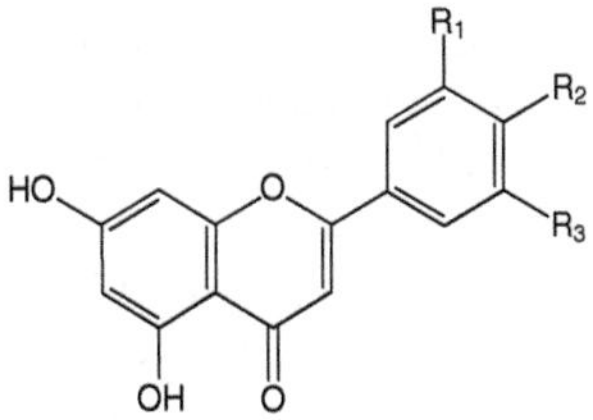

$R_1 = H ; R_2 = OH : Apigenin$
$R_1 = R_2 = OH : Luteolin$

Isoflavones

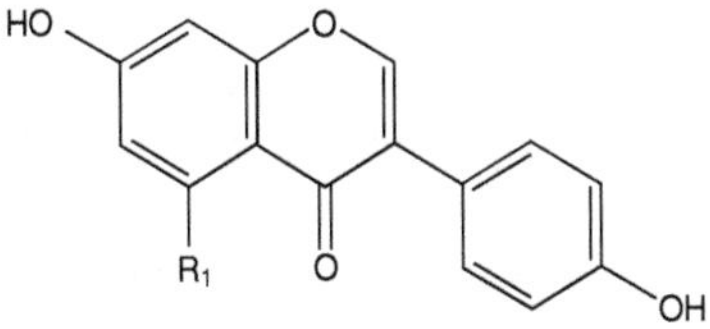

$R_1 = H : Daidzein$
$R_1 = OH : Genistein$

Flavanones

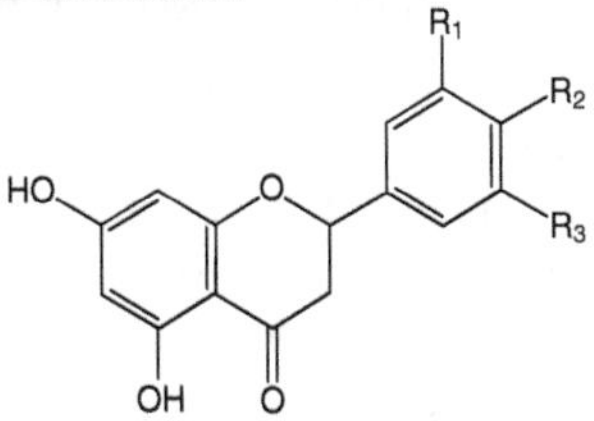

$R_1 = H; R_2 = OH : Narigenin$
$R_1 = R_2 = OH : Eriodictyol$
$R_1 = OH; R_2 = OCH_3 : Hesperetin$

Anthocyanidins

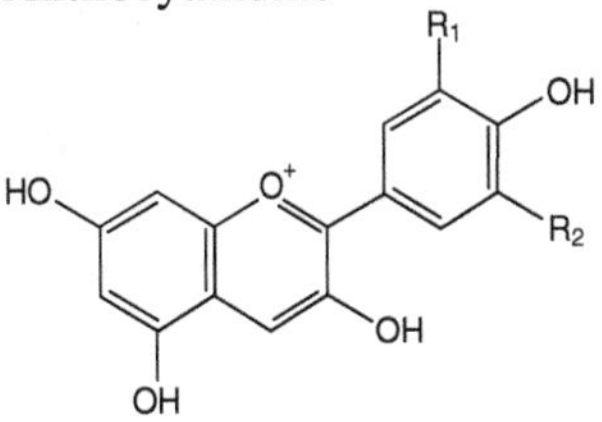

$R_1 = R_2 = H : Pelargonidin$
$R_1 = OH; R_2 = H : Cyanidin$
$R_1 = R_2 = OH : Delphinidin$
$R_1 = OCH_3; R_2 = OH : Petunidin$
$R_1 = R_2 = OCH_3 : Malvidin$

Flavanols

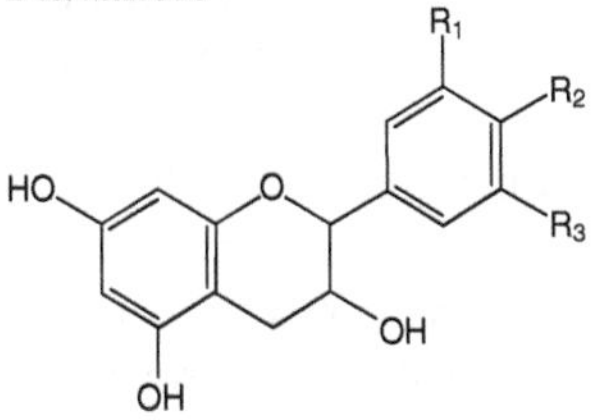

$R_1 = R_2 = OH; R_3 = H : Catechins$
$R_1 = R_2 = R_3 = OH : Gallocatechin$

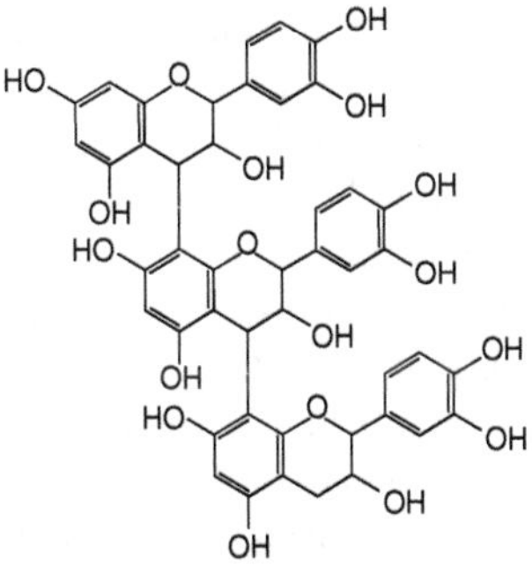

Trimeric procyanidin

FIGURE 5.2 Chemical structure of flavonoids.

5.2.1 PRESENCE OF FLAVONOIDS IN FOODS

Flavonols are the most ubiquitous flavonoids in foods; the main representatives are quercetin and kaempferol. They are generally present at relatively low concentrations of 15 to 30 mg/kg fresh weight. The richest sources are onions (up to 1.2 g/kg fresh weight), curly kale, leeks, broccoli and blueberries. Red wine and tea also contain up to 45 mg flavonols/l. These compounds are present in glycosylated forms. The associated sugar moiety is very often glucose or rhamnose, but other sugars may also be included (e.g., galactose, arabinose, xylose, glucuronic acid). Flavones are much less common than flavonols in fruit and vegetables. Flavones consist mainly of glycosides of luteolin and apigenin. The only important edible sources of flavones identified to date are parsley and celery.[102] In human foods, flavanones are found in tomatoes and certain aromatic plants, such as mint, but they are present in high concentrations only in citrus fruit.[102] The main aglycones are naringenin in grapefruit, hesperetin in oranges, and eriodictyol in lemons. Flavanones are generally glycosylated by a disaccharide at position 7: either a neohesperidose, which imparts a bitter taste (such as naringenin in grapefruit) or a rutinose, which is flavorless. Orange juice contains between 200 and 600 mg hesperidin/l and 15 to 85 mg narirutin/l, and a single glass of orange juice may contain between 40 and 140 mg flavanone glycosides.[99] Because the solid parts of citrus fruit, particularly the albedo (the white spongy portion) and the membrane separating the segments, have a very high flavanone content, the whole fruit may contain up to five times as much as a glass of orange juice.[99]

Isoflavones are flavonoids with structural similarities to estrogens. Although they are not steroids, they have hydroxyl groups in positions 7 and 4' in a configuration analogous to that of the hydroxyls in the estradiol molecule. This confers pseudohormonal properties on them, including the ability to bind to estrogen receptors, and they are consequently classified as phytoestrogens. Isoflavones are found almost exclusively in leguminous plants.[99] Soy and its processed products are the main source of isoflavones in the human diet. The isoflavone content of soy and its manufactured products varies greatly as a function of geographic zone, growing conditions and processing. Soybeans contain 580 to 3800 mg isoflavones/kg fresh weight, and soymilk contains between 30 and 175 mg/l. Flavanols exist in both the monomeric form (catechins) and the polymeric form (proanthocyanidines). Catechins are found in many types of fruits; apricots, which contain 250 mg/kg fresh weight, are the richest fruit source. They are also present in red wine (up to 300 mg/l), but green tea and chocolate are by far the richest sources.[99] An infusion of green tea contains up to 200 mg catechins. Black tea contains fewer monomeric flavanols, which are oxidized during "fermentation" (heating) of tea leaves to more complex condensed polyphenols known as theaflavins (dimers) and thearubigins (polymers). Catechin and epicatechin are the main flavanols in fruit, whereas gallocatechin, epigallocatechin and epigallocatechin gallate are found in certain seeds of leguminous plants, in grapes and, more importantly, in tea.[99] In contrast to other classes of flavonoids, flavanols are not glycosylated in foods. The tea epicatechin is remarkably stable when exposed to heat as long as the pH is acidic; only 15% of this substance is degraded after 7 h in boiling water at pH 5.[99]

Proanthocyanidins, which are also known as condensed tannins, are dimers, oligomers and polymers of catechins that are bound together by links between C4 and C8 (or C6). Through the formation of complexes with salivary proteins, condensed tannins are responsible for the astringent character of fruit (grapes, peaches, kakis, apples, pears, berries, etc.) and beverages (wine, cider, tea, beer, etc.) and for the bitterness of chocolate.[99] This astringency changes over the course of maturation and often disappears when the fruit reaches ripeness; this change has been well explained in the kaki fruit by polymerization reactions with acetaldehyde. Such polymerization of tannins probably accounts for the apparent reduction in tannin content that is commonly seen during the ripening of many types of fruit. It is difficult to estimate the proanthocyanidin content of foods because they have a wide range of structures and weights. Anthocyanins are pigments dissolved in vacuolar sap of the epidermal tissues of flowers and fruit, to which they impart a pink, red, blue or purple color.[99] They exist in different chemical forms, both colored and uncolored, according to pH. Although they are highly unstable in the aglycone form (anthocyanidins) while they are in plants, they are resistant to light, pH and oxidation conditions, which are likely to degrade them. In the human diet, anthocyanins are found in red wine, certain varieties of cereals and certain leafy and root vegetables (aubergines [eggplant], cabbage, beans, onions, radishes), but they are most abundant in fruit.

Cyanidin is the most common anthocyanidin in foods. Food contents are generally proportional to color intensity and reach values up to 2 to 4 g/kg fresh weight in blackcurrants or blackberries. These values increase as the fruit ripens. Anthocyanins are found in the skin of certain types of red fruit and may occur in the flesh (cherries and strawberries) as well. Wine contains 200 to 350 mg anthocyanins/l, and these anthocyanins are transformed into various complex structures as the wine ages.[99] Stilbenes are found in only low quantities in the human diet. One of these, resveratrol, for which anticarcinogenic effects have appeared during screening of medical plants and which has been extensively studied, is found in low quantities in wine (0.3 to 7 mg aglycone/l and 15 mg glycosides/l in red wine). However, because resveratrol is found in such small quantities in the diet, any protective effect of this molecule is unlikely at normal nutritional intake.[99]

In most cases, foods contain complex mixtures of polyphenols, which are often poorly characterized. Apples, for example, contain flavanol monomers (mainly epicatechin) or oligomers (procyanidin B2 mainly), chlorogenic acid and small quantities of other hydroxycinnamic acids, two glycosides of phloretin, several quercetin glycosides and anthocyanins, such as cyanidin 3-galactoside in the skin of certain red varieties. Apples are one of the rare types of food for which fairly precise data on polyphenol composition between varieties of apples have notably been studied. The polyphenol profiles of all varieties of apples are practically identical, but concentrations may range from 0.1 to 5 g total polyphenols/kg fresh weight and may be as high as 10 g/kg in certain varieties of cider apples.[99]

Methods of culinary preparation also have a marked effect on the polyphenol content of foods. For example, simple peeling of fruit and vegetables can eliminate a significant portion of polyphenols because these substances are often present in higher concentrations in the outer parts than the inner parts. Cooking may also have a major effect. Onions and tomatoes lose between 75 and 80% of their initial quercetin content after boiling for 15 min, 65% after cooking in a microwave oven, and 30% after frying. Steam cooking of vegetables, which avoids leaching, is preferable. Potatoes contain up to 190 mg chlorogenic acid/kg, mainly in the skin. Extensive loss occurs during cooking and no remaining phenolic acids were found in french fries or freeze-dried mashed potatoes.[99]

Only partial information is available on the quantities of polyphenols that are consumed daily throughout the world. These data have been obtained through analysis of the main aglycones (after hydrolysis of their glycosides and esters) in the foods most widely consumed by humans. In 1976, Kuhnau[103] calculated that dietary flavonoid intake in the U.S. was 1 g/day and consisted of the following: 16% flavonols, flavones and flavanones; 17% anthocyanins; 20% catechins; and 45% "biflavones." Although these figures were obtained under poorly detailed conditions, they continue to serve as reference data. Certain studies have subsequently provided more precise individual data concerning the intake of various classes of polyphenols. Flavonols have been more extensively studied. Consumption of these substances has been estimated at 20 to 25 mg/day in the U.S., Denmark and Holland.[99] In Italy, consumption ranged from 5 to 135 mg/day, and the mean value was 35 mg/day.[99] The intake of flavanones is similar or possibly higher than that of flavonols, with a mean consumption of 28.3 mg hesperetin/day in Finland.[99]

5.2.2 ABSORPTION AND METABOLISM OF POLYPHENOLS

Metabolism of polyphenols occurs via a common pathway. The aglycones can be absorbed from the small intestine. However, most polyphenols are present in food in the form of esters, glycosides or polymers that cannot be absorbed in their native form. These substances must be hydrolyzed by intestinal enzymes or by the colonic microflora before they can be absorbed. During the course of absorption, polyphenols are conjugated in the small intestine and later in the liver. This process mainly includes methylation, sulfanation and glucuronidation. The conjugation mechanisms are highly efficient and aglycones are generally absent in blood or present in low concentrations after consumption of nutritional doses. Circulating polyphenols are conjugated and extensively bound to albumin and both polyphenols and their derivatives are eliminated chiefly in the urine and bile. Polyphenols are secreted via the biliary route into the duodenum, where they are subjected to the action of bacterial enzymes, especially β-glucuronidase, in the distal segments of the intestine, after which they may be reabsorbed. The entero-hepatic recycling may lead to a longer half-life of polyphenols within the body.

The partitioning of polyphenols and their metabolites between aqueous and lipid phases is largely in favor of the aqueous phase because of their hydrophilicity and binding to albumin. However, in some lipophilic membrane models, some polyphenols penetrate the membrane to various extents. Quercetin showed the deepest interaction, probably because of its ability to assume a planar conformation. At physiologic pH, most polyphenols interact with the polar head groups of phospholipids at the membrane surface via the formation of hydrogen bonds that involve the hydroxyl groups of the polyphenols[99]

5.2.3 BIOCHEMICAL ACTIONS OF POLYPHENOLS

Flavonoids can prevent injury caused by ROS in various ways.[104] One way is the direct scavenging of free radicals.[105-107] Structurally important features defining the reduction potential of flavonoids are believed to be the hydroxylation pattern, especially a 3′,4′-dihydroxy catechol structure in the B-ring, the planarity of the molecule and the presence of 2,3 unsaturation in conjunction with a 4-oxo-function in the C-ring (see Figure 5.1). Thus, flavonoids with an O-dihydroxy catechol group in the B-ring (quercetin, epicatechin, etc.) are more powerful reductants/antioxidants and scavengers of ROS than those having a monohydroxyphenolic structure. Flavonoids are oxidized by radicals resulting in a more stable, less reactive radical. In other words, flavonoids stabilize ROS by reacting with the compound of the radical. Because of the high reactivity of the hydroxyl group of the flavonoids, radicals are made inactive, according to the following equation:

$$\text{Flavonoid (OH)} + R\cdot \rightarrow \text{flavonoid}(O\cdot) + RH$$

where $R\cdot$ is a free radical and $O\cdot$ is an oxygen free radical. Selected flavonoids can directly scavenge superoxide, whereas other flavonoids can scavenge the highly reactive oxygen-derived radical peroxynitrite.[108,109] For example, flavanols are scavengers of superoxide anions,[110] singlet oxygen[111] and lipid peroxy radicals,[112] and they can sequester metal ions by chelation.[113]

It has recently been shown that the flavonoid compounds caffeic acid and (+)-catechin can inhibit peroxynitrite-mediated oxidation of dopamine.[114] Moreover, it has been demonstrated that (—)-epicatechin, (—)-epicatechin gallate and quercetin serve as powerful antioxidants against lipid peroxidation when phospholipid bilayers are exposed to ROS *in vitro*.[107,115] There is also evidence that flavonoids can inhibit the activities of several enzymes, including lipoxygenase,[116-118] cyclooxygenase,[116,117] xanthine oxidase,[119] phospholipase A_2[120] and protein kinases.[121] These biological effects are believed to derive from the antioxidant properties of the related flavonoids.[119] However, increasing evidence suggests that flavonoids might exert modulatory effects in cells independently from classical antioxidant activity through selective actions at different components of a number of protein kinase and lipid kinase signaling cascades, such as phosphoinositide 3-kinase (PI 3-kinase), protein kinase B (Akt/PKB), tyrosine kinases, protein kinase C (PKC), and mitogen-activated protein kinase (MAP kinase).[102]

Flavonoids have the potential to bind to the adenosine triphosphate (ATP)-binding sites of a large number of proteins, including mitochondrial ATPase, calcium plasma membrane ATPase, protein kinase A, PKC and topoisomerase.[102] In addition, interactions with benzodiazepine-binding sites of GABA-A receptors and with adenosine receptors[102] have been shown.

Resveratrol and the citrus flavanones hesperetin and naringenin have been reported to exert inhibitory activity at a number of protein kinases[102] This inhibition is mediated via the binding of the polyphenols to the ATP binding site, presumably causing three-dimensional structural changes in the kinase leading to its inactivity. Flavonoids may also interact with mitochondria, interfere with pathways of intermediary metabolism, and/or down regulate the expression of adhesion molecules.[102] There are a number of additional potential sites where flavonoids may interact with key signaling pathways. For instance, flavonoid-mediated inhibition of oxidative stress-induced apoptosis may occur by preventing the activation of JNK (c-Jun amino-terminal kinase). There is strong evidence linking the activation of JNK to neuronal loss in response to a wide array of proapoptotic stimuli in both developmental and degenerative death signaling.[121,122] A number of flavonoids have been reported to inhibit the activation of JNK, although it is not clear if this is mediated by antioxidant activity or is due to inhibitory actions at signaling molecules.

Much interest has focused recently on the beneficial effects of flavanols, such as epicatechin, epigallocate chin (EGC), and epigallocate chin gallate (EGCG), and there is growing interest that the cytoprotective nature of these polyphenols is based on their interaction within signaling pathways. For example, epicatechin and one of its major *in vivo* metabolites, 3′-O-methyl epicatechin, have been shown to elicit strong cytoprotective effects against oxidative stress in fibroblasts and neurons.[102] In another study, the neuroprotective mechanism of another flavanol, EGCG, against oxidative stress-induced cell death was also found to involve modulation of signaling proteins. Thus, EGCG caused a stimulation of PKC and a modulation of cell survival/cell cycle genes, such as Bax, Bad, Mdm2, Bcl-2, Bcl-w, and Bcl-x.[123,124] Together, these findings suggest that protection is likely to be partly mediated through specific action within signaling pathways, although at this time it remains unclear exactly where such interactions occur within the pathway.

5.2.4 PUTATIVE HEALTH BENEFITS OF FLAVONOIDS

In recent years, there has been an increasing interest in investigating the many positive pharmacological properties of flavonoids. Much of this interest has been spurred by the dietary anomaly referred to as the "French paradox," the apparent compatibility of a high saturated fat diet with a low incidence of coronary atherosclerosis.[125] It was suggested that the polyphenolic substances, such as flavonoids in red wine, can provide protection against coronary heart disease. The natural phytoalexin resveratrol and the flavonoids quercetin and (+)-catechin have been invoked in order to explain the beneficial effects of moderate red wine consumption against coronary heart diseases.[126,127] In addition, epidemiological studies have shown that moderate wine consumption can be protective against neurological disorders, such as age-related macular degeneration[127,128] and AD.[68] Moreover, *in vitro* and *in vivo* preclinical studies have shown the neuroprotective effect of lyophilized red wine,[129] grape polyphenols,[130] quercetin,[131] *trans*-resveratrol[132–134] and (+)-catechin.[135] Taken together, these findings raise the possibility that red wine constituents may be beneficial in the prevention of age-related neurodegenerative disorders. There is also increasing interest for the role of tea (*Camellia sinensis*) in maintaining health and in treating disease. Although tea consists of several components, research has focused on polyphenols, especially those found in green tea. The green tea polyphenols include (—)-epicatechin (EC), (—)-epigallocatechin (EGC), (—)-epicatechin-3-gallate (ECG), (—)-epi-gallocatechin-3-gallate (EGCG). Of these, EGCG generally accounts for greater than 40% of the total.[136] Green tea polyphenols are potent antioxidants.[106] EGCG usually has the greatest antioxidant activity and is the most widely studied polyphenol for disease prevention.[136–138] Many of the putative health benefits of tea are presumed to stem from its antioxidant effects.

The epidemiological evidence indicating the putative role of nutritional antioxidants in the prevention and attenuation of neurodegenerative disorders is receiving experimental confirmation in a number of laboratory studies. Thus, the polyphenol epicatechin was shown to attenuate neurotoxicity induced by oxidized low-density lipoprotein in mouse-derived striated neurons.[138] Tea extracts and EgCG attenuated the neurotoxic action of 6-OHDA in rat PC12 cells, human neuroblastoma SH-SY5Y cells,[137] and was shown to be neuroprotective in a mouse model of PD.[138] Moreover, recent reports have revealed that flavonoids may be neuroprotective in neuronal primary cell cultures. For example, the ginkgo biloba extract, enriched with flavonoids, has been shown to protect hippocampal neurons from nitric oxide or β-amyloid derived, peptide-induced neurotoxicity.[139–141] In addition, the extract of ginkgo biloba, referred to as Egb 761, is one of the most popular plant extracts used in Europe to alleviate symptoms associated with a range of cognitive disorders.[142,143] The mechanism of action of Egb 761 in the central nervous system is only partially understood, but the main effects seem to be related to its antioxidant properties, which require the synergistic action of the flavonoids, the terpenoids (ginkgolides, bilobalide), and the organic acids, principal constituents of Egb 761.[144] These compounds, to varying degrees, act as scavengers of ROS, which have been considered the mediators of the excessive lipid peroxidation and cell damage observed in AD.[145–147]

5.3 ROS, NFκB, AND NEURODEGENERATIVE DISORDERS

The transcription factor NFκB, originally studied in cells of the immune system wherein it regulates cell survival,[148–150] is widely expressed in the nervous system and exists in neurons in both an inducible and a constitutively active form.[151–154] NFκB resides in the cytoplasm in an inactive form consisting of three subunits:

p65, p50 and an inhibitory subunit called IκB.[148,149,154] When IκB is bound to p50/p65, it is inactive; signals that activate NFκB cause dissociation of IκB releasing p50/p65, which then translocates to the nucleus and binds to specific κB DNA consensus sequences in the enhancer region of a variety of κB-responsive genes.[58,60,148,149,154,155]

In neurons, NFκB is activated by various intracellular signals, including cytokines, neurotrophic factors, and neurotransmitters.[58,154,156] Activation of glutamate receptors and membrane depolarization lead to activation of NFκB in hippocampal pyramidal neurons and cerebellar granule neurons in culture.[152,157] The mechanism whereby diverse stimulants lead to the activation of NFκB has been a subject of intense research. Most work has focused on the p50/p65 dimer, the predominant form of NFκB activated in many cells including neurons,[58,60,148] and its association with IB. It is now known that upon stimulation with many NFκB inducers, IκBα is rapidly phosphorylated on two serine residues (S32 and S36), which target the inhibitor protein for ubiquitination and subsequent degradation by the 26S proteasome.[155] Released NFκB dimer can then translocate to the nucleus and activate target genes by binding with high affinity to κB elements in their promoters. The phosphorylation and degradation of IκBα are tightly coupled events, so it is likely that agents that activate NFκB do so by stimulating a specific IκB kinases, or alternatively by inactivating a particular phosphatase. Two IκB kinases (IKKs) termed IKKα and IKKβ have been described in research.[155] IKKα and β have been shown to be activated by important inducers of NFκB, such as IL-1 and TNF, to specifically phosphorylate S32 and S36 of IκBα, and to be crucial for NFκB activation by these cytokines.[155] The IKKs are part of a larger multiprotein complex called the IKK signalsome. It appears that multiple pathways can regulate NFκB, most of which lead to IκB phosphorylation via the IKK-containing signalsome[155] One model has been proposed whereby diverse agents all activate NFκB by causing oxidative stress.[57,149,158] This hypothesis is based on four main lines of evidence:

1. Direct application of H_2O_2 to culture medium activates NFκB in some cell lines.[159–162]
2. In some cell types, ROS have been shown to be increased in response to agents that also activate NFκB.[149,159–163]
3. Virtually all stimuli known to activate NFκB can be blocked by antioxidants, including L-cysteine (a precursor of glutathione), N-acetyl-L-cysteine (NAC), caffeic acid phenethyl ester (CAPE), (–)-epigallocatechin-3-gallate, resveratrol, thiols, dithiocarbamates, vitamin E and its derivatives, and thioredoxin (an important cellular protein oxidoreductase with antioxidant activity).[55,56,127,149,159,164–168]
4. Inhibition or over expression of enzymes that affect the level of intracellular ROS has been shown to modulate the activation of NFκB by some agents.[163,169] Ultimately, this theory led to the proposal of H_2O_2 as the central second messenger in NFκB activation.[163]

A large body of evidence indicates that NFκB is involved in the control of cell survival. The great majority of the available data shows that NFκB exerts an antiapoptotic action. Thus, activation of NFκB can prevent cell death in various culture paradigms.[58,170] Moreover, increasing data suggest that NFκB activation may transduce anti-cell death signals in neurons.[58] For example, TNFα protected cultured hippocampal neurons against death induced by metabolic, excitotoxic and oxidative insults.[58,171] The involvement of NFκB in such neuronal cell death paradigms is suggested by data showing that TNFα induces activation of NFκB in cultured hippocampal neurons against excitotoxic and oxidative insults.[171–173] Moreover, in the PC12 neuronal cell line[174] and in primary sympathetic neurons,[175] activated NFκB has been found to mediate the antiapoptotic effect of nerve growthh factor (NGF). It has also been shown that the resistance of selected clones of PC12 cells to oxidative cell death induced by Aβ and H_2O_2 is mediated by NFκB.[176] An inhibition of NFκB potentiated Aβ peptide-mediated apoptotic damage in primary cultures of cerebellar granule cells,[177] and increased the apoptotic death of PC12 cells induced by autooxidation of dopamine.[178] Similarly, a lack of p50 subunit increased the vulnerability of hippocampal neurons to excitotoxic injury.[179]

Recent studies have shown that NFκB is activated and may play a protective role in neurodegenerative disorders, such as AD,[180] PD[62] and ALS,[64] and severe epileptic seizures.[179] There is also evidence that NFκB plays a pivotal role in the cell survival-promoting action of ADNF9, a nine amino acid activity-dependent neurotrophic factor (ADNF) peptide.[181] In addition, it has recently been reported that NFκB is involved in the neuroprotective effect exerted by subtoxic concentration of N-methyl-D-aspartic acid (NMDA) and can counteract low potassium-induced apoptosis in cultured cerebellar granule neurons.[182,183] Also preconditioning-induced neuroprotection in cultured hippocampal neurons seems to be mediated by activation of NFκB.[184] The mechanism by which NFκB can exert its antiapoptotic effect is still unclear. One possible mechanism would be the transcription of genes encoding trophic factors, antioxidant enzymes and calcium-regulating proteins. One of the first genes shown to be responsive to NFκB was SOD-2, a mitochondrial antioxidant enzyme that protects cells against apoptosis.[180] Other genes induced by NFκB include the cell adhesion molecules, such as ICAM-1,[185] the inducible form of nitric oxide synthase,[186] Bcl-2, Bcl-x, and the Bcl-2 homologue Bfl-1/A1.[61,187,188]

However, in some cases NFκB can promote neuronal death.[189–191] Thus, the neuroprotective effect of acetylsalicylic acid is apparently mediated by inhibition of NFκB.[190] More recently, it was found that NFκB is essential for dopamine-induced apoptosis in PC12 cells.[192] Whether NFκB inhibits or promotes apoptosis might depend on the cell type and the nature of the apoptosis-inducing stimulus.[191] However, the explanation for the conflicting results concerning an antiapoptotic vs. proapoptotic role of NFκB activation still is not clear and has been described as the "Janus faces" of NFκB.[191]

5.4 ALZHEIMER'S DISEASE, OXIDATIVE STRESS, NFκB, AND ANTIOXIDANTS

The incidence rate of Alzheimer's disease (AD), or the number of new cases developing among unaffected individuals over a specified time, increases from approximately 1% annually among people aged 65 to 70 years to approximately 6 to 8% for people over age 85.[193] The rates of disease are slightly higher for women and for African Americans and Caribbean Hispanics.[193] The duration of illness varies considerably from 2 to 20 years. Two population-based studies found that the median survival time for patients with AD was 3 to 4 years.[194,195] The prevalence, or proportion, of individuals surviving with clinically diagnosed AD also varies dramatically with age. Thus, the estimated prevalence of senile dementia in Europe increases with age from 1% in men and women of 60 years of age to 44.7% in the population 90 to 95 years of age.[196] AD is the most common form of dementia, with a prevalence of 0.4% in women and 0.3% in men aged 60 to 69 years.[197] A community-based study has suggested that approximately 4 million persons in the U.S. have contracted AD.[1] AD is a progressive dementing disorder characterized by selective neuronal loss in several areas of the central nervous system. In AD, the progressive memory deficits, cognitive impairments and personality changes are due to progressive dysfunction and death of the neocortex, limbic system, hippocampus and several of the subcortical regions of the brain.

The majority of cases of AD are age-related and, indeed, age is the only reliable risk factor for the nongenetic sporadic forms (85% of all cases) and, therefore, for the majority of cases of this disorder.[2,198] However, molecular genetic analyses suggest that there might be many genes that influence individual susceptibility to AD. The first such susceptibility gene identified was apolipoprotein E for which there are three alleles that encode three different isoforms of apolipoprotein E (E2, E3 and E4). Subjects that produce the E4 isoform are at increased risk of AD.[199] The mechanism by which E4 promotes AD is not well understood, but there is evidence that E4 enhances Aβ aggregation and reduces amyloid precursor protein 42 (APP). In addition, data suggest that E4 might increase the risk of AD by enhancing amyloidogenic processing of certain isoforms of APP, increasing oxidative stress and impairing neuronal plasticity. The characteristic histopathologic alterations in AD are neuritic or senile plaques (SPs) composed largely of amyloid β-peptides (Aβ) and neuronal aggregates of abnormally phosphorylated cytoskeletal proteins (neurofibrillary tangles [NFTs]). A number of data indicate that Aβ is responsible for the neuronal death in AD. Thus, aggregates of Aβ peptides are toxic to neurons in cultures[198,200–202] and can cause cell death by apoptosis[18,30,31,202,203]; however, the exact mechanisms of Aβ-induced neurotoxicity are still unknown.

Several lines of evidence suggest that the overproduction of ROS is implicated in Aβ neurotoxicity:

- Exposure of cultured neurons or neuronal cell lines to Aβ increases the intracellular levels of ROS[2,3,15,204–208] leading to the activation of NFκB.[63]
- Markers of oxidative stress are found to increase in a transgenic mouse model of AD.[147,209]
- Neurotoxicity of Aβ is attenuated by antioxidants, such as vitamin E, the spin-trap compound PBN (α-phenyl-tert-butyl nitrone) and lazaroids,[15,198,200,201,210–212] and/or free radical scavengers.[213]

Thus, in 1992 the protective effect of vitamin E was first described on neurons in culture against Aβ–induced cell death.[201] Following these initial findings, a number of subsequent studies confirmed the role of oxidative stress in the neurotoxic effect of Aβ peptide. For example, Behl et al.[214] found that Aβ can induce the formation of H_2O_2 in hippocampal neurons, which causes peroxidation of cell membranes and ultimately leads to neuronal death. Consistent with these findings, exposure of cultured hippocampal neurons to Aβ induced a significant increase in 4-HNE.[215] Moreover, it has recently been found that the phenolic antioxidant curcumin, which is largely used as a food preservative and herbal medicine in India, reduces oxidative damage and amyloid pathology in a transgenic mouse model of AD.[216] However, in another study, Aβ-induced neurotoxicity in rat hippocampal neurons in culture was not affected by several antioxidants;[217] nevertheless, pretreatment of cultures with Aβ significantly increased the sensitivity of neurons to H_2O_2, suggesting that Aβ can render neurons more susceptible to ROS damage.[217] Some of the proteins oxidatively modified by Aβ–induced oxidative stress include membrane transporters, receptors, GTP-binding proteins (G proteins) and ion channels. Oxidative modifications of tau by 4HNE and other ROS can promote its aggregation and, thereby, may induce the formation of neurofibrillary tangles. Aβ also causes mitochondrial oxidative stress and dysregulation of Ca^{2+} homeostasis, resulting in impairment of the electron transport chain, increased production of superoxide anion radicals and decreased production of ATP.

In agreement with data obtained in experimental models, clinical findings indicate that oxidative stress occurs in AD, as indicated by the finding that higher than normal levels of lipid, protein and DNA oxidation are found in the brains of AD patients.[46,48,145,146,218] Thus, lipid peroxidation, measured as thiobarbituric acid reactive substances (TBARS), was found to be increased in various brain regions of AD patients.[219–221] Moreover, Mecocci et al.[53] found a significant three-fold increase in mitochondrial DNA oxidation in the parietal cortex of AD patients. In addition, immunohistochemical analysis of brain sections from AD patients using an antibody with selectivity for the activated nuclear form of p65 revealed that NFκB was activated in neurons and astrocytes.[63] Cells with activated NFκB were restricted to the close proximity of early plaque stages.[63] Thus, it is possible that Aβ-induced NFκB activation contributes to the pathological changes observed in AD via the induction of proinflammatory and cytotoxic genes or, more likely, that Aβ-induced NFκB activation is part of a cellular defense program.

Based on the preclinical and clinical data indicating the presence of oxidative stress in AD patients, clinical trials were carried out to test the effect of antioxidants in this pathological condition. However, as already indicated above, inconsistent findings were reported in the trials investigating the effects of antioxidant vitamins on cognitive function and dementia. Thus, a controlled clinical trial with *dl*-α-tocopherol (synthetic form: 2000 IU/d) in patients with moderately severe impairment from AD showed some beneficial effects with respect to rate of deterioration of cognitive function.[222] In the same *dl*-α-tocopherol clinical trial, selegiline (10 mg/d), a monoamine oxidase inhibitor, produced beneficial effects similar to that produced by *dl*-α-tocopherol.[222] It is interesting to note that there was no significant difference in effect between the groups receiving a combination of *dl*-α-tocopherol and selegiline and those receiving treatment with the individual agents.[146,222] Several possibilities were proposed to explain the lack of additive effect. One was that selegiline and vitamin E can act by the same mechanism. Indeed, both reduce the levels of free radicals, although by different molecular pathways. Vitamin E protects neurons by destroying formed ROS ("quenching"), whereas selegiline protects neurons by preventing the formation of ROS and by inhibiting oxidative metabolism of catecholamines. Therefore, clinical studies involving vitamin E and selegiline support the concept that ROS are one of the intermediary risk factors for the progression of neurodegeneration in AD.[198] However, in the MRC/BHF Hearth Protection Study, which included 20,536 persons allocated to receive either antioxidant vitamin supplementation (vitamins E and C and β-carotene) or a placebo, no treatment differences were found in the percentage of persons defined as cognitively impaired or in mean cognitive scores after 5 years of treatment.[223] In addition, no difference was found in the number of persons who developed dementia during follow-up.

Another clinical study was conducted among 1059 rural, noninstitutionalized elderly residents of southwestern Pennsylvania, who were participants in the Monongahela Valley Independent Elders Survey.[224] Current use of nutritional supplements containing vitamins A, C, or E, β-carotene, zinc or selenium was measured through self-report. After adjustment for age, education and sex, no significant differences were found in cognitive test performance between antioxidant users and nonusers.[224] However, in the Rotterdam Study, Jama et al.[225] studied 5182 elderly persons and found that dietary and nutritional supplement intake of β-carotene was inversely associated with cognitive impairment, even after adjustment for age, sex, education, smoking, total caloric intake and consumption of other antioxidants. The discrepancy between the results of the study of Mendelsohn et al.[224] and that of Jama et al.[225] could be due to differences in the study populations, such as difference in age distribution or socioeconomic status or the exclusion of demented persons in the Rotterdam study. Although Jama et al.[225] found an association between β-carotene and cognition, they did not find similar results with vitamins E or C. Nevertheless, the data of a protective effect of β-carotene against age-related cognitive impairment were not confirmed in a more recent study.[226] Thus, from the analysis of the data from the Washington Heights-Inwood Columbia Aging Project (WHICAP), results indicated that the risk of AD was not associated with supplement, dietary or total intake of carotenes, vitamin C or vitamin E.[226] In contrast, a recent prospective study has shown a reduced prevalence and incidence of AD in individuals taking vitamins E and C in combination.[227] However, there was no significant reduction in risk of incident AD with vitamin E or vitamin C alone or with a multivitamin. There was also no association between AD risk and use of B-complex vitamins.[227] In two other investigations, an association of high folic acid levels and decreased homocysteine levels with reduced AD risk was found.[228,229] Given the conflicting data reported in many of the trials to date, it is clear that more effort is necessary in the future to try to confirm whether or not there is a relationship between dietary habits (in particular, the amount of polyphenols and other antioxidants intake) and the risk of dementia.

Increasing evidence suggests that diets high in saturated fats may increase the risk of AD, whereas diets rich in mono- and polyunsaturated fatty acids may decrease the risk. Several studies indicate that diets rich in specific long-chain, polyunsaturated fatty acids of the omega-3 series, such as those found in fish, can reduce the risk of AD.[230] Recent studies have extended and confirmed data showing the protective effect of omega-3 fatty acids against AD.[231] Moreover, there is epidemiological data suggesting an association between an inadequate intake of fish oils and a greater than expected incidence of late onset dementia.[232] Interestingly, experimental animal studies support these epidemiological data in that there is evidence that a diet enriched with docosahexaenoic acid (DHA, 22:6n-3) reduces the burden of β-amyloid peptide in a mouse model of AD.[233]

Although the emerging data linking fatty acids to AD are encouraging, the potential of dietary modifications of fat intake to affect disease risk remains to be established. There is also emerging evidence suggesting that cognitively stimulating environments, physical exercise and diets low in energy and fats (cholesterol and saturated fatty acids) may reduce the risk of AD.[193,228,234] Exercise, cognitive stimulation and dietary restriction may each exert a beneficial effect through a similar mechanism involving increased production of brain-derived neurotrophic factor (BDNF).[228,235,236] The possibility that the risk of AD can be reduced by modifications of diet and lifestyle is of considerable interest and suggests the potential for reducing the incidence of AD by preventive strategies similar to those that reduce the risk of cardiovascular disease.

5.5 PARKINSON'S DISEASE, OXIDATIVE STRESS, NFκB, AND ANTIOXIDANTS

Parkinson's disease (PD) is a neurological syndrome manifested by any combination of tremor at rest, rigidity, bradykinesia and loss of postural reflexes. The neuropathological hallmark of PD is the selective degeneration of dopamine (DA) neurons in the nigrostriatal system.[237,238] These neurons synthesize and release

DA, and the loss of dopaminergic influence on other structures in the basal ganglia leads to the classic Parkinsonian symptoms. Moreover, PD is characterized by degeneration of monoamine-containing neurons in the brain stem nuclei (predominantly the locus coeruleus) and is variably associated with pathology in nonnigral systems causing multiple neurotransmitter dysfunctions.[239]

Parkinson's disease develops much less frequently than Alzheimer's disease, ranging from 0.1 to 0.5% annually. Depending on the study, the annual incidence for PD ranges from 0.1 to 0.3% for those over 50 years, to 0.4% for those over 80 years and as high as 2.6% for those 85 to 98 years of age.[240–242] Incidence rates for PD increase with age both in men and women, but the rate in men exceeds that for women by two-fold.[241] The average duration of PD is 9 years. From birth, the lifetime risk of developing PD is about 2% for men and 1.3% for women.[243] Although idiopathic PD is usually sporadic, it is now well established that there is a genetic component to the disease.[244,245] Approximately 5 to 10% of PD patients have a familial form of Parkinsonism with an autosomal-dominant pattern of inheritance.[245] Case control studies have typically indicated a 2- to 14-fold increase in incidence in close relatives of PD patients,[246] and although concordance rates between identical twins are low for overt expression of the disease, they are much higher when subclinical decline in striatal dopaminergic dysfunction is measured by positron emission tomography (PET) imaging (53% in monozygotic twins of PD patients, compared with 13% in dizygotic cases).[247] A specific mutation in exon 4 of the gene encoding α-synuclein has been identified as a causative factor of Parkinsonism in a family from southern Italy.[248] Subsequently, this same mutation was found in other Greek and Brazilian families.[246,249]

Kruger et al.[250] reported a second mutation in a German family. The *parkin* gene mutation was first described in a Japanese family with autosomal recessive, levodopa-responsive disease characterized by degeneration of the substantia nigra and the absence of Lewy bodies.[251] Over 20 different mutations have since been identified[252] and these mutations are now considered to be the most common cause of familial PD. Nevertheless, in sporadic PD, environmental factors have been emphasized.[253] Epidemiological studies have correlated a number of potential factors as those that may increase the risk of developing PD.[254] These include exposure to well water, herbicides, industrial chemicals, wood pulp mills, farming and living in a rural environment. A number of exogenous toxins have been associated with the development of Parkinsonism, including trace metals, cyanide, lacquer thinner, organic solvents, carbon monoxide, and carbon disulfide.[245] There has also been interest in the possible role of endogenous toxins, such as tetrahydroisoquinolines and β-carbolines. However, no specific toxin has been found in the brain of PD patients. The most compelling evidence for an environmental factor in PD relates to the toxin 1-methyl-4-phenyl-1,2,3,6-tetrahydropyridine (MPTP). MPTP is a biproduct of the illicit manufacture of a synthetic meperidine derivative. Some drug addicts who took MPTP developed a syndrome that strikingly resembled PD, both clinically and pathologically.[255,256] MPTP induces toxicity through its conversion in astrocytes to the pyridinium ion (MPP+) in a reaction catalyzed by monoamine oxidase B (MAO-B).[11] MPP+ is then taken up by DA neurons and causes a mitochondrial complex I defect similar to that found in PD.[257] This observation supports the possibility that an environmental factor might cause PD; however, no MPTP-like factor has been identified in PD patients to date.

The principal cytoskeletal pathology of PD is the Lewy body, which in 85 to 100% of cases occurs in many monoaminergic and other subcortical nuclei, spinal cord, sympathetic ganglia, and less frequently in cerebral cortex, myenteric plexuses and adrenal medulla.[237,258–261] Lewy bodies are abnormal intracytoplasmic neuronal inclusions that are considered to be a major anatomic hallmark of PD, although they are seen in pigmented nuclei in various disorders and in aging brains. In the majority of cases, the mechanisms involved in nigral degeneration in PD are unknown, but evidence from studies of postmortem brain tissue suggests the involvement of ROS and oxidative stress.[11,239,262] Oxidative stress may arise from the metabolism of DA with the production of potentially harmful free radical species.[262,263] This may be important as surviving neurons increase DA turnover to compensate for diminishing synaptic transmission.

Circumstantial evidence exists that defects in mitochondrial energy metabolism may cause nigral neuronal degeneration in PD. Thus, MPTP produces dopaminergic neuronal degeneration and Parkinsonian symptoms in humans and nonhuman primates.[264] 1-methyl-4-phenylpyridinium (MPP+), produced by the catabolism of MPTP by monoamine oxidase B (MAO-B) in glia, is selectively taken up into dopaminergic neurons by the DA transporter. Within dopaminergic neurons, MPP+ is concentrated by the electrochemical gradient into mitochondria. MPP+ selectively inhibits NADH CoQ reductase (complex I) of the mitochondrial electron transport chain and induces neuronal degeneration. Evidence exists that similar mitochondrial dysfunction may occur in idiopathic PD; a defect in complex I has been reported in the striatum of patients with PD.[265–268] Similar defects have been found in the platelets,[269] but not skeletal muscle[270] of patients with PD. Reductions have been found in the substantia nigra, but not in other regions of the brain, such as the globus pallidus or cerebral cortex.[271] Therefore, the specificity of mitochondrial impairment may play a role in the degeneration of nigrostriatal dopaminergic neurons. Interestingly, recent evidence indicates that exposure to the complex I inhibitor, rotenone, can cause nigrostriatal dopaminergic degeneration associated with Parkinsonian-like symptoms and accumulation of protein aggregates containing ubiquitin and α-synuclein.[272]

Alterations in pro- and antioxidant molecules have been reported in postmortem tissue from individuals with PD. Increased total iron has been found in the substantia nigra in PD.[263,273–275] Iron could increase oxidative stress by promoting the formation of OH· from H_2O_2 via the Fenton reaction. Reductions in GSH levels in the substantia nigra have also been reported.[186,276–280] These reductions were not detected in other neurodegenerative diseases in which nigral cell loss occurs, suggesting they are specific to PD and not secondary to cell loss alone. Decreases in GSH have also been found in the substantia nigra in individuals with incidental Lewy bodies at postmortem, a potential marker of preclinical PD, suggesting that alterations in GSH are an early event.[281] Reductions in GSH levels could promote and/or be a consequence of oxidative stress. Because GSH is involved in the detoxification of H_2O_2, reductions in GSH could result from increased concentrations of H_2O_2 and in the presence of metals, the highly reactive OH·. The presence of lipid peroxidation and oxidative DNA damage further supports the existence of oxidative stress in PD.[262,282–284]

As already mentioned, the hallmark of PD is a severe reduction of DA in all components of the basal ganglia. DA and its metabolites are depleted in the caudate nucleus, putamen, globus pallidus, nucleus accumbens, the ventral segmental area, and the substantia nigra pars compacta and reticulata. Moderate losses of DA are found in the lateral hypothalamus, medial olfactory region and amygdaloid nucleus.[285] In early Parkinsonism, there appears to be a compensatory increase in DA receptors to accommodate the initial loss of DA neurons.[286,287] As the disease progresses, the number of DA receptors decreases, apparently due to the concomitant degeneration of DA target sites on striated neurons. In the remaining neurons in patients with PD, DA turnover seems greatly increased, judging from the concentrations of homovannilic acid (HVA) in the nerve terminals in the striatum and the cell bodies and dendrites in the substantia nigra,[288] and the ROS production may very well increase as a consequence.

This hypothesis is strengthened by a study showing that the concentrations of GSH decrease when DA turnover increases after reserpine treatment in rats, indicating increased activity of the peroxide scavenging enzyme GSH-Px.[289] If the increase in ROS production (due to increased DA turnover) is not buffered by the scavenging enzymes (SOD, catalase and GSH-Px), the compensatory hyperactivity of the dopaminergic neurons may become self-destructive. Chronic administration of L-DOPA would then only exacerbate the production of destructive ROS.[290,291] The administration of L-DOPA itself has been postulated to enhance the accumulation of ROS.[292,293] Hiramatsu et al.[294] using electron spin resonance spectrometry have shown that 10 mM L-DOPA by itself was inactive, whereas it produced ROS in the presence of 10 mM Fe-diethylenetriaminepantaacetic acid. This effect was blocked by deprenyl, an inhibitor of monoamine oxidase B (MAO-B), which has been advocated as a symptomatic and protective therapy in PD,[295] as well as MPTP-induced Parkinsonism.[296] Another index of oxidative stress in PD might be the evidence of a robust increase of NFκB in the nuclei of dopaminergic neurons in the substantia nigra of PD patients.[62] This clinical finding is consistent with in vitro data showing that oxidative stress induced by C_2-ceramide treatment causes nuclear translocation of NFκB in cultured mesencephalic neurons.[62] More recently, it has been shown that the neurotoxin, 6-OHDA, activates NFκB in PC12 cells by enhancing intracellular ROS levels.[297] Interestingly, in this experimental model, NFκB seems to sustain cell survival by stimulating the expression of the antiapoptotic proteins bcl-2 and bfl-1.[297] Moreover, as already mentioned, the potent green tea polyphenol antioxidant EGCG exerts a neuroprotective effect in a MPTP mouse model of PD.[137]

When induced by the toxins 6-OHDA or MPTP in animal models of PD, nigral cell death seems to involve both necrotic and apoptotic processes. In human PD, there has been some debate about whether key features of apoptosis could be demonstrated, at least when based, alone, on morphological features or terminal deoxynucleotidyl transferase-mediated dUTP-fluorescein nick end labeling (TUNEL).[298,299] However, the recent development of techniques involving double labeling with TUNEL to demonstrate DNA fragmentation in conjunction with cyanine dye that binds to DNA to provide additional structural details. Using this technique, it has been demonstrated that chromatin condensation and DNA fragmentation within the same nuclei in the substantia nigra of PD patients is greater than that seen in normal aging, consistent with the 10-fold higher rate of cell loss seen in patients with the disease.[245,300]

The progressive nature of PD and the fact that neuronal degeneration in the substantia nigra is slow and protracted[301] present opportunities for therapeutic intervention aimed at blocking or slowing down the degenerative process. Recent neuroimaging and autopsy data indicate that there is a preclinical period of 4 to 5 years before symptoms appear. The rate of cell loss and decline of dopaminergic function in the striatum is likely to be on the order of 10% per year, with the disease progressing more rapidly during the early phases than the more advanced stages of the disease.[247,301] Both PET and SPECT (single-photon emission computed tomography) imaging seem to be able to detect a decline in striatal dopaminergic function before clinical symptoms appear,[247] which may make it possible to begin neuroprotective intervention during the preclinical phase.

The largest neuroprotective trial conducted to date, the DATATOP (Deprenyl and Tocopherol Antioxidant Therapy of Parkinsonism) study,[302] involved two putative antioxidant agents, vitamin E and deprenyl.[303–305] Vitamin E had no significant effect at the doses used, but deprenyl slowed the early progression of symptoms and delayed the emergence of disability by an average of 9 months. However, being an MAO-B inhibitor, this drug has symptomatic effects of its own, which has confounded interpretation of the results.[302] Interestingly, animal studies have suggested that the neuroprotective effect is not dependent on MAO-B inhibition *per se*, but rather on an antiapoptotic effect of the metabolite desmethyl-deprenyl, possibly acting on protein translation.[300,306] Before the completion of the large DATATOP study ($n = 800$), an open trial with high dosages of α-tocopherol and ascorbate, administered to a small group of early PD patients ($n = 15$), found that this combination of natural antioxidants delayed by 2.5 years the time necessary to begin the therapy with L-DOPA.[307] There are many alternative antioxidative approaches that may be considered in future clinical trials, including free-radical scavengers, GSH, GSH enhancing agents, ion chelators and drugs that interfere with oxidative metabolism of DA. Interestingly, the classic directly acting DA receptor agonists may belong to the last group; by stimulating DA autoreceptors, these drugs reduce DA synthesis, turnover and release, so that less L-DOPA is needed.[308] In addition, some of these compounds have direct antioxidant effects.[309,310] More recently, the DA receptor agonist, pramipexole, has been used as a monotherapy for the treatment of PD, and it has been shown that it may have neuroprotective effects.[311]

5.6 AMYOTROPHIC LATERAL SCLEROSIS, OXIDATIVE STRESS, NFκB, AND ANTIOXIDANTS

Amyotrophic lateral sclerosis (ALS) is a fatal paralytic neurodegenerative disorder of unknown cause, mainly characterized by a progressive loss of motor neurons in the cerebral cortex, brainstem and spinal cord. ALS is a progressive disease that invariably leads to death within approximately 3 to 5 years from the onset of symptoms.[312] The annual worldwide incidence for ALS ranges between 0.4 and 1.8 per 100,000 people and the prevalence is estimated at 4 to 6 per 100,000, with an overall male predominance.[313] Although most cases are sporadic, about 5 to 10% are familial, with inheritance following an autosomal dominant pattern. About 15 to 20% of patients with familial ALS (FALS), which is clinically indistinguishable from the more common sporadic ALS, carry mutations in the gene encoding for the free radical scavenging enzyme SOD-1.[314,315] Over 50 different SOD-1 mutations have been documented in FALS patients.[316] Transgenic mice have been generated that express mutant forms of SOD-1 found in FALS cases, including gly^{93} → ala (G93A)[317–319] and gly^{37} → arg,[320] which develop motor neuron disease and death within 4 to 6 months if the mutant enzyme is expressed at sufficient levels. Studies of FALS patients with mutations of SOD-1 indicate that SOD-1 activity is decreased 20 to 50%.[315,321] This suggested initially that the disease was due to ROS-induced damage resulting from a structurally defective enzyme with reduced activity.[315] However, no deletions of the SOD-1 gene have been found in FALS families, implying that expression of the mutant protein is required for pathogenesis. Studies in transgenic mice suggest that, rather than causing a loss of function, the mutations of SOD-1 in FALS patients cause a gain of function that results in neuronal degeneration.[319,322] Because transgenic mice expressing wild-type human SOD-1 with comparable elevation of brain SOD activity do not develop motor neuron disease[319,320] and, in fact, show enhanced resistance to oxidative stress,[323,324] the disease is due to expression of the mutant protein and not to elevation of SOD activity in the brain.[325–327]

Several investigators have found increased levels of ROS in animal models of ALS.[328–330] Consistent with animal data, a number of clinical studies indicate that oxidative stress may be involved in the pathology of ALS, as suggested by increased levels of oxidative damage products, such as protein carbonyls, 4-HNE, 8-OHdG and nitrotyrosine.[21,44,51,330–333] In addition, fibroblasts from ALS patients were found to be more sensitive to oxidative stress.[334] Moreover, immunohistochemical studies have shown that NFκB is strongly activated in astrocytes of the spinal cord of ALS patients, probably as a consequence of the oxidative stress.[64] Thus, the occurrence of oxidative stress and activation of NFκB is a common characteristic of AD, PD and ALS. In this regard, it is noteworthy that overlapping syndromes with clinical and pathological features of dementia, ALS and PD have been described.[335] It is also important to mention that degeneration of midbrain DA neurons occurs in a mouse model of ALS.[336]

Various drugs, which can act by reducing oxidative stress, have been used as potential therapeutic agents in transgenic mice expressing the mutated human SOD-1 enzyme. Thus, polyamine- or putrescine-modified catalase, an antioxidant enzyme that removes hydrogen peroxide and has good permeability at the blood–brain barrier, increases the survival of transgenic mice bearing the human mSOD-1[G93A].[337,338] Moreover, the copper chelator and thiol compound penicillamine, the copper chelator trientine, carboxyfullerenes, vitamin E and N-acetylcysteine have been reported to increase the survival time in this mouse model and/or delay the onset of the disease to a small extent.[339–342] The drug riluzole, which inhibits glutamate release at presynaptic terminals, also extends lifespan slightly in human mSOD-1[G93A] transgenic mice.[342] Interestingly, riluzole, which is used clinically in patients with ALS,[343] has been shown to have direct antioxidative effect on cultured cortical neurons.[344] However, no clear evidence for a beneficial effect of α-tocopherol, selegiline, N-acetylcysteine or an antioxidant cocktail has been obtained in humans.[345–347]

Li et al.[348] have recently reported that blockade of caspase-1 and caspase-3 activity by N-benzyloxycarbonyl-Val-Asp-fluoromethylketone (zVAD-fmk) prolongs the survival of transgenic mice expressing the human mSOD-1[G93A] that begin to develop ALS symptoms at the mean age of 3 months. These findings open new perspectives for the use of caspase inhibitors as potential therapeutic agents in the treatment of ALS and other neurodegenerative diseases. However, because of the low oral bioavailability and limited brain penetrance, zVAD-fmk was delivered by intracerebral administration. Thus, the physicochemical characteristics of zVAD-fmk might limit its clinical usefulness. Based on these findings and on the hypothesis that in transgenic mice expressing the human mSOD-1[G93A] an increased formation of ROS occurs, we decided to treat them with lyophilized red wine (which is rich in antioxidant compounds) dissolved in the drinking water that was freely available to the animals. This treatment regimen caused a significant reduction in the overall mortality of the treated mice as compared with control animals. Thus, lyophilized wine prolonged by 6% the survival of mSOD1[G93A] mice.[349]

In the first series of experiments, the onset of treatment was variable and ranged from 43 to 66 days of age for the mice.[349] We have recently repeated the experiments on mSOD1[G93A] mice that were treated with the same concentration of lyophilized red wine, but the treatment was started earlier, i.e., 30 to 40 days from birth. By using this protocol, we have found that administration of lyophilized red wine significantly increased the mean survival time by 15%, as compared with control transgenic mice given drinking water only. The calculated concentration of polyphenolic compounds, expressed as gallic acid equivalent (GAE), was 4824 mg/l. Considering that each mouse drank about 4 ml of liquid daily, it is possible to calculate the daily intake of GAE, which was about 20 mg per mouse. It is tempting to speculate that the mechanism of neuroprotection exerted by lyophilized red wine on mSOD1[G93A] mice might be due to its ability to inhibit caspase-3 activity. This hypothesis is based on *in vitro* experiments showing that lyophilized red wine (5 μg/ml) caused a significant inhibition of caspase-3 activity on primary cultures of rat cerebellar granule neurons.[129] However, it is presently impossible to establish whether the effect of lyophilized red wine on caspase-3 is direct or mediated by inhibition of ROS formation. Furthermore, *ex vivo* experiments aimed at investigating the inhibitory effect of lyophilized red wine on activated caspase-3 in mSOD-1[G93A] mice are necessary to confirm our hypothesis. Unfortunately, treatment with CAPE, curcumin, *trans*-resveratrol, quercetin, hydroxytirosol and EGCG did not cause any significant effect on the survival of mSOD-1[G93A] mice either when given orally in the drinking water or when administered daily intraperitoneally. These findings suggest that treatment with single antioxidant compounds is not an efficient strategy in the therapy of this devastating disease, and the use of a mixture of multiple compounds might be preferable.

5.7 CONCLUSIONS

There is growing evidence that oxidative stress may play an important role in the pathogenesis of AD, PD and ALS. However, in spite of the large body of experimental data showing the protective effect of antioxidants in *in vitro* models of neurodegeneration and in some *in vivo* animal models, there is still limited evidence for a neuroprotective effect of antioxidants in the treatment of neurodegenerative disorders in humans. There may be several reasons for this discrepancy between preclinical and clinical data. Many laboratory studies use models of oxidative stress and investigate rescue by antioxidant agents. These models normally use acute high doses of antioxidants that far exceed those usually ingested via dietary sources.[350] These types of studies are, therefore, unlikely to be comparable to dietary exposure to antioxidants. Moreover, it is conceivable that the therapeutic regimen used so far (e.g., one or two antioxidants) might not be sufficient to halt the neuropathologic process. As pointed out by others, a more efficient strategy would be the use of multiple antioxidants in the treatment of AD, PD and ALS.[146] In this regard, it is important to point out that one possible advantage of the use of extracts of fruits, vegetables or beverages (such as red wine, green tea or ginkgo biloba) in the treatment of neurodegenerative disorders, is that they often contain multiple antioxidant compounds that can potentiate each other. Consistent with this line of reasoning, it has recently been shown that a complex antiaging dietary supplement composed of 31 ingredients, most of them with antioxidant activity, is capable of blocking age-related cognitive decline in transgenic mice expressing high levels of ROS-mediated processes.[351] Particularly important would be the use of lyophilized red wine,[349] which is provided with strong antioxidant capacity.[73,74]

One possible limitation of the neuroprotective strategy (including antioxidant administration) might be consequent to the fact that when overt symptomatology of AD, PD and ALS occurs, a certain amount of neuronal death has already happened. Thus, the neuroprotective agents (including antioxidants) can, at best, only rescue the surviving neurons, an effect which might not be sufficient to attenuate the neurological symptomatology. Nevertheless, recent advances suggest that the goal of curing patients with age-related neurodegenerative disorders is worth pursuing. One reason for optimism is that the extent of neuronal loss in AD and PD patients during the early period of the disease may not be as great as initially thought because many dysfunctional neurons may be able to recover.[350] It is, therefore, important to start the therapeutic intervention at an early stage of the disease process. In this regard, it is interesting to note that some epidemiological studies have shown that dietary habits can influence the incidence of neurodegenerative disorders. In particular, it was found that a diet rich in vitamin E can reduce the risk for PD[69,91] and that moderate wine consumption may decrease the risk for AD.[67,68] However, there are still few and controversial[66,92] epidemiological data on this important point, which might be partly due to the intrinsic difficulties in performing epidemiological surveys regarding the dietary habits of large populations. Nevertheless, it is desirable that future studies aimed at investigating the relationship between dietary antioxidant intake and the relative risk for neurodegenerative disorders such as AD, PD and ALS will shed more light on this very important aspect of public health.

5.8 ACKNOWLEDGMENTS

This work was supported by the Italian MIUR (Ministero Istruzione Università Ricerca) L488/92 project n. s209-p/f. The author is very grateful to Dr. Andreina Poggi for her critical reading of this manuscript.

REFERENCES

1. Evans DA, Funkenstein HH, Albert MS, Scherr PA, Cook NR, Chown MJ, Hebert LE, Hennekens CH, Taylor JO. Prevalence of Alzheimer's disease in a community population of older persons. *JAMA* 1989; 262:2551–2556.
2. Mattson MP. Pathways towards and away from Alzheimer's disease. *Nature* 2004: 430:631–639.
3. Mattson MP, Chan SL, Duan W. Modification of brain aging and neurodegenerative disorders by genes, diet, and behavior. *Physiol Rev* 2002; 82: 637–672.
4. Zhu H, Guo Q, Mattson MP. Dietary restriction protects neurons against the death-promoting action of a presenilin-1 mutation. *Brain Res* 1999; 842:224–229.
5. Bowling AC, Beal MF. Bioenergetic and oxidative stress in neurodegenerative diseases. *Life Sci* 1995; 56:1151–1171.
6. Jenner P. Oxidative damage in neurodegenerative disease. *Lancet* 1994; 344:796–798.
7. Jenner P. Oxidative mechanisms in nigral cell death in Parkinson's disease. *Mov Disord* 1998; 13:24–34.
8. Jenner P, Olanow CW. Oxidative stress and the pathogenesis of Parkinson's disease. *Neurology* 1996; 47(Suppl 3):S161–S170.
9. Olanow CW. A radical hypothesis for neurodegeneration. *Trends Neurosci* 1993; 16:439–444.

10. Halliwell B, Gutteridge JMC. Oxygen radicals and the nervous system. *Trends Neurosci* 1985; 6:22–26.
11. Simonian NA, Coyle JT. Oxidative stress in neurodegenerative diseases. *Annu Rev Pharmacol Toxicol* 1996; 36:83–106.
12. Andersen JK. Oxidative stress in neurodegeneration: cause or consequence? *Nat Med* 2004; 10 Suppl:S18–S25.
13. Jain A, Martensson J, Stole E, Auld PA, Meister A. Glutathione deficiency leads to mitochondrial damage in brain. *Proc Natl Acad Sci USA* 1991; 88:1913–17.
14. Koppal T, Drake J, Yatin S, Jordan B, Varadarajan S, Bettenhausen L, Butterfield DA. Peroxynitrite-induced alterations in synaptosomal membrane proteins: insight into oxidative stress in Alzheimer's disease. *J Neurochem* 1999; 72:310–317.
15. Markesbery WR, Carney JM. Oxidative alterations in Alzheimer's disease. *Brain Pathol* 1999; 9:133–48.
16. Schulz JB, Weller M, Klockgether T. Potassium deprivation-induced apoptosis of cerebellar granule neurons: a sequential requirement for new mRNA and protein synthesis, ICE-like protease activity, and reactive oxygen species. *J Neurosci* 1996; 16:4696–4706.
17. Sée V, Loeffler J-P. Oxidative stress induces neuronal death by recruiting a protease and phosphatase-gated mechanism. *J Biol Chem* 2001; 276:35049–35059.
18. Sastry PS, Rao KS. Apoptosis and the nervous system. *J Neurochem* 2000; 74:1–20.
19. Beal MF. Mitochondria, free radicals, and neurodegeneration. *Curr Opin Neurobiol* 1996; 6:661–666.
20. Beal MF. Oxidative damage in neurodegenerative diseases. *Neuroscientist* 1997, 3:21–27.
21. Beal MF, Ferrante RJ, Browne SE, Matthews RT, Kowall NW, Brown RH Jr. Increased 3-nitrotyrosine in both sporadic and familial amyotrophic lateral sclerosis. *Ann Neurol* 1997, 42:644–654.
22. Castilho RF, Ward MW, Nicholls DG. Oxidative stress, mitochondrial function, and acute glutamate excitotoxity in cultured cerebellar granule cells. *J Neurochem* 1999; 72:1394–1401.
23. Gassem M, Youdim MBH. Free radical scavengers: chemical concepts and clinical relevance. *J Neural Transm* 1999; 56:193–210.
24. Ishikawa Y, Satoh T, Enokido Y, Nishio C, Ikeuchi T, Hatanaka H. Generation of reactive oxygen species, release of L-glutamate and activation of caspases are required for oxygen-induced apoptosis of embryonic hippocampal neurons in culture. *Brain Res* 1999; 824:71–80.
25. Tong L, Toliver-Kinski T, Taglialatela G, Werrbach-Perez K, Wood T, Perez-Polo R. Signal transduction in neuronal death. *J Neurochem* 1998; 71:447–459.
26. Yuan J, Yankner BA. Apoptosis in the nervous system. *Nature* 2000; 407:802–809.
27. Junn E, Mouradian MM. Apoptotic signaling in dopamine-induced cell death: the role of oxidative stress, p38 mitogen-activated protein kinase, cytochrome *c* and caspases. *J Neurochem* 2001, 78:374–383.
28. Martin LJ. Neuronal death in amyotrophic lateral sclerosis is apoptosis: possible contribution of a programmed cell death mechanism. *J Neuropathol Exp Neurol* 1999; 58:459–471.
29. Mochizuki H, Goto K, Mori H, Mizuno Y. Histochemical detection of apoptosis in Parkinson's disease. *J Neurol Sci* 1996; 137:120–123.

30. Nijhawan D, Honarpour N, Wang X. Apoptosis in neural development and disease. *Annu Rev Neurosci* 2000; 23:73–87.
31. Stefanis L, Burke RE, Greene LA. Apoptosis in neurodegenerative disorders. *Curr Opin Neurol* 1997; 10:299–305.
32. Anglade P, Vyas S, Javoy-Agid F, Herrero MT, Michel PP, Marquez J, Prigent-Mouatt A, Ruberg M, Hirsch EC, Agid Y. Apoptosis and autophagy in nigral neurons of patients with Parkinson's disease. *Histol Histopathol* 1997; 12:25–31.
33. Su JH, Anderson AJ, Cummings BJ, Cotman CW. Immunohistochemical evidence for apoptosis in Alzheimer's disease. *NeuroReport* 1994; 5:2529–2533.
34. Rice ME. Ascorbate regulation and its neuroprotective role in the rat brain. *Trends Neurosci* 2000; 23:209–216.
35. McCay PB. Vitamin E: interactions with free radicals and ascorbate. *Annu Rev Nutr* 1985; 5:322–340.
36. Fridovich I. Superoxide dismutases. An adaptation to a paramagnetic gas. *J Biol Chem* 1989; 264:7761–7764.
37. Cohen G, Werner P. Free radicals, oxidative stress, and neurodegeneration. In Calne, D.B. Ed. *Neurodegenerative diseases*. Philadelphia: WB Saunders Co, 1994:139–161.
38. Coyle JT, Puttfarken P. Oxidative stress, glutamate and neurodegenerative disorders. *Science* 1993; 262:689–695.
39. Kruman I, Bruce-Keller AJ, Bredesen D, Waeg G, Mattson MP. Evidence that 4-hydroxynonenal mediates oxidative stress-induced neuronal apoptosis. *J Neurosci* 1997; 17:5089–5100.
40. Selley ML. (E)-4-hydroxy-2-nonenal may be involved in the pathogenesis of Parkinson's disease. *Free Radic Biol Med* 1998; 25:169–174.
41. Yoritaka A, Hattori N, Uchida K, Tanaka M, Stadtman ER, Mizuno Y. Immuno-histochemical detection of 4-hydroxynonenal protein adducts in Parkinson's disease. *Proc Natl Acad Sci USA* 1996; 93:2696–2701.
42. Stadtman ER. Protein oxidation and aging. *Science* 1992; 257:1220–1224.
43. Hensley K, Hall N, Subramian R, Cole P, Harris M, Aksenov M, Aksenova M, Gabbita SP, Wu JF, Carney JM, Lovell M, Markesbery WR, Butterfield DA. Brain regional correspondence between Alzheimer's disease histopathology and biomarkers of protein oxidation. *J Neurochem* 1995; 65:2146–2156.
44. Abe K, Pan LH, Watanabe M, Konno H, Kato T, Hoyama Y. Upregulation of protein-tyrosine nitration in the anterior horn cells of amyotrophic lateral sclerosis. *Neurosci Lett* 1997; 19:124–128.
45. Good PF, Hsu A, Werner P, Perl DP, Olanow CW. Protein nitration in Parkinson's disease. *J Neuropathol Exp Neurol* 1998; 57:338–342.
46. Good PF, Werner P, Hsu A, Olanow CW, Perl DP. Evidence for neuronal oxidative damage in Alzheimer's disease. *Am J Pathol* 1996; 149:21–28.
47. Hensley K, Maidt ML, Yu Z, Sang H, Markesbery WR, Floyd RA. Electrochemical analysis of protein nitrotyrosine and dityrosine in the Alzheimer's brain indicate region-specific accumulation. *J Neurosci* 1998; 18:8126–8132.
48. Smith MA, Richey Harris PL, Sayre LM, Beckman JS, Perry G. Widespread peroxynitrite-mediated damage in Alzheimer's disease. *J Neurosci* 1997; 17:2653–2657.
49. Su JH, Deng GM, Cotman CW. Neuronal DNA damage precedes tangle formation and is associated with upregulation of nitrotyrosine in Alzheimer's brain. *Brain Res* 1997; 774:193–199.

50. Alam ZI, Jenner A, Daniel SE, Lees AJ, Cairns N, Marsden CD, Jenner P, Halliwell B. Oxidative DNA damage in the parkinsonian brain: an apparent selective increase in 8-hydroxyguanine levels in the substantia nigra. *J Neurochem* 1997; 69:1196–1203.

51. Ferrante RJ, Browne SE, Shinobu LA, Bowling AC, Baik MJ, MacGarvey U, Kowall NW, Brown RH Jr, Beal MF. Evidence of increased oxidative damage in both sporadic and familial amyotrophic lateral sclerosis. *J Neurochem* 1997; 69:2064–2074.

52. Gabbita SP, Lovell MA, Markesbery WR. Increased nuclear oxidation in the brain in Alzheimer's disease. *J Neurochem* 1998; 71:2034–2040.

53. Mecocci P, MacGarvey U, Beal MF. Oxidative damage to mitochondrial DNA is increased in Alzheimer's disease. *Ann Neurol* 1994; 36:747–751.

54. Zhang J, Perry G, Smith MA, Robertson D, Olson SJ, Graham DG, Montine TJ. Parkinson's disease is associated with oxidative damage to cytoplasmic DNA and RNA in substantia nigra neurons. *Am J Pathol* 1999; 154:1423–1429.

55. Dalton TP, Shertzer HG, Puga A. Regulation of gene expression by reactive oxygen. *Annu Rev Pharmacol Toxicol* 1999; 39:67–101.

56. Flohé L, Brigelius-Flohé, Saliou C, Traber MG, Packer L. Redox regulation of NF-κB activation. *Free Radic Biol Med* 1997; 22:1115–1126.

57. Li N, Karin M. Is NF-κB the sensor of oxidative stress? *FASEB J* 1999; 13:1137–1143.

58. Mattson MP, Culmsee C, Yu ZF, Camaldola S. Roles of nuclear factor-κB in neuronal survival and plasticity. *J Neurochem* 2000; 74:443–456.

59. Pinkus R, Weiner LM, Daniel V. Role of oxidants and antioxidants in the induction of AP-1, NF-κB, and glutathione s-transferase gene expression. *J Biol Chem* 1996; 271:13422–13429.

60. Mattson MP, Camaldola S. NF-κB in neuronal plasticity and neurodegenerative disorders. *J Clin Invest* 2001; 107:247–254.

61. Tamatani M, Che YH, Matsuzaki H, Ogawa S, Okado H, Miyake S, Mizuno T, Tohyama M. Tumor necrosis factor induces Bcl-2 and bcl-x expression through NF-κB activation in primary hippocampal neurons. *J Biol Chem* 1999; 274:8531–8538.

62. Hunot S, Brugg B, Ricard D, Michel PP, Muriel MP, Ruberg M, Facheux BA. Agid Y, Hirsch EC. Nuclear translocation of NF-κB is increased in dopaminergic neurons of patients with Parkinson's disease. *Proc Natl Acad Sci USA* 1997; 94:7531–7536.

63. Kaltschmidt B, Uherek M, Volk B, Baeuerle PA, Kaltschmidt C. Transcription factor NF-κB is activated in primary neurons by amyloid β peptides and in neurons surrounding early plaques from patients with Alzheimer's disease. *Proc Natl Acad Sci USA* 1997; 94:2642–2647.

64. Migheli A, Piva R, Atzori C, Troost D, Schiffer D. c-Jun, JNK/SAPK kinase and transcription factor NF-κB are selectively activated in astrocytes, but not motor neurons, in amyotrophic lateral sclerosis. *J Neuropathol Exp Neurol* 1997; 56:1314–1322.

65. Deschamps V, Barberger-Gateau P, Peuchant E, Orgogozo JM. Nutritional factors in cerebral aging and dementia: epidemiological arguments for a role of oxidative stress. *Neuroepidemiology* 2001; 20:7–15.

66. Hellenbrand W, Boeing H, Robra B-P, Seidler A, Vieregge P, Nischan P, Joerg J, Oertel WH, Schneider E, Ulm G. Diet and Parkinson's disease II: a possible role for the past intake of specific nutrients. *Neurology* 1996; 47:644–50.
67. Lemeshow S, Letenneur L, Dartigues J-F, Lafont S, Orgogozo J-M, Commenges D. Illustration of analysis taking into account complex survey considerations: the association between wine consumption and dementia in the PAQUID study. *Am J Epidemiol* 1998; 148:298–306.
68. Orgogozo J-M, Dartigues J-F, Lafont S, Letenneur L, Commenges D, Salomon R, Renaud S, Breteler MB. Wine consumption and dementia in the elderly: a prospective community study in the Bordeaux area. *Rev Neurol* 1997; 3:185–192.
69. de Rijk MC, Breteler MMB, den Breeijen JH, Launer LJ, Grobber DE, van der Meché FGA, Hofman A. Dietary antioxidants and Parkinson's disease. *Arch Neurol* 1997; 54:762–765.
70. de Groot H, Rauen U. Tissue injury by reactive oxygen species and the protective effects of flavonoids. *Fundament Clin Pharmacol* 1998; 12:249–255.
71. Leibovici D, Ritchie K, Ledèsert B, Touchon J. The effects of wine and tobacco consumption on cognitive performance in the elderly: a longitudinal study of relative risk. *Int J Epidemiol* 1999; 28:77–81.
72. Cao GH, Russell RM, Lischner N, Prior, RL. Serum antioxidant capacity is increased by consumption of strawberries, spinach, red wine or vitamin C in elderly women. *J Nutr* 1998; 128:2383–2390.
73. Frankel EN, Kanner J, German JB, Parks E, Kinsella JE. Inhibition of oxidation of lipoprotein by phenolic substances in red wine. *Lancet* 1993; 341:454–457.
74. Maxwell S, Cruickshank A, Thorpe G. Red wine and antioxidant activity in serum. *Lancet* 1994; 344:193–194.
75. Ruitenberg A, van Swieten JC, Witteman JCM, Mehta KM, van Duijn CM, Hofman A, Breteler MM. Alcohol consumption and risk of dementia: the Rotterdam study. *Lancet* 2002; 359:281–286.
76. Morris MC, Beckett LA, Scherr PA, Hebert LE, Bennet DA, Fields TS, Evans DA. Vitamin E and and vitamic C supplement use and risk of incident Alzheimer's disease. *Alzheimer Dis Assoc Disord* 1998; 12:121–126.
77. Paleologos M, Cumming RG, Lazarus R. Cohort study of vitamin C intake and cognitive impairment. *Am J Epidemiol* 1998; 148:45–50.
78. Masaki KH, Losonczy KG, Izmirlian G, Foley DJ, Ross GW, Petrovitch H, Havlik R, White LR. Association of vitamin E and C supplement use with cognitive function and dementia in elderly men. *Neurology* 2000; 56:1265–1272.
79. Engelhart MJ, Geerlings MI, Ruitemberg A, van Swieten JC, Hofman A, Witteman JCM, Breteler MMB. Dietary intake of antioxidants and risk of Alzheimer's disease. *JAMA* 2002; 287:3223–3229.
80. Morris MC, Evans DA, Bienias JL, Tangney CC, Bennett DA, Aggarwal N, Wilson RS, Scherr PA. Dietary intake of antioxidant nutrients and the risk of incident Alzheimer's disease in a biracial community study. *JAMA* 2002; 287:3230–3237.
81. Varner AE. Antioxidants and risk of Alzheimer disease. *JAMA* 2002; 288:2265.
82. Jiang Q, Elson-Schwab I, Courtemanche C, Ames BN. γ-Tocopherol and its major metabolite, in contrast to γ-tocopherol, inhibit cyclooxygenase activity in macrophages and epithelial cells. *Proc Natl Acad Sci USA* 2000; 97:11494–11499.

83. in t' Veld BA, Ruitenberg A, Hofman A, Launer LJ, van Duijn CM, Stijnen T, Breteler MM, Stricker BH. Nonsteroidal antiinflammatory drugs and the risk of Alzheimer's disease. *N Engl J Med* 2001; 345(21):1515–1521.

84. Brenner S. Antioxidants and the risk of Alzheimer disease. *JAMA* 2002; 288:2265.

85. Jugdaohsingh R, Anderson SH, Tucker KL, Elliott H, Kiel DP, Thompson RP, Powell JJ. Dietary silicon intake and absorption. *Am J Clin Nutr* 2002; 75:887–93.

86. Anasuya A, Bapurao S, Paranjape PK. Fluoride and silicon intake in normal and endemic fluorotic areas. *J Trace Elem Med Biol* 1996; 10:149–155.

87. Chandra V, Pandav R, Dodge HH, Johnston JM, Belle SH, DeKosky ST, Ganguli M. Incidence of Alzheimer's disease in a rural community in India: the Indo-U.S. study. *Neurology* 2001; 57:985–989.

88. Helmer C, Peuchant E, Letenneur L, Bourdel-Marchasson I, Larrieu S, Dartigues JF, Duborg L, Thomas M-J, Gateau-Barberger P. Association between antioxidant nutritional indicators and the incidence of dementia: results from PAQUID prospective cohort study. *Eur J Clin Pharmacol* 2003; 57:1555–1561.

89. Laurin D, Masaki KH, Foley DJ, White LR, Launer LJ. Midlife dietary intake of antioxidants and risk of late-life incident dementia. The Honolulu-Asia aging study. *Am J Epidemiol* 2004; 159:959–967.

90. Laurin D, Foley DJ, Masaki KH, White LR, Launer LJ. Vitamin E and C supplements and risk of dementia. *JAMA* 2002; 288:2266–2268.

91. Golbe LI, Farrell TM, Davis PH. Case-control study of early life dietary factors in Parkinson's disease. *Arch Neurol* 1998; 45:1350–1353.

92. Logroscino G, Marder K, Cote L, Tang M-X, Shea S, Mayeux R. Dietary lipids and antioxidants in Parkinson's: a population-based, case-control study. *Ann Neurol* 1996; 39:89–94.

93. Perrig WJ, Perrig P, Stahelin HB. The relation between antioxidants and memory performance in the old and very old. *J Am Geriatr Soc* 1997; 45:718–724.

94. Rao AV, Agarwal S. Role of antioxidant lycopene in cancer and hearth disease. *J Am Coll Nutr* 2000; 19:563–569.

95. Rissanen TH, Voutilainen S, Nyyssonen K, Lakka TA, Sivenius J, Salonen R, Kaplan GA, Salonen JT. Low serum lycopene concentration is associated with an excess incidence of acute coronary events and stroke: the Kuopio Ischaemic Hearth Disease Risk Factor Study. *Br J Nutr* 2001; 85:749–754.

96. Keller JN, Guo Q, Holtsberg FW, Bruce-Keller AJ, Mattson MP. Increased sensitivity to mitochondrial toxin-induced apoptosis in neural cells expressing mutant presenilin-1 is linked to perturbed calciun homeostasis and enhanced oxyradical production. *J Neurosci* 1998; 18:4439–4450.

97. Yu ZF, Bruce-Keller AJ, Goodman Y, Mattson MP. Uric acid protects neurons against excitotoxic and metabolic insults in cell culture, and against focal ischemic brain injury in vivo. *J Neurosci Res* 1998; 53:613-625.

98. Joseph JA, Shukitt-Hale B, Denisova NA, Bielinski D, Martin A, McEwen JJ, Bickford PC. Reversal of age-related declines in neuronal signal transduction, cognitive, and motor behavioral deficits with blueberry, spinach, or strawberry dietary supplementation. *J Neurosci* 1999; 19:8114–8121.

99. Manach C, Scalbert A, Morand C, Rémésy C, Jiménez L. Polyphenols: food sources and bioavailability. *Am J Clin Nutr* 2004; 79:727–747.

100. Middleton EJ. Effect of plant flavonoids on immune and inflammatory cell function. *Adv Exp Med Biol* 1998; 439:175–182.

101. Rice-Evans C. Flavonoid antioxidants. *Curr Med Chem* 2001; 8:797–807.

102. Williams RJ, Spencer JPE, Rice-Evans C. Flavonoids: antioxidants or signalling molecules? *Free Radic Biol Med* 2004; 36:838–849.

103. Kuhnau J. The flavonoids. A class of semi-essential food components: their role in human nutrition. *World Rev Nutr Diet* 1976; 24:117–191.

104. Cao G, Sofic E, Prior RL. Antioxidant and prooxidant behavior of flavonoids: structure-activity relationships. *Free Radic Biol Med* 1997; 22:749–60.

105. Hanasaki Y, Ogawa S, Fukui S. The correlation between active oxygen scavenging and antioxidative effects of flavonoids. *Free Radic Biol Med* 1994; 16:845–850.

106. Saija A, Scalese M, Lanza M, Marzullo D, Bonina F, Castelli F. Flavonoids as antioxidant agents: importance of their interaction with biomembranes. *Free Radic Biol Med* 1995; 19:481–486.

107. Salah N, Miller NJ, Paganga G, Tijburg L, Bolwell GP, Rice-Evans C. Polyphenolic flavanols as scavengers of aqueous phase radicals and as chain-breaking antioxidants. *Arch Biochem Biophys* 1995; 322:339–346.

108. Bors W, Heller W, Michel C, Saran M. Flavonoids as antioxidants: determinations of radical-scavenging efficiencies. *Methods Enzymol* 1990; 186:343–355.

109. Nijveldt RJ, van Nood E, van Hoorn DEC, Boelens PG, van Norren K, van Leeuwen PAM. Flavonoids: a review of probable mechanisms of action and potential applications. *Am J Clin Nutr* 2001; 74:418–425.

110. Robak J, Gryglewski RJ. Flavonoids are scavengers of superoxide anions. *Biochem Pharmacol* 1988; 37:837–841.

111. Husain SR, Cillard J, Cillard P. Hydroxyl radical scavenging activity of flavonoids. *Phytochemistry* 1987; 26:2489–2491.

112. Sorata Y, Takahama U, Kimura M. Protective effect of quercetin and rutin on photosensitized lysis of human erythrocites in the presence of hematoporphyrin. *Biochim Byophys Acta* 1984; 799:313–317.

113. Takahama U. Inhibition of lipoxygenase-dependent peroxidation by quercetin: mechanisms of antioxidative function. *Phytochemistry* 1985; 24:1443–1446.

114. Kerry N, Rice-Evans C. Inhibition of peroxynitrite-mediated oxidation of dopamine by flavonoid and phenolic antioxidants and their structural relationship. *J Neurochem* 1999; 73:247–253.

115. Terao J, Piskula M, Yao Q. Protective effect of epicatechin, epicatechin gallate, and quercetin on lipid peroxidation in phopholipid bilayers. *Arch Biochem Biophys* 1994; 308:278–284.

116. Hoult JRS, Moroney MA, Payà M. Action of flavonoids and coumarins on lipoxygenase and cyclooxigenase. *Meth Enzymol* 1994; 234:443–455.

117. Laughton MJ, Evans PJ, Moroney MA, Hoult JRC, Halliwell B. Inhibition of mammalian 5-lipoxygenase and cyclooxygenase by flavonoids and phenolic dietary additives: relationship to antioxidant activity and to ion-reducing ability. *Biochem Pharmacol* 1991; 42:1673–1681.

118. Ratty AK, Sunamoto J, Das NP. Interaction of flavonoids with 1,1diphenyl-2-picryhydrazinyl free radical, liposomal membranes and soybean lipoxygenase-1. *Biochem Pharmacol* 1988; 37:989–995.

119. Cotelle N, Bernier JL, Catteau JP, Pommery J, Wallet JC, Gaydou EM. Antioxidant properties of hydroxy-flavones. *Free Radic Biol Med* 1996; 20:35–43.

120. Gil B, Sanz MJ, Terencio MC, Ferrandiz ML, Bustos G, Payà M, Gunasegaran R, Alcaraz MJ. Effects of flavonoids on Naja naja and human recombinant synovial phospholipase A2 and inflammatory responses in mice. *Life Sci* 1994; 54:333–338.

121. Cushman M, Nagaratham D, Burg DL, Geahlen RL. Synthesis and protein-tyrosine kinase inhibitory activities of flavonoid analogues. *J Med Chem* 1991; 34:798–806.

122. Mielke K, Herdegen T. JNK a p38 stress kinases: degenerative effectors of signal-transduction-cascades in the nervous system. *Progr Neurobiol* 2000; 61:45–60.

123. Davis RJ. Signal transduction by JNK group of MAP kinases. *Cell* 2000; 103:239–252.

124. Levites Y, Amit T, Youdim MB, Mandel S. Involvement of protein kinase C activation and cell/survival/cell cycle genes in green tea polyphenol (–)-epigallo-catechin 3 gallate neuroprotective action. *J Biol Chem* 2002; 277:30574–30580.

125. Renaud S, De Lorgeril M. Wine, alcohol, platelets, and the French paradox for coronary heart disease. *Lancet* 1992; 339:1523–1526.

126. Pace-Asciak CR, Hahn S, Diamandis EP, Soleas G, Goldberg DM. The red wine phenolics trans-resveratrol and quercetin block human platelet aggregation and eicosanoid synthesis: implications for protection against coronary heart disease. *Clin Chim Acta* 1995; 235:207–209.

127. Tsai SH, Lin-Shiau SY, Lin JK. Suppression of nitric oxide synthase and the down-regulation of the activation of NF-κB in macrophages by resveratrol. *Br J Pharmacol* 1999; 126:673–680.

128. Obisesan TO, Hirsh, R, Kosoko O, Carlson L, Parrott M. Moderate wine consumption is associated with decreased odds of developing age-related macular degeneration in NHANES-1. *J Am Ger Soc* 1998; 46:1–7.

129. De Ruvo C, Amodio R, Algeri S, Martelli N, Intilangelo A, D'Ancona GM, Esposito E. Nutritional antioxidants as antidegenerative agents. *Int J Dev Neurosci* 2000; 18:359–366.

130. Sun GY, Xia J, Draczynska-Lusiak B, Simonyi A, Sun AY. Grape polyphenols protect neurodegenerative changes induced by chronic ethanol administration. *NeuroReport* 1999; 10:93–96.

131. Shutenko Z, Henry Y, Pinard E, Seylaz J, Potier P, Berthet F, Girard P, Sercombe R. Influence of the antioxidant quercetin *in vivo* on the level of nitric oxide determined by electron paramagnetic resonance in rat brain during global ischemia and reperfusion. *Biochem Pharmacol* 1999; 57:199–208.

132. Chanvitayapongs S, Draczynska-Lusiak B, Sun AY. Amelioration of oxidative stress by antioxidants and resveratrol in PC12 cells. *Neuroreport* 1997; 8:1499–1502.

133. Karlsson J, Emgård M, Brundin P, Burkitt MJ. *trans*-Resveratrol protects embryonic mesencephalic cells from *tert*-butyl hydroperoxide: electron paramagnetic resonance spin trapping evidence for a radical scavenging mechanism. *J Neurochem* 2000; 75:141–150.

134. Virgili M, Contestabile A. Partial neuroprotection of *in vivo* excitotoxic brain damage by chronic administration of the red wine antioxidant agent, trans-resveratrol in rats. *Neurosci Lett* 2001; 281:123–126.

135. Inanami O, Watanabe Y, Syuto B, Nakano M, Tsuji M, Kuwabara M. Oral administration of (–)catechin protects against ischemia-reperfusion-induced neuronal death in the gerbil. *Free Radic Res* 1998; 29:359–365.

136. Hara Y. Influence of tea catechins on digestive tract. *J Cell Biochem* 1997; 27(Suppl):52-58.

137. Levites Y, Weinreb O, Maor G, Youdim MBH, Mandel S. Green tea polyphenol (–)-epigallocatechin-3-gallate prevents *N*-methyl-4-phenyl-1,2,3,6-tetrahydropyridine-induced dopaminergic neurodegeneration. *J Neurochem* 2001; 78:1073–1082.

138. Levites Y, Youdim MBH, Maor G, Mandel S. Attenuation of 6-hydroxydopamine (6-OHDA)-induced nuclear factor-kappaB (NF-κB) activation and cell death by tea extracts in neuronal cultures. *Biochem Pharmacol* 2002; 63:21–29.

139. Schroeter H, Williams RJ, Matin R, Iversen L, Rice-Evans CA. Phenolic antioxidants attenuate neuronal cell death following uptake of oxidized low-density lipoprotein. *Free Radic Biol Med* 2000; 29:1222–1233.

140. Bastianetto, S.; Ramassamy, C.; Dore, S.; Christen, Y.; Poirier, J.; Quirion, R. The Ginkgo biloba extract (Egb 761) protects hippocampal neurons against cell death induced by beta-amyloid. *Eur J Neurosci* 2000, 12:1882–1890.

141. Bastianetto S, Zheng W-H, Quirion R. The Ginkgo biloba extract (Egb 761) protects and rescues hippocampal cells against nitric oxide-induced toxicity: involvement of its flavonoid constituents and protein kinase C. *J Neurochem* 2000; 74:2268–2277.

142. Cott J. Natural product formulations in Europe for psychotropic indication. *Psychopharmacol Bull* 1995; 31:745–751.

143. Le Bars P, Katz MM, Berman N, Itil TM, Freedman AM, Schatzberg AF. A placebo-controlled, double blind, randomized trial of an extract of ginkgo biloba for dementia. *JAMA* 1997; 278:1327–1332.

144. Kleijnen J, Knipschild P. Ginkgo biloba. *Lancet* 1992; 340:1136–1139.

145. Pappolla MA, Omar RA, Kim KS, Robakis NK. Immunohistochemical evidence of antioxidative stress in Alzheimer's disease. *Am J Pathol* 1992; 140:621–628.

146. Prasad KD, Cole WC, Hovland AR, Prasad KC, Nahreini P, Kumar B, Edward-Prasad J, Andreatta CP. Multiple antioxidants in the prevention and treatment of neurodegenerative disease: analysis of biologic rationale. *Curr Opin Neurol* 1999; 12:761–770.

147. Smith MA, Hirai K, Hsiao K, Pappolla MA, Harris PLR, Siedlak SL, Tabaton M, Perry G. Amyloid-β deposition in Alzheimer's transgenic mice is associated with oxidative stress. *J Neurochem* 1998; 70:2212–2215.

148. Baeuerle PA, Baltimore D. NF-κB: ten years after. *Cell* 1996; 87: 13–20.

149. Baeuerle PA, Henkel T. Function and activation of NF-κB in the immune system. *Annu Rev Immunol* 1994; 12:141–79.

150. Siebenlist U, Franzoso G, Brown K. Structure, regulation and function of NF-κB. *Annu Rev Cell Biol* 1994; 10:405–455.

151. Kaltschmidt C, Kaltschmidt B, Baeuerle PA. Brain synapses contain inducible forms of the transcription factor NF-κB. *Mech Dev* 1993; 43:135–147.

152. Kaltschmidt C, Kaltschmidt B, Baeuerle PA. Stimulation of ionotropic glutamate receptors activates transcription farctor NF-κB in primary neurons. *Proc Natl Acad Sci USA* 1995; 92:9618–9622.

153. Kaltschmidt C, Kaltschmidt B, Neumann H, Wekerle H, Baeuerle PA. Constitutive NF-κB activity in neurons. *Mol Cell Biol* 1994; 14:3981–3992.

154. O'Neill LAJ, Kaltschmidt C. NF-κB: a crucial transcription factor for glial and neuronal cell function. *Trends Neurosci* 1997; 20:252–258.

155. Bowie A, O'Neill LAJ. Oxidative stress and nuclear factor-κB: a reassessement of the evidence in the light of recent discoveries. *Biochem Pharmacol* 2000, 59:13–23.

156. Carter, BD, Kaltschmidt C, Kaltschmidt B, Offenhauser N, Bohm-Matthei R, Baeuerle PA, Barde YA. Selective activation of NF-κB by nerve growth factor through the neurotrophin receptor p75. *Science* 1996; 272:542–545.

157. Guerrini L, Blasi F, Denis-Donini S. Synaptic activation of NF-κB by glutamate in cerebellar granule neurons *in vitro*. *Proc Natl Acad Sci USA* 1995; 92: 9077–9081.

158. Meyer M, Schreck R, Baeuerle PA. H_2O_2 and antioxidants have opposite effects on activation of NF-κB and AP-1 in intact cells: AP-1 as secondary antioxidant-responsive factor. *EMBO J* 1993; 12:2005–2015.

159. Schreck R, Albermann K, Baeuerle PA. Nuclear factor κB: an oxidative stress-responsive transcription factor of eukaryotic cells (a review). *Free Radic Res Commun* 1992; 17:221–237.

160. Schreck R, Baeuerle PA. A role for oxygen radicals as second messengers. *Trends Cell Biol* 1991; 1:39–42.

161. Schreck R, Meier B, Männel DN, Dröge W, Baeuerle PA. Dithiocarbamates as potent inhibitors of nuclear factor κB activation in intact cells. *J Exp Med* 1992; 175:1181–1194.

162. Schreck R, Rieber P, Baeuerle PA. Reactive oxygen intermediates as apparently widely used messengers in the activation of the NF-κB transcription factor and HIV. *EMBO J* 1991; 8:2247–2258.

163. Schmidt KN, Amstad P, Cerutti P, Baeuerle PA. The roles of hydrogen peroxide and superoxide as messengers in the activation of transcription factor NF-kappa B. *Chem Biol* 1995; 2:13–22.

164. Lin Y-L, Lin J-K. (–)-Epigallocatechin-3-gallate blocks the induction of nitric oxide synthase by down-regulating lipopolysaccharide-induced activity of transcription factor nuclear factor-κB. *J Neurochem* 2001; 52:465–472.

165. Natarajan K, Singh S, Burke TR Jr, Grunberger D, Aggarwal BB. Caffeic acid phenethyl ester is a potent and specific inhibitor of activation of nuclear transcription factor NF-κB. *Proc Natl Acad Sci USA* 1996; 93:9090–9095.

166. Schenk H, Klein M, Erdbrügger W, Dröge W. Distinct effects of thioredoxin and antioxidants on the activation of transcription factors NF-κB and AP-1. *Proc Natl Acad Sci USA* 1994; 91:1672–1676.

167. Yang F, Oz HS, Barve S, De Villiers WJS, McClain CJ, Varilek GW. The green tea polyphenol (–)-epigallocatechin-3-gallate blocks nuclear factor-κB by inhibiting IκB kinase activity in the intestinal epithelial cell line IEC-6. *Mol Pharmacol* 2001; 60:528–533.

168. Amodio R, De Ruvo C, Di Matteo V, Poggi A, Di Santo A, Martelli N, Lorenzet R, Rotilio D, Cacchio M, Esposito E. Caffeic acid phenethyl ester blocks apoptosis in cerebellar granule cells. *Int J Devl Neurosci* 2003; 21:379–398.

169. Manna SK, Zhang HJ, Yan T, Oberly LW, Aggarwal BB. Overexpression of manganese superoxide dismutase suppresses tumor necrosis factor-induced apoptosis and activation of nuclear transcription factor-κB and activated protein-1. *J Biol Chem* 1998; 273:13245–13254.

170. Beg AA, Baltimore D. An essential role for NF-κB in preventing TNF-α-induced cell death. *Science* 1996; 274:782–787.

171. Barger SW, Hörster D, Furukawa K, Goodman Y, Krieglestein J, Mattson MP. Tumor necrosis factors α and β protect neurons against amyloid β-peptide toxicity: evidence for involvement of a κB-binding factor and attenuation of peroxide and Ca^{2+} accumulation. *Proc Natl Acad Sci USA* 1995; 92:9328–3232.

172. Barger SW, Mattson MP. Induction of neuroprotective κB-dependent transcription by secreted forms of the Alzheimer's β-amyloid precursor. *Mol Brain Res* 1996; 40:116–126.

173. Goodman Y, Mattson MP. Ceramide protects hippocampal neurons against excitotoxic and oxidative insults, and amyloid β-peptide toxicity. *J Neurochem* 1996; 66:869–872.

174. Taglialatela G, Robinson R, Perez-Polo JR. Inhibition of nuclear factor κB (NFκB) activity induces nerve growth factor-resistant apoptosis in PC12 cells. *J Neurosci Res* 1997; 47:155–162.

175. Maggiwar SB, Sarmiere PD, Dewhurst S, Freeman RS. Nerve growth factor-dependent activation of NF-κB contributes to survival of sympathetic neurons. *J Neurosci* 1998; 18:10356–10365.

176. Lezoualc'h F, Sagara Y, Holsboer F, Behl C. High constitutive NF-κB activity mediates resistance to oxidative stress in neuronal cells. *J Neurosci* 1998; 18:3224–32.

177. Kaltschmidt B, Uherek M, Wellmann H, Volk B, Kaltschmidt C. Inhibition of NF-κB potentiates amyloid β-mediated neuronal apoptosis. *Proc Natl Acad Sci USA* 1999; 96:9409–9414.

178. Lee H-J, Kim S-H, Kim K-W, Um J-H, Lee HW, Chung B-S, Kang C-D. Anti-apoptotic role of NF-κB in the auto-oxidized dopamine-induced apoptosis of PC12 cells. *J Neurochem* 2001; 76:602–609.

179. Yu ZF, Zhou D, Bruce-Keller AJB, Kindy MS, Mattson MP. Lack of the p50 subunit of nuclear factor-κB increases the vulnerability of hippocampal neurons to excitotoxic injury. *J Neurosci* 1999; 19:8856–8865.

180. Mattson MP, Goodman Y, Luo H, Fu W, Furukawa K. Activation of NF-κB protects hippocampal neurons against oxidative stress-induced apoptosis: evidence for induction of manganese superoxide dismutase and suppression of peroxynitrite production and protein tyrosine nitration. *J Neurosci* Res 1997; 49:681–697.

181. Glazner GW, Camandola S, Mattson MP. Nuclear factor-κB mediates the cell survival-promoting action of activity-dependent neurotrophic factor peptide-9. *J Neurochem* 2000; 75:101–108.

182. Koulich E, Nguyen T, Johnson K, Giardina CA, D'Mello SR. NF-κB is involved in the survival of cerebellar granule neurons: association of IκB phosphorylation with cell survival. *J Neurochem* 2001; 76:1188–1198.

183. Lipsky RH, Xu K, Zhu D, Kelly C, Terhakopian A, Novelli A, Martini AM. Nuclear factor κB is a critical determinant in *N*-methyl-D-aspartate receptor-mediated neuroprotection. *J Neurochem* 2001; 78:254–264.

184. Ravati A, Ahlemeyer B, Becker A, Klumpp S, Krieglstein J. Preconditioning-induced neuroprotection is mediated by reactive oxygen species and activation of the transcription factor nuclear factor-κB. *J Neurochem* 2001; 78:909–919.

185. Lee SJ, Hou J, Benveniste EN. Transcriptional regulation of intercellular adhesion molecule-1 in astrocytes involves NF-κB and C/EPB isoforms. *J Neuroimmunol* 1998; 92:196–207.

186. Taylor BS, de Vera ME, Ganster RW, Wang Q, Shapiro RA, Morris SM Jr, Billiar TR, Geller DA. Multiple NF-κB enhancer elements regulate cytokine induction of the human inducible nitric oxide synthase gene. *J Biol Chem* 1998; 273:15148–15156.

187. Glasgow JN, Wood T, Perez-Polo JR. Identification and characterization of nuclear factor-κB binding sites in the murine *bcl-x* promoter. *J Neurochem* 2000; 75:1377–1389.

188. Zong WX, Edelstein LC, Chen C, Bash J, Gelinas C. The prosurvival Bcl-2 homolog Bfl-1/A is a direct transcriptional target of NF-κB that blocks TNFα-induced apoptosis. *Genes Dev* 1999; 13:382–387.

189. Grilli M, Memo M. Possible role of NF-κB and p53 in the glutamate-induced pro-apoptotic neuronal pathway. *Cell Death Differ* 1999; 6:22–27.

190. Grilli M, Pizzi M, Memo M, Spano P. Neuroprotection by aspirin and sodium salicylate through blockade of NF-κB activation. *Science* 1996; 274:1383–1385.

191. Lipton SA. Janus faces of NF-κB: neurodestruction versus neuroprotection. *Nat Med* 1997; 3:20–21.

192. Panet H, Barzilai A, Daily D, Melamed E, Offen D. Activation of nuclear transcription factor kappa B (NF-κB) is essential for dopamine-induced apoptosis in PC12 cells. *J Neurochem* 2001; 77:391–398.

193. Mayeux P. Epidemiology of neurodegeneration. *Annu Rev Neurosci* 2003; 26:81–104.

194. Helmer C, Joly P, Letenneur L, Commenges D. Mortality with dementia: results from a French perspective. *Am J Epidemiol* 2001; 154: 642–648.

195. Wolfson C, Wolfson DB, Asgharian M, M'Lan CE, Ostbye T, Rockwood K, Hogan DB; Clinical Progression of Dementia Study Group. A reevaluation of the duration of survival after the onset of dementia. *N Engl J Med* 2001; 344:1111–1116.

196. Hofman A, Rocca WA, Brayne C, Breteler MMB, Clarke M, Cooper B, Copeland JRM, Dartigues JF, Da Silva Droux A, Hagnell O, Heeren TJ, Engeland K, Jonker C, Lindesay J, Lobo A, Mann AH, Molsa PK, Morgan K, O'Connor DW, Sulkava R, Kay DWK, Amaducci L. The prevalence of dementia in Europe: a collaborative study of 1980–1990 findings. *Int J Epidemiol* 1991; 20:736–748.

197. Rocca WA, Hofman A, Brayne C, Breteler M, Clarke M, Copeland JRM, Dartigues JF, Engedal K, Hagnell O, Heeren TJ, Jonker C, Lindesay J, Lobo A, Mann AH, Molsa PK, Morgan K, O'Connor DW, Da Silva Droux A, Sulkawa R, Kay DWK, Amaducci L. Frequency and distribution of Alzheimer's disease in Europe: a collaborative study of 1980–1990 prevalence findings. *Ann Neurol* 1991; 30:381–390.

198. Behl C. Alzheimer's disease and oxidative stress: implications for novel therapeutic approaches. *Prog Neurobiol* 1999; 57:301–323.

199. Roses AD. A model for susceptibility polymorphism for complex diseases: apolipoprotein E and Alzheimer's disease. *Neurogenetics* 1997; 1:3–11.

200. Behl C. Vitamin E and other antioxidants in neuroprotection. *Int J Vitam Nutr Res* 1999; 69:213–219.

201. Behl C, Davis JB, Cole GM, Schubert D. Vitamin E protects nerve cells from amyloid β protein toxicity. *Biochem Biophys Res Commun* 1992; 186:944–950.

202. Loo D, Copani A, Pike C, Whittemore E, Walencewicz A, Cotman CW. Apoptosis is induced by β-amyloid in cultured central nervous system neurons. *Proc Natl Acad Sci USA* 1993; 90:7951–7955.

203. Ekinci FJ, Linsley M-D, Shea TB. β-Amyloid-induced calcium influx induces apoptosis by oxidative stress rather than τ phopshorilation. *Brain Res Mol Brain Res* 2000; 76:389–395.

204. Guo Q, Christakos S, Robinson N, Mattson MP. Calbindin blocks the pro-apoptotic actions of mutant presenilin-1: reduced oxidative stress and preserved mitochondrial function. *Proc Natl Acad Sci USA* 1998; 95:3227–3232.

205. Guo Q, Fu W, Holtsberg FW, Steiner SM, Mattson MP. Superoxide mediates the cell-death-enhancing action of presenilin-1 mutations. *J Neurosci Res* 1999; 56:457–470.

206. Guo Q, Sebastian LS, Sopher BL, Miller MW, Ware CB, Martin GM, Mattson MP. Increased vulnerability of hippocampal neurons from presenilin-1 mutant knock-in mice to amyloid β-peptide toxicity: central roles of superoxide production and caspase activation. *J Neurochem* 1999; 72:1019–1029.

207. Keller JN, Pang Z, Geddes JW, Begley JG, Germeyer A, Wang G, Mattson MP. Impairment of glucose and glutamate transport and induction of mitochondrial oxidative stress and dysfunction in synaptosomes by amyloid β-peptide: role of the lipid peroxidation product 4-hydroxynonenal. *J Neurochem* 1997; 69:273–284.

208. Markesbery WR. Oxidative stress hypothesis in Alzheimer's disease. *Free Radic Biol Med* 1997; 23:134–147.

209. Pappolla MA, Chyan Y-J, Omar RA, Hsiao K, Perry G, Smith MA, Bozner P. Evidence of oxidative stress and *in vivo* neurotoxicity of β-amyloid in a transgenic mouse model of Alzheimer's disease: a chronic oxidative paradigm for testing antioxidant therapies *in vivo*. *Am J Pathol* 1998; 152:871–877.

210. Goodman Y, Mattson MP. Secreted forms of β-amyloid precursor protein protect hippocampal neurons against amyloid β-peptide-induced oxidative injury. *Exp Neurol* 1994; 128:1–12.

211. Harris ME, Hensley K, Butterfield A, Leedle R, Carney JM. Direct evidence of oxidative injury produced by the Alzheimer's β-amyloid peptide (1-40) in cultured hippocampal neurons. *Exp Neurol* 1995; 131:193–202.

212. Lucca E, Angeretti N, Forloni G. Influence of cell culture conditions on the protective effect of antioxidants against β-amyloid toxicity: studies with lazaroids. *Brain Res* 1997; 764:293–298.

213. Hensley K, Carney JM, Mattson MP, Aksenova M, Harris M, Wu JF, Floyd RA, Butterfield DA. A model for β-amyloid aggregation and neurotoxicity based on free radical generation by the peptide: relevance to Alzheimer's disese. *Proc Natl Acad Sci USA* 1994; 91:3270–3274.

214. Behl C, Davis JB, Lesley R, Schubert D. Hydrogen peroxide mediates amyloid β protein toxicity. *Cell* 1994; 77:817–822.

215. Mark RJ, Lovell MA, Markesbery WR, Uchida K, Mattson MP. A role of 4-hydroxynonenal, an aldehydic product of lipid peroxidation, in disruption of ion homeostasis and neuronal death induced by β-peptide. *J Neurochem* 1997; 255–264.

216. Lim GP, Chu T, Yang F, Beech W, Frautschy SA, Cole GM. The curry spice curcumin reduces oxidative damage and amyloid pathology in an Alzheimer transgenic mouse. *J Neurosci* 2001; 21:8370–8377.

217. Lockhart BP, Benicourt C, Junien JL, Privat A. Inhibitors of free radical formation fail to attenuate direct beta-amyloid 25-35 peptide-mediated neurotoxicity in rat hippocampal cultures. *J Neurosci Res* 1994; 4:494–505.

218. Aksenov MY, Aksenova MV, Butterfield DA, Geddes JW, Markesbery WR. Protein oxidation in the brain in Alzheimer's disease. *Neuroscience* 2001; 103:273–283.

219. Balazs L, Leon M. Evidence of an oxidative challenge in the Alzheimer's brain. *Neurochem Res* 1994; 19:1131–1137.
220. Lovell MA, Ehmann WD, Butler SM, Markesbery WR. Elevated thiobarbituric acid-reactive substances and antioxidant enzyme activity in the brain in Alzheimer's disease. *Neurology* 1995; 45:1594–1601.
221. Subbarao MA, Richadson JS, Ang LC. Autopsy samples of Alzheimer's cortex show increased peroxidation *in vitro*. *J Neurochem* 1990; 55:342–345.
222. Sano M, Ernesto C, Thomas RG, Klauber M, Schafer K, Grundman M, Woodbury P, Growdon J, Cotman CW, Pfeiffer E, Schneider LS. A controlled trial of selegiline, alpha-tocopherol, or both as treatments for Alzheimer's disease. *N Engl J Med* 1997; 336:1216–1222.
223. Heart Protection Study Collaborative Group. MRC/BHF Heart Protection Study of antioxidant vitamin supplementation in 20,536 high-risk individuals: a randomised placebo-controlled trial. *Lancet* 2002; 60:23–33.
224. Mendelsohn AB, Belle SH, Stoehr GP, Ganguli M. Use of antioxidant supplements and its association with cognitive function in a rural elderly cohort. The MoVIES project. *Am J Epidemiol* 1998; 148:38–44.
225. Jama WJ, Launer LJ, Witterman JCM, den Breeijen JH, Breteler MMB, Grobee DE, Hofman A. Dietary antioxidants and cognitive function in a population-based sample of older persons. The Rotterdam Study. *Am J Epidemiol* 1996; 144:275–280.
226. Luchsinger JA, Tang M-X, Shea S, Mayeux R. Antioxidant vitamin intake and risk of Alzheimer disease. *Arch Neurol* 2003; 60:203–208.
227. Zandi PP, Anthony JC, Khachaturian AS, Stone SV, Gustafson D, Tschanz JT, Norton MC, Welsh-Bohmer KA, Breitner JCS, for the Cache Study Group. Reduced risk of Alzheimer disease in users of antioxidant vitamin supplement. *Arch Neurol* 2004; 61:82–88.
228. Mattson MP. Gene-diet interaction in brain aging and neurogenerative disorders. *Ann Intern Med* 2003; 139:441–444.
229. Wang HX, Wahlin A, Basun H, Fastbom J, Winblad B, Fratiglioni L. Vitamin B(12) and folate in relation to the development of Alzheimer's disease. *Neurology* 2001; 56:1188–1194.
230. Kalmijn S. Fatty acid intake and the risk of dementia and cognitive decline: a review of clinical and epidemiological studies. *J Nutr Health Aging* 2000; 4:202–207.
231. Bourre JM. Dietary omega-3 fatty acids and psychiatry: mood, behaviour, stress, depression, dementia and aging. *J Nutr Health Aging* 2005; 9:31–38.
232. Whalley LJ, Starr JM, Deary IJ. Diet and dementia. *J Br Menopause Soc* 2004; 10:113–117.
233. Lim GP, Calon F, Morihara T, Yang F, Teter B, Ubeda O, Salem N Jr, Frautschy SA, Cole GM. A diet enriched with the omega-3 fatty acid docosahexaenoic acid reduces amyloid burden in an aged Alzheimer's mouse model. *J Neurosci* 2005; 25:3032–3040.
234. Pope SK, Shue VM, Beck C. Will a healthy lifestyle help prevent Alzheimer's disease? *Annu Rev Public Health* 2003; 24:111–132.
235. Young D, Lawlor PA, Leone P, Dragunow M, During MJ. Environmental enrichment inhibits spontaneous apoptosis, prevents seizures and is neuroprotective. *Nat Med* 1999; 5:448–453.

236. Lee J., Duan W, Mattson MP. Evidence that brain-derived neuritrophic factor is required for basal neurogenesis and mediates, in part, the enhancement of neurogenesis by dietary restriction in the hippocampus of adult mice. *J Neurochem* 2002, 82:1367–1375.

237. Jellinger K. Pathology of Parkinson's disease. In Calne DB, Ed. *Handbook of Experimental Pharmacology*, vol 8. Berlin: Springer, 1989. p. 47–112.

238. Scherman D, Desnos C, Darchen F, Pollak P, Javoy-Agid F, Agid Y. Striatal dopamine deficiency in Parkinson's disease: role of aging. *Ann Neurol* 1989; 26:551–557.

239. Ebadi M, Srinivasan SK, Baxi MD. Oxidative stress and antioxidant therapy in Parkinson's disease. *Progr Neurobiol* 1996; 48:1–19.

240. Bower JH, Maragonore DM, McDonnell SK, Rocca WA. Incidence and distribution of Parkinsonism in Olmsted County, Minnesota, 1976-1990. *Neurology* 1999; 52:1214–1220.

241. Baldereschi M, Di Carlo A, Rocca WA, Vanni P, Maggi S, Perissinotto E, Grigoletto F, Amaducci L, Inzitari D. Parkinson's disease and Parkinsonism in a longitudinal study: two-fold higher incidence in men. ILSA Working Group. Italian Longitudinal Study on Aging. *Neurology* 2000; 55:1358–1563.

242. de Rijk MC, Launer LJ, Berger K, Breteler MM, Dartigues JF, Baldereschi M, Fratiglioni L, Lobo A, Martinez-Lage J, Trenkwalder C, Hofman A. Prevalence of Parkinson's disease in Europe: a collaborative study of population-based cohorts. Neurologic Diseases in the Elderly Research Group. *Neurology* 2000; 54 (11 Suppl 5): S21–S23.

243. Elbaz A, Bower JH, Maraganore DM, McDonnell SK, Peterson BJ, Ahlskog JE, Schaid DJ, Rocca WA. Risk tables for Parkinsonism and Parkinson's disease. *J Clin Epidemiol* 2002; 55:25–31.

244. Golbe L. The genetics of Parkinson's disease: a reconsideration. *Neurology* 1990; 40:7–14.

245. Olanow CW, Tatton WG. Etiology and pathogenesis of Parkinson's disease. *Annu Rev Neurosci* 1999; 22:123–144.

246. Gasser T. Genetics of Parkinson's disease. *Ann Neurol* 1998; 44:S53–S57.

247. Brooks DJ. The early diagnosis of Parkinson's disease. *Ann Neurol* 1998; 44(Suppl), S19–S31.

248. Polymeropoulos MH, Lavedan C, Leroy E, Ide SE, Dehejia A, Dutra A, Pike B, Root H, Rubenstein J, Boyer R, Stenroos ES, Chandrasekharappa S, Athanassiadou A, Papapetropoulos T, Johnson WG, Lazzarini AM, Duvoisin RC, Di Iorio G, Golbe LI, Nussbaum RL. Mutation in the alpha-synuclein gene identified in families with Parkinson's disease. *Science* 1997; 276:2045–2007.

249. Teive HA, Raskin S, Iwamoto FM, Germiniani FM, Baran MH, Werneck LC, Allan N, Quagliato E, Leroy E, Ide SE, Polymeropoulos MH. The G209A mutation in the alpha-synuclein gene in Brazilian families with Parkinson's disease. *Arq Neuropsiquiatr* 2001; 59:722–724.

250. Kruger R, Kuhn W, Muller T, Woitalla D, Graeber M, Kosel S, Przuntek H, Epplen JT, Schols L, Riess O. Ala30Pro mutation in the gene encoding alpha-synuclein in Parkinson's disease. *Nat Genet* 1998; 18:106–108.

251. Kitada T, Asakawa S, Hattori N, Matsumine H, Yamamura Y, Minoshima S, Yokochi M, Mizuno Y, Shimizu N. Mutations in the parkin gene cause autosomal recessive juvenile Parkinsonism. *Nature* 1998; 392:605–608.

252. Lim KL, Dawson VL, Dawson TM. The genetics of Parkinson's disease. *Curr Neurol Neurosci Rep* 2002; 2:439–446.
253. Langston JW Epidemiology versus genetics in Parkinson's disease: progress in resolving an age-old debate. *Ann Neurol* 1998; 44:(Suppl) S45–S52.
254. Tanner CM, Langston J.W. Do environmental toxins cause Parkinsons's disease? A critical review. *Neurology* 1990; 40:17–30.
255. Hornykiewicz O. Aging and neurotoxins as causative factors in idiopathic Parkinson's disease — a critical analysis of the neurochemical evidence. *Prog Neuropsychopharmacol Biol Psychiatry* 1989; 13:319–328.
256. Langston JW, Ballard PA, Tetrud JW, Irwin I. Chronic Parkinsonism in humans due to a product of meperidine analog synthesis. *Science* 1983; 219:979–980.
257. Nicklas WJ, Vyas I, Heikkila RE. Inhibition of NADH-linked oxidation in brain mitochondria by 1-methyl-4-phenyl-pyridine, a metabolite of the neurotoxin 1-methyl-4-phenyl-1,2,5,6-tetrahydropyridine. *Life Sci* 1985; 36:2503–2508.
258. Forno L. The Lewy body in Parkinson's disease. *Adv Neurol* 1986; 45:35–43.
259. Hornykiewicz O. Neurochemical pathology and the etiology of Parkinson's disease: basic facts and hypothetical possibilities. *Mt Sinai J Med* 1988; 55:11–20.
260. Jellinger K. An overview of morphological changes in Parkinson's disease. *Adv Neurol* 1986; 45:1–16.
261. Louis ED, Goldman JE, Powers JM, Fahn S. Parkinsonism features of eight pathologically diagnosed cases of diffuse Lewy body disease. *Mov Disord* 1995; 10:188–194.
262. Jenner P, Dexter DT, Sian J, Schapira AHV, Marsden CD. Oxidative stress as a cause of nigral cell death in Parkinson's disease and incident Lewy body disease. *Ann Neurol* 1992; 32:582–587.
263. Dexter DT, Carayon A, Javoy-Agid F, Agid Y, Wells SE, Jenner P, Marsden C. Alterations in the levels of iron, ferritin and other trace metals in Parkinson's disease and other neurodegenerative diseases affecting the basal ganglia. *Brain* 1991; 114:1953–1975.
264. Tipton KF, Singer TP. Advances in our understanding of the mechanisms of the neurotoxicity of MPTP and related compounds. *J Neurochem* 1993; 61:1191–1206.
265. Bindoff LA, Birch-Machin M, Cartlidge NEF, Parker WD Jr, Turnbull DM. Mitochondrial function in Parkinson's disease. *Lancet* 1989; 2:49.
266. Hattori N, Tanaka M, Ozawa T, Mizuno Y. Immunohistochemical studies on complexes I, II, III, and IV of mitochondria in Parkinson's disease. *Ann Neurol* 1991; 30:563–571.
267. Parker WD Jr, Boyson SJ, Park JK. Abnormalities of the electron transport chain in idiopathic Parkinson's disease. *Ann. Neurol* 1989; 26:719–723.
268. Schapira AHV, Cooper JM, Dexter D, Clark JB, Jenner P, Marsden CD. Mitochondrial complex I deficiency in Parkinson's disease. *J Neurochem* 1990; 54:823–827.
269. Krige D, Carroll MT, Cooper JM, Marsden CD, Schapira AHV. Platelet mitochondrial function in Parkinson's disease. *Ann Neurol* 1992; 32:782–788.
270. DiMonte DA, Sandy MS, Jewell SA, Adornato B, Tanner CM, Langston JW. Oxidative phosphorylation by intact muscle mitochondria in Parkinson's disease. *Neurodegeneration* 1993; 2:275–281.

271. Schapira AHV, Mann VM, Cooper JM, Dexter D, Daniel SE, Jenner P, Clark JB, Marsden CD. Anatomic and disease specificity of NADH CoQ$_1$ reductase (complex I) deficiency in Parkinson's disease. *J Neurochem* 1990; 55:2142–2145.

272. Betarbet R, Sherer TB, Mackenzie G, Garcia-Osuna M, Panov AV, Greenamyre T. Chronic systemic pesticide exposure reproduces features of Parkinson's disease. *Nat Neurosci* 2000; 3:1301–1306.

273. Dexter DT, Wells FR, Lees AJ, Agid F, Agid P, Jenner P, Marsden CD. Increased nigral iron content and alterations in other metal ions occurring in the brain in Parkinson's disease. *J Neurochem* 1989; 52:1830–1836.

274. Hirsch EC, Brandel J-P, Galle P, Javoy-Agid F, Agid Y. Iron and aluminum increase in the substantia nigra of patients with Parkinson's disease: an x-ray microanalysis. *J Neurochem* 1991; 56:446–451.

275. Riederer P, Sofic E, Rausch W-D, Schmidt B, Reynolds GP, Jellinger K, Youdim BH. Transition metals, ferritin, glutathione, and ascorbic acid in Parkinsonian brains. *J Neurochem* 1989; 52:515–520.

276. Pearce RKB, Owen A, Daniel S, Jenner P, Marsden CD. Alterations in the distribution of glutathione in the substantia nigra in Parkinson's disease. *J Neural Transm* 1997; 104:661–677.

277. Perry TL, Godin D, Hansen S. Parkinson's disease: a disorder due to nigral glutathione deficiency? *Neurosci Lett* 1982; 33:305–310.

278. Sian J, Dexter DT, Lees AJ, Daniel S, Agid Y, Javoy-Agid F, Jenner P, Marsden CD. Alterations in glutathione levels in Parkinson's disease and other neurodegenerative disorders affecting basal ganglia. *Ann Neurol* 1994; 36:348–355.

279. Sian J, Dexter DT, Lees AJ, Daniel S, Jenner P, Marsden CD. Glutathione-related enzymes in brain in Parkinson's disease. *Ann Neurol* 1994; 36:356–361.

280. Sofic E, Lange KW, Jellinger K, Riederer P. Reduced and oxidized glutathione in the substantia nigra of patients with Parkinson's disease. *Neurosci Lett* 1992; 142:128–130.

281. Dexter DT, Sian J, Rose S, Hindmarsh JG, Mann VM, Cooper JM, Wells FR, Daniel SE, Lees AJ, Schapira AHV, Jenner P, Marsden CD. Indices of oxidative stress and mitochondrial function in individuals with incidental Lewy body disease. *Ann Neurol* 1994; 35:38–44.

282. Dexter DT, Carter CJ, Wells FR, Javoy-Agid F, Agid Y, Lees A, Jenner P, Marsden CD. Basal lipid peroxidation in substantia nigra is increased in Parkinson's disease. *J Neurochem* 1989; 52:381–389.

283. Dexter DT, Holley AE, Flitter WD, Slater TF, Wells FR, Daniel S, Lees AJ, Marsden CD. Increased levels of lipid hydroperoxides in the Parkinsonian substantia nigra: an HPLC and ESR study. *Mov Disord* 1994; 9:92–97.

284. Sanchez-Ramos J, Overik E, Ames BN. A marker of oxyradical-mediated DNA damage (8-hydroxy-2'deoxyguanosine) is increased in nigro-striatum of Parkinson's disease brain. *Neurodegeneration* 1994; 3:197–204.

285. Yurek DM, Sladek JR. Dopamine cell replacement: Parkinson's disease. *Annu Rev Neurosci* 1990; 13:415–440.

286. Hagglund J, Aquilonius SM, Erkernas SM, Harving P, Lundquist H, Gullberg P, Langstrom B. Dopamine receptor properties in Parkinson's disease and Huntington's chorea evaluated by positron emission tomography using C-N-methyl-spiperone. *Acta Neurol Scand* 1987; 75:87–94.

287. Rinne UK, Rinne JO, Laasko K, Laihinen A, Lonnberg P. Brain receptor changes in Parkinson's disease in relation to the disease process and treatment. *J Neural Transm* 1983; 18:279–286.

288. Agid Y, Ruberg M, Javoy-Agid F, Hirsch E, Raisman-Vozari R, Vyas S, Faucheux B, Michel P, Kastner A, Blanchard V, Damier P, Villares J, Zhang P. Are dopaminergic neurons selectively vulnerable to Parkinson's disease? *Adv Neurol* 1993; 60:148–164.

289. Spina MB, Cohen G. Dopamine turnover and glutathione oxidation: implications for Parkinson's disease. *Proc Natl Acad Sci USA* 1989; 86:1398–1400.

290. Mena MA, Pardo B, Casarejos MJ, Fahn S, de Yebenes JG. Neurotoxicity of levodopa on catecholamine-rich neurons. *Mov Disord* 1992; 7:23–31.

291. Spencer Smith T, Parker WD Jr, Bennett JP Jr. L-DOPA increases nigral production of hydroxyl radicals *in vivo*: potential L-DOPA toxicity? *NeuroReport* 1994; 5:1006–1011.

292. Graham DG, Tiffany SM, Bell WR, Gutknecht WF. Autoxidation versus covalent binding of quinones as the mechanism of toxicity of dopamine, 6-hydroxydopamine, and related compounds toward C1300 neuroblastoma cells *in vitro*. *Mol Pharmacol* 1978; 14:644–653.

293. Wick M, Byers L, Frey E. L-DOPA: selective toxicity for melanoma cells *in vitro*. *Science* 1977; 197:468–469.

294. Hiramatsu M, Kohno M, Mori A, Shiraga H, Pfeiffer RF, Ebadi M. An ESR study of 6-hydroxydopamine: generated hydroxy radicals and superoxide anions in brain. *Neurosciences* 1994; 20:129–138.

295. Golbe LL, Langston JW, Shoulson I. Selegiline and Parkinson's disease: protective and symptomatic consideration. *Drugs* 1990; 39:646–651.

296. Heikkila RE, Manzino L, Duvoisin RC, Cabbat FS. Protection against the dopaminergic neurotoxicity of 1-methyl-4-phenyl-1,2,3,6-tetrahydropyridine by monoamine oxidase inhibitors. *Nature* 1984; 311:467–469.

297. Blum D, Torch S, Nisoou M-F, Verna J-M. 6-hydroxydopamine-induced nuclear factor-kappaB activation in PC12 cells. *Biochem Pharmacol* 2001; 62:473–481.

298. Burke R.E, Kholodilov NG. Programmed cell death: does it play a role in Parkinson's disease? *Ann Neurol* 1998; 44:S126–S133.

299. Tatton NA, Maclean-Fraser A, Tatton WG, Perl DP, Olanow CW. A fluorescent double-labeling method to detect and confirm apoptotic nuclei in Parkinson's disease. *Ann. Neurol* 1998; 44(Suppl):S142–S148.

300. Marsden CD, Olanow CW. The causes of Parkinson's disease are being unraveled and rational neuroprotective therapy is close to reality. *Ann Neurol* 1998; 44(Suppl):S189–S196.

301. Fearnley JM, Lees AJ. Aging and Parkinson's disease: substantia nigra regional selectivity. *Brain* 1991; 114:2283–2301.

302. Parkinson Study Group. Mortality in DATATOP: a multicenter trial in early Parkinson's disease. *Ann Neurol* 1998; 43:318–325.

303. Shoulson I. DATATOP: a decade of neuroprotective inquiry. *Ann Neurol* 1998; 44:S160–S166.

304. The Parkinson's Study Group. Effects of tocopherol and deprenyl on the progression of disability in early Parkinson's disease. *N Engl J Med* 1993; 328:176–183.

305. Wu R-M, Chiueh CC, Pert A, Murphy DL. Apparent antioxidant effect of l-deprenyl on hydroxyl radical formation and nigral injury elicited by MPP+ *in vivo*. *Eur J Pharmacol* 1993; 243:241–247.

306. Keller WC. Neuroprotection for Parkinson's disease. *Ann Neurol* 1998; 44(Suppl):S155–S159.

307. Fahn S. An open trial of high-dosage antioxidants in early Parkinson's disease. *Am J Clin Nutr* 1991; 53:380S–382S.

308. Ogawa N, Tanaka K, Asanuma M, Kawai M, Masumizu T, Kohno M, Mori A. Bromocriptine protects mice against 6-hydroxydopamine and scavenges hydroxyl free radicals *in vitro*. *Brain Res* 1994; 657:207–213.

309. Olanow CW, Jenner P, Brooks D. Dopamine agonists and neuroprotection in Parkinson's disease. *Ann Neurol* 1998; 44(Suppl):S167–S174.

310. Schapira AHV. Neuroprotection and dopamine agonists. *Neurology* 2002; 58(Suppl 1):S9–S18.

311. Sawada H, Ibi M, Kihara T, Urushitani M, Akaike A, Kimura J, Shimohama S. Dopamine D2-type agonism protect mesencephalic neurons from glutamate neurotoxicity: mechanisms of neuroprotective treatment against oxidative stress. *Ann Neurol* 1998; 44:110–119.

312. Rowland LT. Amyotrophic lateral sclerosis. *Curr Opin Neurol* 1994; 7:310–315.

313. Tandan R, Bradley WG. Amyotrophic lateral sclerosis: part 1. Clinical features, pathology, and ethical issues in management. *Ann Neurol* 1985; 18:271–280.

314. Cudkowicz ME, McKenna-Yasek D, Sapp PE, Chin W, Geller B, Hayden DL, Schoenfeld DA, Hosler BA, Horvitz HR, Brown RH. Epidemiology and mutations in superoxide dismutase in amyotrophic lateral sclerosis. *Ann Neurol* 1997; 41:210–221.

315. Deng HX, Hentati A, Tainer JA, Iqbal Z, Cayabyab A, Hung W-Y, Getzoff ED, Hu P, Herzfeldt B, Roos RP, Warner C, Deng G, Soriano E, Smyth C, Parge HE, Ahmed A, Roses AD, Hallewell RA, Pericak-Vance M, Siddique T. Amyotrophic lateral sclerosis and structural defects in Cu,Zn superoxide dismutase. *Science* 1993; 261:1047–1051.

316. Siddique T, Nijhawan D, Hentati A. Molecular genetic basis of familial ALS. *Neurology* 1996; 47(Suppl):27–35.

317. Dal Canto M, Gurney ME. Neuropathological changes in two lines of mice carrying a transgene for mutant human Cu,Zn SOD, and in mice overexpressing wild type human SOD: a model of familial amyotrophic lateral sclerosis. *Brain Res* 1995; 676:25–40.

318. Ghadge GD, Lee JP, Bindokas VP, Jordan J, Ma L, Miller RJ, Roos RP. Mutant superoxide dismutase-1-linked familial amyotrophic lateral sclerosis: molecular mechanisms of neuronal death and protection. *J Neurosci* 1997; 17:8756–8766.

319. Gurney ME, Pu H, Chiu AY, Dal Canto MC, Polchow CY, Alexander DD, Caliendo J, Hentati A, Kwon YW, Deng H-X, Chen W, Zhai P, Sufit RL, Siddique T. Motor neuron degeneration in mice that express a human Cu, Zn superoxide dismutase mutation. *Science* 1994; 264:1772–1775.

320. Wong PC, Pardo CA, Borchelt DR, Lee MK, Copeland NG, Jenkins NA, Sisodia SS, Cleveland DW, Price DL. An adverse property of familial ALS-linked SOD-1 mutations causes motor neuron disease characterized by vacuolar degeneration of mitochondria. *Neuron* 1995; 14:1105–1116.

321. Bowling AC, Schulz JB, Brown RH Jr, Beal MF. Superoxide dismutase activity, oxidative damage, and mitochondrial energy metabolism in familial and sporadic amyotrophic lateral sclerosis. *J Neurochem* 1993; 61:2322–2325.

322. Rabizadeh S, Gralla EB, Borchelt DR, Gwinn R, Valentine JS, Sisodia S, Wong P, Lee M, Hahn H, Bredesen DE. Mutations associated with amyotrophic lateral sclerosis convert superoxide dismutase from an antiapoptotic gene to a proapoptotic gene: studies in yeast and neural cells. *Proc Natl Acad Sci USA* 1995; 92:3024–3028.

323. Lee MH, Hyum D-H, Halliwell B, Jenner P. Effect of overexpression of wild-type mutant Cu/Zn-superoxide dismutases on oxidative stress and cell death induced by hydrogen peroxide, 4-hydroxynonenal or serum deprivation: potentiation of injury by ALS-related mutant superoxide dismutases and prevention by Bcl-2. *J Neurochem* 2001; 78: 209–220.

324. Przedborski S, Jackson-Lewis V, Kostic V, Carlson E, Epstein CJ, Cadet JL. Superoxide dismutase, catalase, and glutathione peroxidase activities in copper/zinc-superoxide dismutase transgenic mice. *J Neurochem* 1992; 58:1760–1767.

325. Borchelt D.R, Lee MK, Slunt HS, Guarnieri M, Xu Z-S, Wong PC, Brown RH, Price DL, Sisodia SS, Cleveland DW. Superoxide dismutase 1 with mutations linked to familial amyotrophic lateral sclerosis possess significant activity. *Proc Natl Acad Sci USA* 1994; 91:8292–8296.

326. McCord JM. Mutant mice, CuZn superoxide dismutase, and motor neuron degeneration. *Science* 1995; 266:1586–1587.

327. Wiedau-Pazos M, Goto JJ, Rabizadeh S, Gralla EB, Roe JA, Lee MK, Valentine JS, Bredesen DE. Altered reactivity of superoxide dismutase in familial amyotrophic lateral sclerosis. *Science* 1996; 271:515–517.

328. Bogdanov M, Ramos LE, Xu Z, Beal FM. Elevated "hydroxyl radical" generation *in vivo* in an animal model of amyotrophic lateral sclerosis. *J Neurochem* 1998; 71:1321–24.

329. Hall ED, Andrus PK, Oostveen JA, Fleck TJ, Gurney ME. Relationship of oxygen radical-induced lipid peroxidative damage to disease onset and progression in a transgenic model of familial ALS. *J Neurosci Res* 1998; 53:66–77.

330. Liu D, Wen J, Liu J, Li L. The roles of free radicals in amyotrophic lateral sclerosis: reactive oxygen species and elevated oxidation of protein, DNA, and membrane phospholipids. *FASEB J* 1999; 13:2318–2328.

331. Bogdanov M, Brown RH, Matson W, Smart R, Hayden D, O'Donnell H, Beal MF, Cudkowicz M. Increased oxidative damage to DNA in ALS patients. *Free Radic Biol Med* 2000; 29:652–658.

332. Crow JP, Sampson JB, Zhuang Y, Thompson JA, Beckman JS. Decreased zinc affinity of amyotrophic superoxide dismutase mutants leads to enhanced catalysis of tyrosine nitration by peroxynitrite. *J Neurochem* 1997; 69:1936–1944.

333. Pedersen WA, Fu W, Keller JN, Markesbery WR, Appel S, Smith RG, Kasarkis E, Mattson MP. Protein modification by the lipid peroxidation product 4-hydroxynonenal in the spinal cords of amyotrophic lateral sclerosis patients. *Ann Neurol* 1998; 44:819–824.

334. Aguirre T, Van Den Bosch L, Goetshalckx K, Tilkin P, Mathijs G, Cassiman JJ, Robberecht W. Increased sensitivity of fibroblasts from amyotrophic lateral sclerosis patients to oxidative stress. *Ann. Neurol.* 1998; 43:452–457.

335. Hudson AJ. Amyotrophic lateral sclerosis and its association with dementia, Parkinsonism and other neurological disorders: a review. *Brain* 1981; 104:217–247.

336. Kostic V, Gurney ME, Deng H-X, Siddique T, Epstein CJ, Przedborski S. Midbrain dopaminergic neuronal degeneration in a transgenic mouse model of familial amyotrophic lateral sclerosis. *Ann Neurol* 1997; 41:497–504.

337. Poduslo JF, Whelan SL, Curran GL, Wengenack TM. Therapeutic benefit of polyamine-modified catalase as a scavenger of hydrogen peroxide and nitric oxide in familial amyotrophic lateral sclerosis transgenics. *Ann Neurol* 2000; 48:943–947.

338. Reinholz MM, Merkle CM, Poduslo JF. Therapeutic benefits of putrescine-modified catalase in a transgenic mouse model of familial amyotrophic lateral sclerosis. *Exp Neurol* 1999; 159:204–216.

339. Andreassen OA, Dedeoglu A, Friedlich A, Ferrante KL, Hughes D, Szabo C, Beal MF. Effects of an inhibitor of poly(ADP-ribose) polymerase, desmethylselegiline, trientine, and lipoic acid in transgenic ALS mice. *Exp Neurol* 2001; 168:419–424.

340. Andreassen OA, Dedeoglu A, Klivenyi P, Beal MF, Bush AI. N-acetyl-L-cysteine improves survival and preserves motor performance in an animal model of familial amyotrophic lateral sclerosis. *Neuroreport* 2000; 11:2491–243.

341. Dugan LL, Lovett EG, Quick KL, Lotharius J, Lin TT, O'Malley KL. Fullerene-based antioxidants and neurodegenerative disorders. *Parkinsonism Relat Disord* 2001; 7:243–246.

342. Gurney ME, Cutting FB, Zhai P, Doble A, Taylor C, Andrus PK, Hall ED. Benefit of vitamin E, riluzole, and gabapentin in a transgenic model of familial amyotrophic lateral sclerosis. *Ann Neurol* 1996; 39:147–157.

343. Bensimon G, Lacomblez L, Meininger V and the ALS/riluzole study group. A controlled trial of riluzole in amyotrophic lateral sclerosis. *N Engl J Med* 1994; 330:585-591.

344. Koh J-Y, Kim D-K, Hwang JY, Kim YI, Seo JH. Antioxidative and proapoptotic effects of riluzole on cultured cortical neurons. *J Neurochem* 1999; 72:716–723.

345. Desnuelle C, Dib M, Garrel C, Favier A. A double-blind, placebo-controlled randomized clinical trial of alpha-tocopherol (vitamin E) in the treatment of amyotrophic lateral sclerosis. ALS riluzole-tocopherol Study Group. *Amyotroph Lateral Scler Other Motor Neuron Disord.* 2001; 2:9–18.

346. Lange DJ, Murphy PL, Diamond B, Appel V, Lai EC, Younger DS, Appel SH. Selegiline is ineffective in a collaborative double-blind, placebo-controlled trial for treatment of amyotrophic lateral sclerosis. *Arch Neurol* 1998; 55:93–96.

347. Vyth A, Timmer JG, Bossuyt PM, Louwerse ES, de Jong JM. Survival in patients with amyotrophic lateral sclerosis, treated with an array of antioxidants. *J Neurol Sci* 1996; 139 Suppl:99–103.

348. Li M, Ona VO, Guégan C, Chen M, Jackson-Lewis V, Andrews LJ, Olszewski AJ, Stieg PE, Lee J-P, Przedborski S, Friedlander RM. Functional role of caspase-1 and caspase-3 in an ALS transgenic mouse model. *Science* 2000; 288:335–339.

349. Esposito E, Rossi C, Amodio R, Di Castelnuovo A, Bendotti C, Rotondo T, Algeri S, Rotilio D. Lyophilized red wine administration prolongs survival in an animal model of amyotrophic lateral sclerosis. *Ann Neurol* 2000; 48:686–687.

350. Sano M. Do dietary antioxidants prevent Alzheimer's disease? *Lancet Neurol* 2002; 1:342.

351. Lemon JA, Boreham DR, Rollo CD. A dietary supplement abolishes age-related cognitive decline in transgenic mice expressing elevated free radical processes. *Exp Biol Med* 2003; 228:800–810.

352. Gash DM, Zhang Z, Gerhardt G. Neuroprotective and neurorestorative properties of GDNF. *Ann Neurol* 1998; 44:S121–S125.

6 Nutrients and Herbals in the Pharmacotherapy of Unipolar/Major Depression

Matthew Chronowic

CONTENTS

6.1 INTRODUCTION

Approximately 7% of the North American population is currently affected by mood disorders.[1] The bouts of depression and mania that characterize these conditions cause a great deal of morbidity and increase the risk of mortality, ranking these disorders among the top 10 causes of disability.[1] Therefore, effective treatment options are of the utmost importance to increase quality of life for these individuals, as well as to increase the labor capacity of the work force. Originally the domain of the psychiatrist, the pharmacotherapy of these disorders is now often in the hands of the general physician. This requires considerable knowledge of the disease processes and appropriate pharmacotherapy choices by healthcare professionals.

Understanding the biological basis of these mood disorders has been a difficult process and a good deal of research continues in this area today. As our understanding has grown, so too has the wide range of pharmaceuticals available to treat these disorders. With such a broad spectrum of pharmaceuticals to choose from, it is not only important to understand how the drugs may interact with one another, but also to understand how nutrition and diet can affect pharmacotherapy. Nutritional augmentation of a drug regimen could have the potential to decrease the dose of medication required, subsequently lessening the adverse side effects that are common to most pharmaceuticals. Conversely, nutrition also has the capacity to affect the metabolism of drugs, resulting in a lesser or greater efficacy, which would require compensatory dosing by the prescribing physician. Therefore, it is the aim of this chapter to present some of the observed drug–nutrient interactions that have been noted in the pharmacotherapy of unipolar depression.

6.2   UNIPOLAR DEPRESSION

The most prominent hypothesis of the etiology of unipolar depression, or major depressive disorder, is the idea that a deficit of monoamine neurotransmission underlies the disorder; specifically a lack of norepinephrine and serotonin (5-hydroxytryptamine or 5-HT) neurotransmission. Despite being relatively few in number (<1 in 200,000), monoaminergic neurons send axonal branches throughout the brain and likely act through G-protein coupled receptors to alter overall brain activity.[1] Our current understanding of the disease does extend beyond this simple model, but it is evident that pharmacologically elevating monoamines do have the capacity to elevate mood in many individuals affected by this disorder.[2] Furthermore, it is mainly in the context of this simple model that we understand the mechanistic basis of the current pharmaceuticals used to treat depression.

The first class of drugs developed to treat unipolar depression was the monoamine oxidase inhibitors (MAOIs), introduced in the mid 1950s. As the name suggests, these drugs have the capacity to inhibit the enzyme, monoamine oxidase. This enzyme, found at high concentrations in neurons and liver cells, degrades monoamine neurotransmitters. By inhibiting this process, the amount of monoamine neurotransmitters is increased in the synaptic cleft, resulting in a subsequent increase in monoaminergic neurotransmission. However, this class of drugs can be quite dangerous if combined with substances that further increase the amount of serotonin in the synaptic cleft, leading to a condition known as the serotonin syndrome.[2] This syndrome is characterized by altered mental status, agitation, diaphoresis, hyperthermia, and hypertonicity, putting the individual in grave danger.[2] Clinically, this syndrome causes mental, autonomic, and neurological disorders that appear very suddenly, often less than 24 hours after the offending substance is taken.[3] Also, there are a number of foods that must be avoided when taking MAOIs, which, if consumed, could result in hypertensive crisis. This will be discussed in greater detail below. Due to the significant risks associated with these pharmaceuticals, they are often a last line of defense used in treatment-resistant depression. The current MAOIs in use are phenelzine and tranylcypromine.[2]

Also brought onto the market in the 1950s were the tricyclic antidepressants, which are a major class of drugs used to treat depression. This class of drugs works by nonselectively blocking the reuptake of monoamines. Reuptake is a mechanism that prevents over-stimulation of the postsynaptic neuron by bringing neurotransmitters back into the presynaptic neuron. By nonselectively blocking monoamine reuptake, the concentrations of serotonin, norepinephrine, epineph- rine, and dopamine are all increased in the synaptic cleft. Consequently, a number of different monoamine receptors are activated both in the brain and many other tissues where receptors are expressed. This lack of selectivity explains why the tricyclic antidepressants are associated with a plethora of side effects: drowsiness, dry mouth, urinary retention, constipation, blurred vision, low blood pressure, weight gain, and cardiac effects.[2] The current tricyclic antidepressants in use include amitriptyline, clomipramine, desipramine, nortriptyline, and imipramine.[2]

A major development in unipolar depression pharmacotherapy was the intro- duction of selective serotonin reuptake inhibitors (SSRIs) in the 1980s. This class of drugs also works by inhibiting the reuptake of neurotransmitters; however, it differs from tricyclic antidepressants in that it is selective only for serotonin. By binding only to the serotonin reuptake transporter protein, there is an increase in serotonin in the synaptic cleft, but the other monoamine concentrations remain unchanged. This property of the SSRIs results in fewer side effects than the tricyclic antidepressants, although several are still observed, including nausea, nervousness, insomnia, sexual dysfunction, and headache.[2] Given the increased selectivity and decreased severity of side effects, SSRIs (fluoxetine, sertraline, paroxetine, citalopram, and escitalopram) are usually the first-line therapy in unipolar depression.[2]

Similar to the SSRIs, another class of drugs named the serotonin and nore- pinephrine reuptake inhibitors (SNRIs), which block the reuptake of both sero- tonin and norepinephrine, were developed for the treatment of unipolar depres- sion. The SNRIs still have fewer side effects than tricyclic antidepressants and are more efficacious in some individuals than the SSRIs. However, there is some risk of hypertension as well as other side effects with the SNRIs (venlafaxine and duloxetine), which requires the doctor's consideration when prescribing.[2]

Finally, the last class of drugs used for the treatment of unipolar depression is the atypical antidepressants. They fall outside the four aforementioned catego- ries due to differences in both structure and function. Some operate by weakly inhibiting reuptake of specific neurotransmitters, some by inhibiting neurotrans- mitter receptors directly, whereas the mechanisms of others still remain to be clarified. These mechanisms will be elaborated upon as needed in the following sections. In line with the other classes of drugs, the atypical antidepressants, mirtazapine, bupropion and trazodone, are also associated with a range of side effects.[2]

There are a few problems with the monoamine theory of unipolar depression. First of all, it cannot account for the fact that antidepressant drugs produce their biochemical effects within minutes or hours, yet the onset of therapeutic benefit usually takes weeks. Furthermore, the severity of the depressive state and the amount of monoamine depletion do not necessarily correlate.[4] Our knowledge of intracellular signaling has drastically improved over the past decade, and accumulating evidence seems to suggest that protein phosphorylation is part of the long-term mechanism of antidepressants.[4] Evidence has shown that various antidepressants can alter both the activity and translocation of second-messenger regulated protein kinases; in particular, protein kinase C (PKC), cyclic AMP-dependent protein kinase (PKA), and Ca^{2+}/calmodulin-dependent protein kinase II (CaMKII).[4] Increasing activation of protein kinases allows for increased phosphorylation of certain subcellular components (of particular interest are microtubule-associated protein 2 [MAP2] and synaptotagmin) that may consequently affect cytoskeleton remodeling, a process involved in neurotransmitter release.[4] This new theory of the mechanistic basis of antidepressant action continues to develop at a rapid pace and shows great promise at aiding in the development of more effective antidepressants as well as furthering our understanding of the etiology of the disease.

Another theory that accounts for the temporal discrepancy between the biochemical and clinical effects of antidepressants is the idea that these compounds decrease N-methyl-D-aspartate (NMDA) receptor function. This is supported by the observation that chronic (14 day) administration, but not acute (1 day), of 17 different antidepressants produces adaptive changes in the binding of radioligand to NMDA receptors in a mouse model.[5] This is an interesting finding as it corresponds quite well with the time course required for the clinical benefit of antidepressants.

It is in the context of these mechanisms that the interaction of nutritional and dietary components with unipolar depression drugs will be examined.

6.2.1 AMINO ACIDS

With the monoamine hypothesis of unipolar depression in mind, the most logical point to begin the discussion of nutrient–drug interactions is with amino acids. The essential amino acid tryptophan is the dietary precursor to the monoamine—serotonin. On the other hand, the monoamines norepinephrine, epinephrine, and dopamine are synthesized from the amino acid tyrosine. The first inclination is to suspect that more amino acid precursor could give rise to more monoamine synthesis, and subsequently resolve the deficit in monoaminergic neurotransmission seen in unipolar depression. Furthermore, considering that most antidepressants inhibit serotonin reuptake as part of their mechanism,[6] one would think that having more amino acid precursors available would provide a more suitable environment for pharmacotherapy to work. Unfortunately, the relationship is not so simple.

There have been many studies conducted to determine if baseline amino acid status is correlated to pharmacotherapy success. In these studies, it is common to use a ratio of tryptophan over the sum of all other large, neutral amino acids (Trp/LNAA). The sum of plasma LNAA is typically obtained by adding valine, isoleucine, leucine, tyrosine, and phenylalanine together. This Trp/LNAA ratio is used because tryptophan competes with the other LNAA to get across the blood–brain barrier (BBB). Hence, an excess of other LNAAs will hinder tryptophan's uptake into the brain, causing a subsequent decrease in serotonin synthesis. A similar ratio is used for tyrosine (Tyr/LNAA) when the study is concerned with noradrenergic neurotransmission, except that tryptophan replaces tyrosine in the denominator.

The baseline Trp/LNAA ratio has been shown to be inversely proportional to improvement on the tricyclic antidepressants, amitriptyline and clomipramine, with a Trp/LNAA ratio below the group mean predicting a better treatment response.[7] In addition, the same study also showed that the plasma concentration of tryptophan was inversely proportional to the clinical response to the SSRIs, citalopram, and paroxetine.[7] Another study using a mixture of SSRIs (fluvoxamine, fluoxetine, and citalopram), along with SNRIs (amitriptyline and clomipramine), and a tricyclic antidepressants (TCA) (nortriptyline), showed that the Trp/LNAA ratio during the first week of therapy could be used to predict clinical efficacy of the group as a whole.[8] However, no such relationship was observed when examining treatment of major depression with the MAOI, moclobemide.[9] The Tyr/LNAA has also shown some utility in predicting the response to treatment with the TCA, nortriptyline, with the baseline ratio similarly being inversely correlated to subsequent clinical improvement on the medication.[10] Unfortunately, not all results are in agreement with the above trends. In one of the larger studies conducted in this area ($n = 147$), baseline Trp/LNAA and Tyr/LNAA ratios were not correlated with the 6-month treatment outcome of depressed subjects placed on fluoxetine or nortriptyline.[11] It was initially hoped that a clear pattern of plasma amino acid status could suggest the best choice for pharmacotherapy. However, the mixed nature of the results has made this exceedingly difficult.

It has been suggested that the ability of the 5-HT postsynaptic receptors to adapt to serotonin availability is more important than the availability of precursor amino acids.[11] This could also mean that a reduction in receptor plasticity is a marker of treatment resistance in depression.[12] If this were the case, then the baseline amino acid profile could be a more meaningful predictor of treatment response in those individuals who have a greater ability to regulate their 5-HT receptors. On the other hand, those individuals who lack such plasticity would likely be those that do not respond well to increasing monoamine precursors via diet, or by increasing monoamines directly using antidepressants.

An interesting observation is that subjects given the TCA antidepressant, clomipramine, for 6 months had their plasma tryptophan concentration reduced to 28% of its initial value over the treatment period, but this value was still only 68% of the initial value 3 months after successful pharmacotherapy was completed.[13] This was interpreted as a rebound phenomenon due to the fact that antidepressants commonly inhibit the liver tryptophan pyrrolase enzyme, which is the first enzyme in the kynurenine pathway and, therefore, determines how much tryptophan is degraded.[13] Once pharmacotherapy ceases, this enzyme loses its inhibition and resumes the degradation of tryptophan. Such a process could possibly contribute to the relapse that is common in the treatment of unipolar depression, and monitoring of plasma amino acid levels could become increasingly important. More research is needed to look at the possibility of modulating plasma tryptophan levels in order to deter relapse.

A commonly used experimental methodology in this field is to cause an acute depletion of either tryptophan or tyrosine by giving an amino acid drink devoid of either tryptophan or tyrosine and phenylalanine, respectively. A tryptophan-free mixture will induce protein synthesis in the liver, but all of the required tryptophan will be taken from the plasma causing a rapid depletion of the circulating levels. The same is true when a drink devoid of tyrosine and phenylalanine is used. The acute depletion of tyrosine has been shown to have little effect on a small group of subjects who had responded successfully to pharmacotherapy, the majority of whom had been on SSRIs.[14] This suggested that the status of dopaminergic neurotransmission was not of critical importance to SSRI pharmacotherapy.[14] However, acute tryptophan depletion has been shown to cause relapse in successful responders to the SSRI, fluoxetine, but to a much lesser extent in responders to the TCA, desipramine.[15] Not only does this provide the mechanism of action of these drugs, but it also suggests that closely moderating plasma levels of the serotonin precursor, tryptophan, may be more important to preventing relapse in subjects that have responded successfully to SSRIs than to TCAs. More studies are needed to confirm such an observation, but knowing that tryptophan plasma levels are more crucial in responders to a certain type of medication could suggest a novel method of preventing relapse. In addition, because subjects were randomized to each treatment group in this study, it suggests that the response to acute tryptophan depletion is more related to the type of antidepressant used, and not to patient variables.[15]

In stark contrast to these results, a small study ($n = 14$) showed that currently depressed patients receiving the SSNRI, venlafaxine, improved in clinical outcome when they were subjected to acute tryptophan depletion.[16] The authors hypothesized that an initial decrease in serotonergic neurotransmission that typically occurs after administration of SSRIs may be prevented by acute tryptophan depletion.[16] This suggests that the stage of pharmacotherapy that an individual is in might determine how they respond to acute tryptophan depletion.

There are a few different nutritional supplements that have been co-administered with conventional antidepressant medications in an effort to improve monoaminergic neurotransmission in unipolar depression. These supplements include L-tryptophan, 5-hydroxytryptophan (5-HTP), and α-lactalbumin. Tryptophan is acted upon by the enzyme tryptophan hydroxylase, which converts it to 5-HTP.[6] The 5-HTP is subsequently acted upon by L-amino acid decarboxylase to form serotonin.[6] α-lactalbumin is a whey protein that is high in tryptophan, which is not a characteristic found in many proteins. Supplementation focuses on monoamine precursors because serotonin itself lacks the ability to cross the blood–brain barrier, hence making supplementation ineffective.

One study has shown that co-administration of tryptophan with the SSRI, fluoxetine, caused a significant decrease in clinical symptoms of unipolar depression in the first week of pharmacotherapy, but at no later points in time.[17] This is an important observation considering that side effects of antidepressants begin immediately with clinical response beginning after approximately 2 weeks, which makes the initial phase of treatment notoriously difficult.[17] It should be noted that the over-the-counter sale of L-tryptophan was banned in the U. S. by the U.S. Food and Drug Administration (USFDA) in 1990 as a result of a number of deaths related to a contaminated batch.[6] This batch caused at least 38 deaths due to eosinophilia myalgia syndrome.[6] However, α-lactalbumin supplementation is still available over-the-counter and may be a worthwhile alternative.

There is much interest in using the -lactalbumin protein to increase serotonergic activity in the brain. One study showed that a 2-day experimental diet supplemented with α-lactalbumin could decrease depressive feelings under stress in subjects that were stress-vulnerable.[18] This is likely due to the fact that, when combined with a regular diet, α-lactalbumin has the capacity to increase the Trp/LNAA ratio.[19] It still remains to be determined if α-lactalbumin co-administered with antidepressants has a beneficial effect, but there is some evidence for the utility of 5-HTP in this regard.

5-HTP may be more efficacious than L-tryptophan, or α-lactalbumin, as it bypasses the tryptophan hydroxylase enzyme in serotonin synthesis, which is the rate-limiting step, and, in addition, it cannot be shunted into niacin or protein production.[20] A review of the literature suggesting that 5-HTP is effective in treating unipolar depression showed that only a few studies were of sufficient quality to show "statistical superiority to placebo" and they were mostly augmentation studies.[6] In light of this observation, it is clear that more studies looking at the augmentation of classical antidepressant pharmacotherapy with 5-HTP are warranted. It has been suggested that the advent of the SSRIs in the 1980s caused a loss of interest in 5-HTP as a treatment, but in light of the augmentation studies perhaps it should be reconsidered as a treatment option.[6]

Both clinicians, as well as patients, need to be aware of the remote possibility of serotonin syndrome in regards to co-administration of more than one compound. The most commonly reported substances involved in causing this syndrome are the MAOIs in combination with L-tryptophan or fluoxetine, but there has been a reported case of an over-the-counter cough medicine causing serotonin syndrome in a man with vascular disease.[21] However, there have been no reports of serotonin syndrome with the use of 5-HTP as a monotherapy, or in augmentation studies with antidepressants.[6] Despite these promising results, patients should probably only use 5-HTP under the supervision of their clinician.

Ultimately, the efficacy of L-tryptophan, 5-HTP, and α-lactalbumin to augment traditional pharmacotherapy in unipolar depression likely depends on a number of factors. First, the type of drug being used may determine whether or not modulating monoaminergic precursors has any beneficial effect. Second, individual variation, such as 5-HT receptor plasticity and the relative abundance of precursor amino acids already available, could also determine whether more monoamine precursor would be of any clinical benefit. Furthermore, the degree of inhibition of the liver enzyme tryptophan pyrrolase may very well determine how much tryptophan is being catabolized and, hence, how much is needed in the diet. Finally, the involvement of serotonergic deficits, noradrenergic deficits, or both in unipolar depression etiology could ultimately determine the utility of the amino acid precursors to monoamines. As our understanding of the biological and molecular etiology of depression becomes clearer, it is likely that examination of the above factors in individual patients could suggest which pharmacotherapy may be the most effective, and whether augmentation with monoamine precursors would have any therapeutic benefit.

6.2.2 FOLATE, VITAMIN B_{12}, AND HOMOCYSTEINE

There is accumulating evidence that a deficiency in one-carbon metabolism may be linked to unipolar depression, as well as the clinical response to pharmacotherapy. Vitamin B_{12} and folic acid (folate) are integral to maintaining appropriate one-carbon metabolism and, therefore, may play a role in the prevention and treatment of unipolar depression (see Chapters 2, 8, and 9 for detailed figures).

One-carbon metabolism centers on the methylation cycle, which involves the production of S-adenosylmethionine (SAM) from the amino acid methionine. SAM contains a reactive methyl group making it a crucial methyl donor in the human body. The number of substrates that SAM is responsible for methylating is extremely large and includes nucleic acids, proteins, phospholipids, myelin, polysaccharides, choline, catecholamines, and numerous other small molecules.[22] With this list in mind, it is easy to see that a reduced capacity for one-carbon metabolism could have a plethora of consequences. Once SAM donates its methyl group it becomes S-adenosylhomocysteine (SAH), which is reversibly hydrolysed to homocysteine. Homocysteine can then have three possible fates: either directed towards the transulfuration pathway, converted back to SAH, or recycled back to methionine via the enzyme methionine synthase. Conversion of homocysteine back to methionine allows for the formation of more SAM and the subsequent methylation of numerous substrates. However, methionine synthase requires Vitamin B_{12} as a cofactor and methyltetrahydrofolate, a metabolite of dietary folate, as a substrate. The production of methyltetrahydrofolate requires the enzyme methyltetrahydofolate reductase (MTHFR), giving it an indirect role in the recycling of homocysteine back to methionine. One polymorphism of the MTHFR gene (677C > T) has been extensively studied and appears to result in a 25% average increase of homocysteine levels, depending on folate status of the individual.[22] The reason for this is that this polymorphism codes for a thermolabile form of the MTHFR protein, resulting in reduced enzyme activity and, hence, a decreased ability to form methyltetrahydrofolate.[22] The status of a number of the components of this cycle may ultimately have an influence on the etiology of unipolar depression as well as the capacity for pharmacotherapy to work.

In an ethnically diverse sample of the U.S. population of approximately 3000 individuals, those who met the criteria for a lifetime diagnosis of unipolar depression had lower concentrations of folate in serum and red blood cell samples than subjects who had never been depressed.[23] Furthermore, numerous studies have examined baseline levels of compounds involved in the methylation cycle to see if they correlate with the subsequent response to pharmacotherapy. The three main compounds of interest, vitamin B_{12}, folate, and homocysteine, are those which could potentially be modulated in order to better accommodate treatment of unipolar depression. One study showed that low folate levels prior to 8 weeks of treatment with fluoxetine predicted a poor treatment outcome in outpatients with unipolar depression, but homocysteine and vitamin B_{12} levels were unrelated.[24] In 2002, a literature review was conducted to examine the relationship between homocysteine and neuropsychiatric disorders and, based on the five studies that were included examining unipolar depression, the authors concluded that a significant proportion of depressed patients had either elevated total homocysteine levels or low levels of folate or vitamin B_{12}.[25] Unfortunately, no consistent relationship could be found for any one of the three compounds. Furthermore, it was concluded that there is preliminary evidence that both folate and homocysteine levels have some capacity to predict antidepressant treatment efficacy.[25]

The following year a prospective study showed that 6-month treatment outcome in subjects with unipolar depression being treated with a wide variety of antidepressants was associated with baseline vitamin B_{12} status, but only weakly, and likely not independently from baseline folate status.[26] Higher levels of vitamin B_{12} were associated with a better treatment outcome in this study, but the wide variety of medications in the study limits the specificity of the results.[26] Furthermore, an archival study of inpatients in a geriatric psychiatric unit suggested that elevated homocysteine and low folate, but not vitamin B_{12}, were associated with radiological markers of neuropathology.[27] Of particular interest was the fact that none of the patients in the study were clinically deficient in folate.[27] This could suggest that a reevaluation of what defines a functionally significant folate deficiency may be in order, at least in regards to certain organs and particular health-status groups.[27] Overall, it is difficult to be certain that baseline measures of any one compound associated with one-carbon metabolism can predict treatment response in major depression, but it is possible that interplay between folate, homocysteine, and vitamin B_{12} could predict response.

The status of one-carbon metabolism may also have the ability to predict treatment resistance and possibility of relapse in subjects with unipolar depression. One study showed that low folate status predicted further treatment resistance in subjects with unipolar depression who did not respond to initial treatment with fluoxetine.[28] These subjects, who participated in a 4-week, double-blind augmentation trial with either a fluoxetine dose increase, fluoxetine augmented with lithium, or fluoxetine augmented with desipramine, showed a strong relationship between low baseline folate status and further treatment resistance.[28] However, elevated homocysteine levels and low vitamin B_{12} levels were not associated.[28] Furthermore, this group also showed that low baseline serum folate levels, but not elevated homocysteine or low vitamin B_{12} levels, were associated with increased risk of relapse during the continuation phase of fluoxetine pharmacotherapy.[29] This study examined 71 patients, who had previously remitted from unipolar depression for at least 3 weeks while undergoing fluoxetine treatment and were followed for a subsequent 28 weeks to be monitored for depressive relapse.[29] These studies suggest that low folate status might have the ability to predict treatment resistance as well as possibility of relapse, in addition to its possible ability to predict treatment outcome, as noted above. If this is substantiated by further research, folate status could prove to be a valuable clinical indicator.

There are a few points of detail that should be considered while contemplating the above relationships. The first of which is the possibility that macrocytic anemia could be a predictor of poor treatment response in unipolar depression, as it is often caused by either a folate or vitamin B_{12} deficiency. However, one study found that neither macrocytosis nor anemia could predict antidepressant refractoriness, in addition to not being able to predict low serum folate or vitamin B_{12}.[30] Based on these results, it does not appear that macrocytosis or anemia is useful in predicting treatment response. Another important finding is that the relationship between low folate levels and an increased incidence of unipolar depression may not exist in all populations. For instance, it was shown that 117 newly admitted Chinese inpatients with unipolar depression had normal levels of folate, and that folate levels could not predict outcome on standard assessments of depression.[31] However, both the subjects and controls were found to have a high intake of green vegetables.[31] Therefore, the utility of serum folate levels to predict incidence of depression might be limited in populations with a high intake of green vegetables. Whether or not this relationship extends the likelihood of a favorable response to pharmacotherapy remains to be determined.

A few studies have been undertaken to investigate the use of supplemental folate in augmenting the traditional pharmacotherapy of unipolar depression. It was shown that the addition of 15 mg daily folate to the standard treatments of 123 subjects, having either major depression or schizophrenia, with borderline or deficient folate status, resulted in significant clinical and social improvements in both groups over the course of a 6-month period.[32] Later, a study was conducted to see if subjects with unipolar depression, randomly assigned to treatment with 20 mg of fluoxetine plus 500 µg of folic acid or a similar looking placebo, responded differently.[33] Interestingly, only the female subjects receiving folate showed a significantly greater improvement compared to placebo, as well as a significant decrease in plasma homocysteine levels.[33] It was suggested that the dose of folic acid needed to enhance pharmacotherapy in males could be higher than what was given in the study and should be sufficient to decrease plasma levels of homocysteine.[33] It is clear that more research needs be done in order to determine the optimum doses for different subjects.

Folinic acid, which is metabolized to methylfolate in the body, may have some capacity to improve treatment in SSRI-refractory individuals with unipolar depression. In a study of 22 subjects with major depression, who had either partial response or were nonresponders to an SSRI, the addition of folinic acid at 15 to 30 mg daily was modestly effective at improving response to SSRI treatment.[34] Of those who completed the trial, 31% of subjects achieved a 50% or greater reduction in the Hamilton Depression Rating Scale, and 19% of subjects achieved clinical remission.[34] This study was not placebo-controlled, but certainly shows the need for more research investigating the use of folate to augment traditional antidepressant treatment in subjects refractory to SSRI treatment.

A systemic review of the literature investigating the role of folate for the treatment of unipolar depression found only two randomized, controlled studies involving a combined total of 151 people that assessed the use of folate to augment traditional pharmacotherapy.[35] However, the combined data from these two studies showed that the addition of folate to treatment reduced Hamilton Depression Rating Scores on average by 2.65 points, and there was no evidence of problems with tolerability.[35] These are promising results, yet more studies are needed to confirm them to determine appropriate dosing for different individuals and to elucidate what baseline characteristics influence the required dose.

There have been a number of proposed mechanisms suggesting how one-carbon metabolism may influence brain function, and these mechanisms could help explain how folate augmentation improves the efficacy of traditional pharmacotherapy. These mechanisms are reviewed by Coppen and Bolander-Gouaille.[22] The first possible explanation is that a decreased recycling of homocysteine back to SAM decreases the body's methylation capacity, which could impair production of neurotransmitters and membrane phospholipids. Both of these effects could alter the molecular environment in which antidepressants work. The second possible explanation is that a disturbed one-carbon metabolism will result in reduced levels of tetrahydrobiopterin (BH_4), a compound that is dependent on folate for its turnover. BH_4 is a cofactor for the enzymes tryptophan hydroxylase and tyrosine hydroxlyase, which represent the rate-limiting steps in serotonin, and dopamine/norepinephrine synthesis, respectively. Therefore, a reduction in BH_4 levels could also mean a reduced capacity for synthesis of neurotransmitters. Finally, it is also possible that reduced levels of BH_4, a potent antioxidant, and increased levels of homocysteine, a molecule that could cause vascular injury via several oxidative mechanisms, could together result in cellular injury leading to cerebral dysfunction. At this point it is not clear which of these mechanisms play a role in the pathogenesis of depression, or in the subsequent success of pharmacotherapy. However, it could very well be possible that more than one of these mechanisms is involved.

Currently, it appears that disturbed one-carbon metabolism plays a role in the pathogenesis and treatment efficacy of depression. However, to what extent it is involved and the exact mechanism of this interaction still remains to be elucidated. More research is needed to determine the appropriate dosing for augmentation of traditional pharmacotherapy as well as to determine what baseline characteristics influence this relationship. Furthermore, the individual roles of folate, vitamin B_{12}, and homocysteine in the disease process and treatment potential need to be further investigated. Currently, it appears that modulating folate levels has the greatest capacity to help prevent and treat unipolar depression, but it may be possible that the modulation of all three compounds could be the most beneficial. Nevertheless, the modulation of one-carbon metabolism remains a very promising avenue of research for unipolar depression.

6.2.3 S-ADENOSYLMETHIONINE

The use of S-adenosylmethionine (SAM) in the treatment of unipolar depression makes perfect sense considering the previous section discussing one-carbon metabolism and its possible relationship to this disease. It functions as a cofactor in the rate-limiting steps of the tryptophan hydroxylase and tyrosine hydroxylase reactions, which are responsible for the production of serotonin and dopamine/norepinephrine, respectively.[36] Theoretically, by providing exogenous SAM, one should be able to improve the capacity for methylation reactions that are necessary for neurotransmitter synthesis, along with a myriad other reactions. However, the function of SAM might extend beyond its role in methylation reactions.

As a monotherapy, SAM has shown some clinical utility. One open, multicenter study showed that in 145 patients with unipolar depression, the parenteral administration of 400 mg/day SAM for 15 days caused scores of depression to decrease after both 7 days and 15 days.[37] This is an important finding as most traditional antidepressants have a 2-week lag period, during which there is no clinical benefit. This rapid onset of action of SAM treatment is a common finding, with improvement seen anywhere from 2 days to 2 weeks after treatment begins.[36] A number of studies have compared the efficacy of SAM monotherapy to traditional antidepressants. One small study comparing intravenous administration of SAM at 400 mg/day with oral administration of the tricyclic antidepressant, imipramine, found that SAM produced superior results at the end of the first week and, by the end of the study, 66% of the patients in the SAM group and only 22% of the patients in the imipramine group had a clinically significant improvement.[38] Later, two multicenter studies, each with approximately 300 subjects with unipolar depression, were conducted simultaneously to compare 1600 mg/day SAM given orally and 400 mg/day given intramuscularly, both to 150 mg imipramine/day given orally.[39] The clinical responses for the SAM and imipramine arms did not differ, but significantly fewer side effects were observed in subjects treated with SAM.[39] Overall, in six of the eight studies that have compared SAM with tricyclic antidepressants, SAM was of equivalent efficacy, and in one study it was superior to imipramine.[36] These are promising results for SAM as a monotherapy, considering that it seems to be well tolerated with few side effects and has an onset of action that is faster than traditional antidepressants. In addition to these clinical trials, electroencephalogram/event-related potential mapping identified SAM as an antidepressant when given intravenously at 800 mg/day.[40]

Unfortunately, there are far fewer studies that have looked at augmenting traditional pharmacotherapy of unipolar depression with SAM. It has been shown that combining orally administered imipramine with 200 mg/day of intramuscularly administered SAM caused an earlier decrease in depressive symptoms than subjects who received a placebo along with imipramine.[41] When the research surrounding the use of SAM in the treatment of unipolar depression was reviewed in 2002, there were only two augmentation studies included and they both showed that combining SAM with tricyclic antidepressants resulted in an earlier onset of action than tricyclic antidepressants alone.[36] These are promising results, but they certainly emphasize the need for more placebo-controlled studies investigating the use of SAM to augment traditional pharmacotherapies. Furthermore, accurate dosing information, as well as the use of SAM to augment other types of antidepressants, such as the SSRIs, still needs to be investigated.

There are a few theories proposed to explain SAM's ability to lessen clinical signs of unipolar depression sooner than traditional antidepressants. The first is that SAM can increase synapsin I, which regulates the number of vesicles that are available to be exocytosed from the presynaptic neuronal terminal.[42] This is supported by the fact that administration of 100 mg/kg/day of SAM for 12 days in Sprague-Dawley rats induced changes in calcium/calmodulin-dependent protein kinase II (CaMKII) activity and increased synapsin I levels in the hippocampus and frontal cortex nerve terminals.[42] Synapsin I is a substrate for CaMKII, so both of these results could be interpreted to mean that SAM has the ability to modulate neurotransmitter release. This could account for its rapid mode of action that is commonly observed in human trials. Furthermore, again in the rat model, SAM treatment prevented the 5-HT_{1A} receptor upregulation that normally accompanies acute administration of imipramine.[43] This could also help explain the quick response time seen in patients treated with SAM. More research needs to be conducted to clarify SAM's mode of action, but it is likely that it has the capacity to modify intraneuronal signaling mechanisms.

Overall, it appears that SAM may have some capacity to treat unipolar depression as well as augment traditional pharmacotherapy; however, more clinical studies are needed to confirm this. The current body of evidence suffers from the fact that a wide range of doses (200 to 1600 mg/day) and a variety of methods of administration (oral, intramuscular, and intravenous) have been used.[36] Furthermore, having an additional diagnosis of bipolar disorder might contraindicate the use of SAM, as it has been shown to increase anxiety, mania, and hypomania in subjects with bipolar depression.[36] SAM has also been criticized for the lack of evidence investigating its long-term side effects and toxicity,[44] as well as the lack of information describing drug interactions. All of these areas require further study if SAM is to be commonly used for unipolar depression. Furthermore, there is concern that over-the-counter SAM supplements may have varying amounts of active compound in them, as it is very unstable at room temperature when exposed to air.[44] Nevertheless, SAM remains a potential treatment strategy for unipolar depression and augmentation of traditional pharmacotherapy, but needs further investigation into appropriate dosing, long-term toxicity, drug interactions, and stability when stored.

6.2.4 ZINC

Some studies have shown that plasma zinc levels in depressed subjects are significantly lower than levels in healthy controls,[45] yet this relationship was not statistically significant in other studies.[46] However, regardless of baseline zinc levels, both these studies showed that plasma zinc levels significantly increased after successful treatment with antidepressants.[45,46] Furthermore, in a rat model, treatment with citalopram and imipramine as well as electroconvulsive shock therapy, all elevated hippocampal zinc concentrations.[47] These studies suggest that zinc may have a role in the pharmacotherapy of unipolar depression.

A number of studies have investigated the use of zinc supplementation to augment traditional antidepressant efficacy. One study showed that zinc ($ZnSO_4$) at a dose of 30 mg/kg and/or imipramine at 30 mg/kg reduced the immobility time in the forced swim test, also known as Porsolt's test, in both mice and rats.[48] Furthermore, a combination of zinc and imipramine at ineffective doses (1 and 5 mg/kg, respectively) was clinically effective in rats.[48] Research has suggested that the state of immobility in the forced swim test reflects lowered mood in rats and is improved with antidepressant treatment as well as electroconvulsive shock therapy.[49] Therefore, the aforementioned study may suggest that augmentation of traditional pharmacotherapy with zinc may have the capacity to improve treatment of unipolar depression. This notion was further supported by the finding that low, otherwise ineffective doses of imipramine and citalopram, administered together with low, ineffective doses of zinc were effective in decreasing immobility times in mice subjected to the forced swim test.[50] In addition to these findings, it has been shown that the use of zinc hydroaspartate alone has antidepressant properties in both the forced swim test as well as the olfactory bulbectomy animal models of depression.[51] Furthermore, there was a concomitant rise in serum levels of zinc in association with the antidepressant-like effects, and no tolerance was developed following chronic treatment.[51] These results all support a role for zinc status in the treatment of unipolar depression.

In addition to the research conducted in animal models of depression, there is some preliminary evidence showing zinc augmentation of traditional pharmacotherapy in humans. One small ($n = 14$), placebo-controlled, double-blind study showed that zinc supplementation was able to augment the treatment of unipolar depression with tricyclic antidepressants as well as SSRIs.[52] Subjects in the zinc supplementation group showed a significant decrease in both Hamilton Depression Rating Scale and Beck Depression Inventory measures of clinical symptoms after 6 and 12 weeks of supplementation, as compared with placebo supplementation.[52] These preliminary findings are encouraging and emphasize the need for additional clinical intervention trials of zinc and conventional antidepressants.

The mechanistic basis of zinc's action in the treatment of unipolar depression is an area of great interest. One line of evidence suggests that the chronic administration of antidepressants ultimately results in a region-specific dampening of N-methyl-D-aspartate (NMDA) receptor function, and conversely, the administration of compounds that reduce transmission at NMDA receptors act as antidepressants.[53] In accordance with this theory, it has been shown that zinc has the capacity to modulate binding of NMDA receptor agonists and antagonists to NMDA receptors in the forced swim test, resulting in antidepressant-like effects.[54] Furthermore, it has been shown that there is a significant decrease in the potency of zinc to inhibit binding at NMDA receptors in the hippocampal tissue of suicide victims; a group with a high likelihood of suffering from depression.[55] This interaction of zinc with NMDA receptors requires further research, as animal models of depression are somewhat controversial, and not all suicide subjects had a diagnosis of depression.[55]

It has been suggested that it is possible that zinc may reduce NMDA receptor function via single or multiple mechanisms, but experiments to reveal the exact nature of zinc's influence on the NMDA receptor are currently being conducted.[56] The observed actions of zinc include a direct antagonism of the NMDA receptor, the ability to act on the AMPA receptor, and also to inhibit group I metabotropic glutamate receptor function, all of which may ultimately affect NMDA receptor function (reviewed in Nowak[56]).

In addition to the work on NMDA receptors, it has been shown that zinc has the ability to potentiate the action of acetylcholine on the nicotinic acetylcholine receptors (nAChRs), and fluoxetine has the ability to inhibit acetylcholine's action.[57] Furthermore, when the two substances are combined, fluoxetine is able to greatly reduce or even abolish the potentiating action of zinc.[57] How this action of zinc is involved in the etiology and treatment of depression, and whether it is related to the NMDA mechanism in some way, still remains to be elucidated.

Another interesting finding is that zinc was able to enhance 5-HT uptake in certain areas of adult rat brain, and that zinc reversed the inhibition of 5-HT uptake exerted by fluoxetine, imipramine, and 6-nitroquipazine.[58] This recent finding suggests that zinc may very well play a role in modulating serotonergic neurotransmission. Whether this is related to its ability to inhibit NMDA receptor function, or interact with nAChRs, requires additional study.

Overall, it appears as though zinc has the capacity to augment pharmacotherapy in animal models of depression as well as in a preliminary trial in human subjects. Although the mechanistic basis of this still requires much investigation, zinc has shown some ability to modulate NMDA receptor activity, nAChR activity, and influences 5-HT uptake. It is possible one or more of these mechanisms may explain zinc's capacity to augment antidepressant pharmacotherapy, but much more work is needed to clarify these relationships.

6.2.5 St. John's Wort (*Hypericum perforatum*)

While it does not promote growth and, as such, cannot be classified as a nutrient, St. John's wort is included in this chapter as it is commonly taken by individuals suffering from unipolar depression, either as a monotherapy or in combination with other antidepressant compounds. However, individuals taking this extract should be aware of the spectrum of drugs with which it can interact. This chapter will discuss only the interactions related to antidepressants, but for a more complete list of drug interactions associated with St. John's wort, see Zhou.[59] Evidence of the efficacy of St. John's wort in the treatment of major depression is inconsistent, as reported by a recent meta-analysis.[60] Nevertheless, it is still extremely popular for the treatment of depression, possibly because of the misinformed and commonly held notion that all "natural" compounds are safe and superior to pharmaceuticals.

A review of the literature suggests that co-administration of St. John's wort with the tricyclic antidepressant, amitriptyline, results in decreased plasma levels of the drug as well as two of its metabolites.[59] Therefore, co-supplementation of St. John's wort with amitriptyline can have drastic effects on the plasma concentration of the drug, reducing its capacity for effective treatment. Cytochrome P450 3A4 (CYP 3A4), which is found in the liver and intestine, plays a role in two different steps of amitriptyline metabolism.[61,62] A literature review showed that St. John's wort had the capacity to induce both hepatic and intestinal CYP 3A4 expression,[59] which likely results in increased clearance of amitriptyline. Obviously, healthcare practitioners need to be aware of this important interaction when treating subjects with unipolar depression.

In addition to its capacity to increase clearance of the tricyclic antidepressant amitriptyline, St. John's wort may also contribute to induction of the serotonin syndrome when taken along with an SSRI. A number of case reports have linked co-consumption of St. John's wort and an SSRI with symptoms typical of the serotonin syndrome.[63-65] A number of biologically active components of St. John's wort, including hyperforin, adhyperforin, and procyanidins, have the capacity to inhibit synaptosomal uptake of neurotransmitters.[66] St. John's wort can be considered a nonselective reuptake inhibitor as it has the capacity to inhibit reuptake of serotonin, dopamine, and norepinphrine, as well as GABA and glutamate. In the case of the latter two substances, these are not typically affected by other antidepressants.[67] Therefore, the combination of SSRI treatment, which also inhibits the reuptake of serotonin, with St. John's wort could have the capacity to cause an accumulation of excess serotonin in the synaptic cleft, resulting in serotonin syndrome. Due to our limited knowledge of the safety of combining SSRIs with St. John's wort, it has been suggested that combining these two substances should be avoided.[59]

It is crucial that healthcare practitioners, as well as patients being treated with antidepressants, be aware of the interactions between amitriptyline, SSRIs, and St. John's wort. Combining these substances can not only have negative effects on the outcome of pharmacotherapy, but could also be life threatening. Furthermore, St. John's wort interacts with a multitude of other drugs, some of which unipolar depressed patients may be taking for other health problems. Clearly its use must be carefully monitored by this population.[59]

6.2.6 GINKGO BILOBA AND PANAX GINSENG

The use of herbal supplements and alternative medicines for various reasons is becoming increasingly popular. Therefore, it is worthwhile to note a few possible

interactions between certain herbal supplements and particular traditional antidepressant drugs.

There has been one case report that described an elderly woman with Alzheimer's
disease who went into a coma while taking a low dose of trazodone, an atypical
antidepressant, and Ginkgo biloba.[68] The underlying mechanism behind this remains
unclear, but it may be related to the ability of Ginkgo biloba to enhance gamma-
aminobutyric acid (GABA)-related neuronal activity in the brain, and/or its capacity
to increase CYP 3A4 activity, which results in increased formation of the active
metabolite of trazodone.[69] This is supported by the fact that bilobalide, a constituent
of Ginkgo biloba, has been shown to increase GABA levels, possibly by its ability
to increase levels of glutamic acid decarboxylase in mouse brain.[70] Furthermore, it
is supported by the observation that administration of Ginkgo biloba extract to rats
has the ability to enhance the expression of certain cytochrome P450 enzymes.[71]
More research is needed to investigate the interaction between Ginkgo biloba and
trazodone in order to determine if such a combination is capable of inducing coma
and, if so, what mechanism underlies this.

A review of the literature in this area also found several case reports describing
a possible interaction between Panax ginseng and the MAOI, phenelzine, resulting
in mania.[69] The mechanism underlying this potential interaction is not currently
understood, but it has been speculated that it may relate to the psychoactive effects
of ginseng.[69] Such psychoactive effects include the ability of a ginseng saponin
to block human nicotinic acetylcholine receptors (nAChRs)[72] as well as the ability
of a different saponin to inhibit NMDA receptors in cultured rat hippocampal
neurons.[73] A better understanding of Panax ginseng's psychotropic effects could
help to explain the potential for this herbal product to induce mania when taken
simultaneously with phenelzine.

Due to the increasing popularity of herbal supplements and their likely concomitant use with various drugs, it is of the utmost importance that healthcare
practitioners report all potential interactions with medications. As we improve
our understanding of the effects that these herbal compounds have on the central
nervous system and drug-metabolizing enzymes, it will become more clear as to
how their concomitant use with antidepressant medications could result in
unwanted complications.

6.2.7 VITAMIN B$_6$

There is a fairly well-established relationship between treatment with the MAOI,
phenelzine and vitamin B$_6$ deficiency. Over the years, there have been a number
of reports describing vitamin B$_6$ deficiency associated with phenelzine use.[74–76]
One open treatment study detected no effects of phenelzine on vitamin B$_6$ levels,
but these results may have been confounded by concomitant use of vitamin
supplements by the subjects.[77]

Despite finding an average 54% reduction of vitamin B$_6$ levels in subjects
treated with phenelzine as compared to a control group, one study did not find
a correlation between the pyridoxal phosphate (active form of vitamin B$_6$ in the

body) level and daily dose.[76] This indicates that there could be other factors involved, yet still suggests that phenelzine use can induce a vitamin B_6 deficiency. However, administration of a pyridoxine supplement along with phenelzine has alleviated the symptoms of vitamin B_6 deficiency in patients.[74,75]

The suspected reason for the vitamin B_6 deficiency associated with phenelzine use, as discussed in Malcolm et al.,[76] is the nonenzymatic formation of a pyridoxalhydrazone complex involving the two compounds. This could result in a rapid decrease in plasma levels of pyridoxal phosphate after taking phenelzine. As is the case for the other supplements listed above, healthcare practitioners as well as patients need to be aware of this relationship in order to avoid deficiencies of vitamin B_6 while taking phenelzine.

6.2.8 TYRAMINE

Tyramine is a monoamine derived from the amino acid tyrosine and can be found in many foods. The enzyme, monoamine oxidase, is responsible for the oxidative deamination of tyramine and, hence, its metabolism. It has been well established that individuals being treated with a MAOI can have a hypertensive crisis if they consume large amounts of tyramine. When an individual is taking a MAOI drug, MAO-A type in the gut wall and liver is inhibited, allowing tyramine from the diet to enter the circulation.[78] Tyramine has vasopressor activity of its own, but also promotes the release norepinephrine from nerve terminals, both of which contribute to an increase in blood pressure.[78] The hyperadrenergic state induced by consumption of large quantities of tyramine while taking a MAOI is commonly referred to as "the cheese reaction" and can result in a number of symptoms. This condition can take three different forms as reviewed by Brown et al.[78] The most common is characterized by a sudden, severe headache, along with pallor, chills, and neck stiffness; the second form relates almost exclusively to the cardiovascular system and is characterized by sudden palpitations, hypertension, chest pain, apprehension, headache, pallor, and collapse; the third and most devastating manifestation of the condition is characterized by intracerebral hemorrhage and death.[78]

A diet has been devised in order to assure that individuals taking MAOI drugs do not consume large amounts of tyramine. This diet has gone through extensive refining in order to be as unrestrictive as possible, helping to ensure compliance with medications. Foods that are to be avoided on this diet, due to their high levels of tyramine, include aged cheese, aged or cured meats, any potentially spoiled meat/poultry/fish, broad (fava) bean pods, marmite (concentrated yeast extract), sauerkraut, soy sauce and soy bean condiments, and tap beer.[79] However, pizza bought from large-chain commercial outlets appears to be safe, even with double-cheese and double-pepperoni.[80] Nevertheless, it has been suggested that caution be exercised if ordering from smaller pizza outlets or if purchasing a gourmet pizza that could contain aged cheeses.[80] By receiving accurate dietary advice about the MAOI diet, patients taking this class of drug should be able to prevent potentially lethal hypertensive crises.

6.2.9 OMEGA-3 FATTY ACIDS

In recent years, much attention has been given to the role that polyunsaturated fatty acids (PUFAs) may play in mood disorders. This stems from the observation that some epidemiology has shown that frequent fish consumption, which is indicative of a high intake of the omega-3 fatty acids eicosapentaenoic acid (EPA) and docosahexaenoic acid (DHA), is associated with a lower incidence of depressive symptoms in the general population.[81] Furthermore, some studies have shown that subjects with unipolar depression have lower serum levels of omega-3 fatty acids and a compensatory increase in omega-6 fatty acids, when compared to nondepressed controls.[82] Such observations have stimulated investigations into the potential roles that PUFAs may play in disease etiology, therapy, and antidepressant augmentation.

A number of studies have investigated the efficacy of adding omega-3 PUFAs to the traditional antidepressant treatment of unipolar depression. One study showed that adding EPA, at a dose of 1 g/day, to the pharmacotherapy of 70 subjects who remained depressed while on traditional antidepressants, was effective in treating their depression.[83] Similarly, adding the ethyl ester of EPA, to the maintenance antidepressant therapy of 20 subjects who continued to have depressive episodes, caused significant clinical benefit compared to augmentation with placebo, by the third week of treatment.[84]

When the literature in this area was recently reviewed, four of seven randomized, double-blind, placebo-controlled trials investigating the use of omega-3 fatty acids to treat depression (five studies of unipolar depression, one of bipolar, and one of postpartum depression) showed a significant improvement in depression with administration of at least 1 g/day of EPA.[85] Results for the administration of DHA were not as promising, and it remains to be determined whether EPA alone is equally as effective as a combination of DHA and EPA.[85] It should be noted that in the four studies that demonstrated positive findings, subjects were concurrently treated with traditional antidepressants or mood stabilizing agents, but in only one of the three null trials were the subjects receiving concurrent treatment.[85] Therefore, it could not be ascertained whether the benefit of the omega-3 supplementation was independent of the standard antidepressant treatment that subjects were undergoing.[85] Furthermore, it was not clear whether treatment with omega-3 PUFAs benefited all subjects with depression or only those with a particularly low concentration of these fatty acids.[85]

One concern about research in this area is the loss of blinding that may occur due to a fishy aftertaste that is sometimes noted by subjects.[85] Should a subject note such a taste, it is quite possible that this will affect how they perceive their condition. Hence, this could add an element of confounding to this area of research if it is not controlled.

There is much speculation on how it is that omega-3 polyunsaturated fatty acids participate in the etiology and treatment of unipolar depression and control of mood.[85] One theory suggests that mood disorders may be caused by impaired phospholipid metabolism and impaired fatty-acid related signal transduction.[86]

Another suggests that omega-3 fatty acids have some capacity to regulate serotonergic neurotransmission.[87] Thirdly, it has been noted that unipolar depression is associated with an acute phase response, with increased secretions of proinflammatory eicosanoids, and excessive secretion of proinflammatory cytokines.[88] Therefore, by limiting the available omega-3 fatty acids, the relative abundance of omega-6 PUFAs is increased (including arachidonic acid), which leads to excess synthesis of proinflammatory eicosanoids. (For further discussion and metabolic pathway descriptions, see Chapter 4.) Each of these mechanisms represents a large area of study currently undergoing intensive research. How, and to what extent, each of these mechanisms is involved in the therapeutic benefit of omega-3 fatty acids in unipolar depression requires much clarification. However, it is possible, and even likely, that these mechanisms are integrated or that more than one mechanism contributes to the beneficial properties of these fatty acids. Overall, the omega-3 fatty acids show promise in the augmentation of traditional antidepressant treatments for unipolar depression. Nevertheless, more research is required

6.3   CONCLUSION

It appears that there are a number of nutrients that may have the capacity to interact with current antidepressants in a positive manner. A better understanding of these relationships could theoretically allow for nutritional modifications, or the use of dietary supplements, which could improve the efficacy of unipolar depression pharmacotherapy. Furthermore, such dietary alterations could decrease the required dose of traditional antidepressants resulting in a consequent lessening of negative side effects. In addition, there are a number of dietary components that can cause various detrimental effects when combined with antidepressants. A clear understanding of these relationships is important for healthcare practitioners when prescribing unipolar depression medications in order to avoid any unnecessary suffering for the patient.

Understanding the mechanistic basis of the beneficial nutrient–drug interactions is of the utmost importance for their utilization in the pharmacotherapy of individuals suffering from unipolar depression. However, many of these interactions are currently explained by seemingly disparate mechanisms, which is a good indication that much more research is needed in this area. Conversely, understanding the mechanistic basis of the detrimental nutrient–drug interactions could help prevent adverse side effects from occurring as well as help improve our understanding of the etiology of the condition.

While the "monoamine theory of unipolar depression" has proved at least partly useful in developing treatments for unipolar depression, it has also left much room for improvement. It is likely that pharmacotherapy will advance greatly as we attain a better understanding of the molecular and cellular basis of this condition. Furthermore, such an understanding will also allow for enhanced utilization of dietary modifications that assist in pharmacotherapy, and avoidance of dietary components that could result in unwanted side effects.

TABLE 6.1
Summary of Nutrients and Herbals in the Pharmacotherapy of Unipolar/Major Depression

Nutrient or Herbal Supplement	Molecular Target or Suspected Activity	Possible Confounders or Possible Negative Interactions
Tryptophan	Amino acid precursor to serotonin	*Confounders:* Other large neutral amino acids compete to get across blood–brain barrier Tryptophan can be shunted into niacin or protein production (5-HTP cannot) The type of drug being taken can determine efficacy of tryptophan Subject variation: 5-HT receptor plasticity, the relative abundance of precursor amino acids already available, stage of pharmacotherapy Degree of inhibition of the liver enzyme tryptophan pyrrolase The relative importance of serotonin and norepinephrine deficits in depression etiology *Negative Interaction:* Theoretically, use of any serotonin precursor along with a drug that increases serotonin in the synaptic cleft could possibly cause serotonin syndrome
Tyrosine	Amino acid precursor to norepinephrine, epinephrine, and dopamine	Similar to above
5-HTP	Precursor to serotonin, but bypasses the tryptophan hydroxylase step that tryptophan must go through to become 5-HTP	Similar to above
α-Lactalbumin	A whey protein high in tryptophan, which provides precursor for serotonin synthesis	Similar to above
Folate, vitamin B₁₂, (and homocysteine)	Methionine synthase requires B₁₂ as a cofactor and methyltetrahydrofolate as a substrate *Possible consequences of disturbed one-carbon metabolism:*	*Confounders:* MTHFR polymorphisms can have an indirect effect of homocysteine recycling The association between low folate status and incidence of depression may not exist in populations with high intake of green vegetables

TABLE 6.1 (CONTINUED)
Summary of Nutrients and Herbals in the Pharmacotherapy of Unipolar/Major Depression

Nutrient or Herbal Supplement	Molecular Target or Suspected Activity	Possible Confounders or Possible Negative Interactions
Folate, vitamin B_{12}, (and homocysteine) (*continued*)	1. Decreased recycling of homocysteine decreases the body's methylation capacity, which could impair production of neurotransmitters and membrane phospholipids 2. Decreased production of tetrahydrobiopterin (BH_4), which is a cofactor for tryptophan hydroxylase and tyrosine hydroxylase (rate-limiting steps in monoamine synthesis) 3. Decreased BH_4 (antioxidant) and increased homocysteine (a potential prooxidant) could result in cellular injury leading to cerebral dysfunction	Dose of folate needed to augment pharmacotherapy may be higher in males than females (it may have to be high enough to decrease homocysteine levels) Interactions between folate, B_{12}, and homocysteine may make interpretations of results difficult
SAM	1. Needed in the tryptophan hydroxylase and tyrosine hydroxylase reactions and, hence, may affect synthesis of neurotransmitters 2. Might be able to increase synapsin I, which regulates the number of vesicles available to be exocytosed from the presynaptic neuronal terminal 3. Has the capacity to prevent 5-HT_{1A} receptor upregulation, which is normally caused by certain antidepressants	*Confounders*: A wide range of doses and routes of administration have been used in studies Over-the-counter supplements may contain varying amounts of active compound *Negative Interactions*: May increase anxiety, mania, and hypomania in individuals with bipolar Not much is known about long-term side effects and toxicity

Zinc	Has the capacity to modulate binding of receptor agonists and antagonists to NMDA receptors by three potential mechanisms: 1. Direct antagonism of NMDA receptor 2. Ability to act on AMPA receptor 3. Ability to inhibit group I metabotropic glutamate receptor Appears to have the ability to potentiate the action of acetylcholine on nAChRs Shown to enhance 5-HT uptake in certain areas of rat brain and reverse inhibition of uptake caused by certain antidepressants	*Confounders:* Animal models of depression are controversial Suicide victims used in certain studies did not all have a diagnosis of unipolar depression before death
St. John's wort	Induces hepatic and intestinal levels of CYP3A4, which increases the metabolism of amitriptyline Is a nonselective reuptake inhibitor and, therefore, may cause serotonin syndrome when combined with an SSRI	*Negative Interactions:* Interacts with a large number of different drugs used for various conditions
Ginkgo biloba	Bilobalide may increase GABA levels in the brain by increasing glutamic acid decarboxylase levels May increase CYP 3A4 activity resulting in increased conversion of trazodone to its active metabolite	*Negative Interaction:* Suspected to have caused a coma in an elderly woman with Alzheimer's disease, when taken along with trazodone
Panax ginseng	Ginseng sapoins observed to block nAChRs Ability to inhibit NMDA receptors	*Negative Interaction:* When taken with phenelzine, it may result in mania
Vitamin B_6	B_6 and phenelzine nonenzymatically form a complex, resulting in a loss of available B_6	*Negative Interaction:* Phenelzine treatment observed to cause B_6 deficiency *Confounders:* Mixed results of the studies might be the result of concomitant use of vitamin supplements in some studies

TABLE 6.1 (CONTINUED)
Summary of Nutrients and Herbals in the Pharmacotherapy of Unipolar/Major Depression

Nutrient or Herbal Supplement	Molecular Target or Suspected Activity	Possible Confounders or Possible Negative Interactions
Tyramine	Monoamine oxidase (MAO) is needed for the oxidative deamination of tyramine When MAO is blocked, tyramine enters the circulation Tyramine has vasopressor activity and also releases norepinephrine from nerve terminals The end result is an increase in blood pressure	*Negative Interaction*: A hypertensive crisis may result if foods high in tyramine are consumed by an individual taking an MAOI drug
Omega-3 PUFAs (EPA and DHA)	Three theories suggest how fatty acids may relate to mood disorders: 1. Mood disorders may be caused by impaired phospholipids metabolism and impaired fatty-acid related signal transduction 2. Omega-3 fatty acids may have the ability to regulate serotonergic neurotransmission 3. Limitation of omega-3 PUFAs leads to excess omega-6 PUFAs, which are the precursors to proinflammatory eicosanoids	*Confounders*: EPA, DHA, and the combination of EPA + DHA may have differing efficacies Patient variables, such as baseline fatty acid profiles, may also determine efficacy Loss of blinding may occur in supplementation studies due to a fishy aftertaste after consuming the fish oil

REFERENCES

1. Kalia M. Neurobiological basis of depression: an update. *Metab Clin Exp* 2005; 54, pt. Suppl.(5): 24–27.
2. To SE, Zepf RA, and Woods AG. The symptoms, neurobiology, and current pharmacological treatment of depression. *J Amer Assoc Neurosci Nurse* 2005; 37(2): 102–107.
3. Birmes P, Coppin D, Schmitt L, and Lauque D. Serotonin syndrome: a brief review. *Can Med Assoc J* 2003; 168(11): 1439–1442.
4. Popoli M, Brunello N, Perez J and Racagni G. Second messenger-regulated protein kinases in the brain: their functional role and the action of antidepressant drugs. *J Neurochem* 2000; 74(1): 21–33.
5. Skolnick P, Layer RT, Popik P, Nowak G, Paul IA and Trullas R. Adaptation of N-methyl-D-aspartate (NMDA) receptors following antidepressant treatment: implications for the pharmacotherapy of depression. *PharmacoPsych* 1996; 29(1): 23–26.
6. Turner EH, Loftis JM and Blackwell AD. Serotonin a la carte: supplementation with the serotonin precursor 5-hydroxytryptophan. *Pharmacol Ther* 2006; 109(3): 325–338.
7. Møller SE. 5-HT uptake inhibitors and tricyclic antidepressants: relation between trytophan availability and clinical response in depressed patients. *Eur J Neuropsychopharmacology* 1990; 1(1): 41–44.
8. Lucini V, Lucca A, Catalano M and Smeraldi E. Predictive value of tryptophan/large neutral amino acids ratio to antidepressant response. *J Affect Disord* 1996; 36(3-4): 129–133.
9. Møller SE. Plasma amino acid profiles in relation to clinical response to moclobemide in patients with major depression. *J Affect Disord* 1993; 27(4): 225–231.
10. Møller SE, Ødum K, Kirk L, Bjerre M, Fog-Møller F and Knudsen A. Plasma tyrosine/neutral amino acid ratio correlated with clinical response to nortriptyline in endogenously depressed patients. *J Affect Disord* 1985 9(3): 223–229.
11. Porter RJ, Mulder RT, Joyce PR and Luty SE. Tryptophan and tyrosine availability and response to antidepressant treatment in major depression. *J Affect Disord* 2005; 86(2-3): 129–134.
12. Porter RJ, Mulder RT and Joyce PR. Baseline prolactin and L-tryptophan availability predict response to antidepressant treatment in major depression. *Psychopharmacology* (Berl) 2003; 165(3): 216.
13. Fekkes D, Timmerman L and Pepplinkhuizen L. Effects of clomipramine on plasma amino acids and serotonergic parameters in panic disorder and depression. *Europ Neuropsychopharma* 1997; 7(3): 235–239.
14. Mctavish SFB, Mannie ZN and Cowen PJ. Tyrosine depletion does not cause depressive relapse in antidepressant-treated patients. *Psychopharmacology* (Berl) 2004; 175(1): 124.
15. Delgado PL, Miller HL, Salomon RM, Licinio J, Krystal JH, Moreno FA, Heninger GR, Charney DS. Tryptophan-depletion challenge in depressed patients treated with desipramine or fluoxetine: implications for the role of serotonin in the mechanism of antidepressant action. *Biol Psych* 1999; 46(2): 212–220.

16. Booij L, Van der Does AJW, Haffmans PMJ and Riedel WJ. Acute tryptophan depletion in depressed patients treated with a selective serotonin-noradrenalin reuptake inhibitor: augmentation of antidepressant response? *J Affect Disord* 2005; 86(2-3): 305–311.

17. Levitan RD, Shen J, Jindal R, Driver HS, Kennedy SH and Shapiro CM. Preliminary randomized double-blind placebo-controlled trial of tryptophan combined with fluoxetine to treat major depressive disorder: antidepressant and hypnotic effects. *J Psychiatr Neurosci* 2000; 25(5): 439.

18. Markus CR, Olivier B, Panhuysen GE, Van Der Gugten J, Alles MS, Tuiten A, Westenberg HG, Fekkes D, Koppeschaar HF, de Haan EE. The bovine protein alpha-lactalbumin increases the plasma ratio of tryptophan to the other large neutral amino acids, and in vulnerable subjects raises brain serotonin activity, reduces cortisol concentration, and improves mood under stress. *Am J Clin Nutr* 2000; 71(6): 1536–1544.

19. Beulens JWJ, Bindels JG, de Graaf C, Alles MS and Wouters-Wesseling W. Alpha-lactalbumin combined with a regular diet increases plasma Trp–LNAA ratio. *Physiol Behav* 2004; 81(4): 585–593.

20. Birdsall TC. 5-Hydroxytryptophan: a clinically-effective serotonin precursor. *Alternat Med Rev* 1998; 3(4): 271–280.

21. Skop BP, Finkelstein JA, Mareth TR, Magoon MR and Brown TM. The serotonin syndrome associated with paroxetine, an over-the-counter cold remedy, and vascular disease. *Am J Emerg Med* 1994; 12(6): 642–644.

22. Coppen A, Bolander-Gouaille C. Treatment of depression: time to consider folic acid and vitamin B_{12}. *J Psychopharma* 2005; 19(1): 59.

23. Morris MS, Fava M, Jacques PF, Selhub J and Rosenberg IH. Depression and folate status in the U.S. population. *Psychother Psychosom* 2003; 72(2): 80–89.

24. Fava M, Borus JS and Alpert JE. Folate, vitamin B12, and homocysteine in major depressive disorder. *Am J Psych* 1997; 154: 426–428.

25. Reutens S, Sachdev P. Homocysteine in neuropsychiatric disorders of the elderly. *Int J Geriatr Psych* 2002; 17(9): 859.

26. Hintikka J, Tolmunen T, Tanskanen A and Viinamaki H. High vitamin B_{12} level and good treatment outcome may be associated in major depressive disorder. BMC Psych [electronic resource] 2003; 3: 17. E-pub: 2003 Dec 02.

27. Scott TM, Tucker KL, Bhadelia A, Benjamin B, Patz S, Bhadelia R, Liebson E, Price LL, Griffith J, Rosenberg I, Folstein MF. Homocysteine and B vitamins relate to brain volume and white-matter changes in geriatric patients with psychiatric disorders. *Amer J Geriatr Psych* 2004; 12(6): 631–638.

28. Papakostas GI, Petersen T, Mischoulon D, Green CH, Nierenberg AA, Bottiglieri T, Rosenbaum JF, Alpert JE, Fava M. Serum folate, vitamin B12, and homocysteine in major depressive disorder, Part 1: predictors of clinical response in fluoxetine-resistant depression. *J Clin Psych* 2004; 65(8): 1090–1095.

29. Papakostas GI, Petersen T, Mischoulon D, Green CH, Nierenberg AA, Bottiglieri T, Rosenbaum JF, Alpert JE, Fava M. Serum folate, vitamin B12, and homocysteine in major depressive disorder, Part 2: predictors of relapse during the continuation phase of pharmacotherapy. *J Clin Psych* 2004; 65(8): 1096–1098.

30. Mischoulon D, Burger JK, Spillmann MK, Worthington JJ, Fava M and Alpert JE. Anemia and macrocytosis in the prediction of serum folate and vitamin B_{12} status, and treatment outcome in major depression. *J Psychosom Res* 2000; 49(3): 183–187.

31. Lee S, Wing YK and Fong S. A controlled study of folate levels in Chinese inpatients with major depression in Hong Kong. *J Affect Disord* 1998; 49(1): 73–77.

32. Godfrey PS, Toone BK, Carney MW, Flynn TG, Bottiglieri T, Laundy M, Chanarin I, Reynolds EH. Enhancement of recovery from psychiatric illness by methylfolate. *Lancet* 1990; 336(8712): 392–395.

33. Coppen A, Bailey J. Enhancement of the antidepressant action of fluoxetine by folic acid: a randomised, placebo controlled trial. *J Affect Disord* 2000; 60(2): 121–130.

34. Alpert JE, Mischoulon D, Rubenstein GEF, Bottonari K, Nierenberg AA and Fava M. Folinic acid (leucovorin) as an adjunctive treatment for SSRI-refractory depression. *Annal Clin Psych* 2002; 14(1): 33–38.

35. Taylor MJ, Carney S, Geddes J and Goodwin G. Folate for depressive disorders. Cochrane database of systematic reviews (Online: Update Software) 2003; (2): CD003390.

36. Mischoulon D, Fava M. Role of S-adenosyl-L-methionine in the treatment of depression: a review of the evidence. *Amer J Clin Nutr* 2002; 76(5): 1158S–61S.

37. Fava M, Giannelli A, Rapisarda V, Patralia A and Guaraldi GP. Rapidity of onset of the antidepressant effect of parenteral S-adenosyl-l-methionine. *Psych Res* 1995; 56(3): 295–297.

38. Bell KM, Plon L and Bunney WE. S-adenosylmethionine treatment of depression: a controlled clinical trial. *Am J Psych* 1988; 145: 1110–1114.

39. Delle Chiaie R, Pancheri P and Scapicchio P. Efficacy and tolerability of oral and intramuscular S-adenosyl-L-methionine 1,4-butanedisulfonate (SAMe) in the treatment of major depression: comparison with imipramine in 2 multicenter studies. *Am J Clin Nutr* 2002; 76(5): 1172S–1176S.

40. Saletu B, Anderer P, Di Padova C, Assandri A and Saletu-Zyhlarz GM. Electrophysiological neuroimaging of the central effects of S-adenosyl-L-methionine by mapping of electroencephalograms and event-related potentials and low-resolution brain electromagnetic tomography. *Am J Clin Nutr* 2002; 76(5): 1162S–71S.

41. Berlanga C, Ortega-Soto Hé A, Ontiveros M and Senties Hé. Efficacy of S-adenosyl-L-methionine in speeding the onset of action of imipramine. *Psych Res* 1992; 44(3): 257–262.

42. Consogno E, Tiraboschi E, Iuliano E, Gennarelli M, Racagni G and Popoli M. Long-term treatment with s-adenosylmethionine induces changes in presynaptic cam kinase II and synapsin I. *Biol Psych* 2001; 50(5): 337–344.

43. Bellido I, Gomez-Luque A, Plaza A, Rius F, Ortiz P and Sanchez de la Cuesta, F. S-adenosyl-l-methionine prevents 5-HT$_{1A}$ receptors up-regulation induced by acute imipramine in the frontal cortex of the rat. *Neurosci Lett* 2002; 321(1-2): 110–114.

44. Young SN. Are SAMs and 5-HTP safe and effective treatments for depression? *J Psychiatr Neurosci* 2003; 28(6): 471.

45. McLoughlin IJ, Hodge JS. Zinc in depressive disorder. *Acta Psychiatr Scand* 1990; 82(6): 451–453.

46. Narang RL, Gupta KR, Narang AP and Singh R. Levels of copper and zinc in depression. *Indian J Physiol Pharmacol* 1991; 35(4): 272–274.

47. Nowak G, Schlegel-Zawadzka M. Alterations in serum and brain trace element levels after antidepressant treatment: part I. Zinc. *Biol Trace Elem Res* 1999; 67(1): 85–92.

48. Kroczka B, Branski P, Palucha A, Pilc A and Nowak G. Antidepressant-like properties of zinc in rodent forced swim test. *Brain Res Bull* 2001; 55(2): 297–300.
49. Porsolt RD, Anton G, Blavet N and Jalfre M. Behavioural despair in rats: a new model sensitive to antidepressant treatments. *Eur J Pharmacol* 1978; 47(4): 379–391.
50. Szewczyk B, Branski P, Wieronska JM, Palucha A, Pilc A and Nowak G. Interaction of zinc with antidepressants in the forced swimming test in mice. *Pol J Pharmacol* 2002; 54(6): 681–685.
51. Nowak G, Szewczyk B, Wieronska JM, Branski P, Palucha A, Pilc A, Sadlik K, Piekoszewski W. Antidepressant-like effects of acute and chronic treatment with zinc in forced swim test and olfactory bulbectomy model in rats. *Brain Res Bull* 2003; 61(2): 159–164.
52. Nowak G, Siwek M, Dudek D, Zieba A and Pilc A. Effect of zinc supplementation on antidepressant therapy in unipolar depression: a preliminary placebo-controlled study. *Pol J Pharmacol* 2003; 55(6): 1143–1147.
53. Skolnick P. Antidepressants for the new millennium. *Eur J Pharmacol* 1999; 375(1-3): 31–40.
54. Rosa AO, Lin J, Calixto JB, Santos ARS and Rodrigues ALú S. Involvement of NMDA receptors and l-arginine-nitric oxide pathway in the antidepressant-like effects of zinc in mice. *Behav Brain Res* 2003; 144(1-2): 87–893.
55. Nowak G, Szewczyk B, Sadlik K, Piekoszewski W, Trela F, Florek E, Pilc A. Reduced potency of zinc to interact with NMDA receptors in hippocampal tissue of suicide victims. *Pol J Pharmacol* 2003; 55(3): 455–459.
56. Nowak G, Szewczyk B. Mechanisms contributing to antidepressant zinc actions. *Pol J Pharmacol* 2002; 54(6): 587–592.
57. Garcia-Colunga J, Vazquez-Gomez E and Miledi R. Combined actions of zinc and fluoxetine on nicotinic acetylcholine receptors. *Pharmacogenomics J* 2004; 4(6): 388–393.
58. García-Colunga J, Reyes-Haro D, Godoy-García IU and Miledi R. Zinc modulation of serotonin uptake in the adult rat corpus callosum. *J Neurosci Res* 2005; 80(1): 145.
59. Zhou S, Chan E, Pan S, Huang M and Lee EJ. Pharmacokinetic interactions of drugs with St. John's wort. *J Psychopharmacol* 2004; 18(2): 262.
60. Linde K, Mulrow CD, Berner M and Egger M. St. John's wort for depression. *Cochrane Database Syst Rev* 2005; (2)(2): CD000448.
61. Venkatakrishnan K, Schmider J, Harmatz JS, Ehrenberg BL, von Moltke LL, Graf JA, Mertzanis P, Corbett KE, Rodriguez MC, Shader RI, Greenblatt DJ. Relative contribution of CYP3A to amitriptyline clearance in humans: *in vitro* and *in vivo* studies. *J Clin Pharmacol* 2001; 41(10): 1043–1054.
62. Venkatakrishnan K, von Moltke LL and Greenblatt DJ. Nortriptyline E-10-hydroxylation *in vitro* is mediated by human CYP2D6 (high affinity) and CYP3A4 (low affinity): implications for interactions with enzyme-inducing drugs. *J Clin Pharmacol* 1999; 39(6): 567–577.
63. Gordon JB. SSRIs and St. John's wort: possible toxicity? *Amer Fam Physician* 1998; 57(5): 950, 953.
64. Barbenel D, Yusufi B, O'Shea D and Bench C. Mania in a patient receiving testosterone replacement post-orchidectomy taking St. John's wort and sertraline. *J Psychopharmacol* 2000; 14(1) :84.

65. Spinella M, Eaton LA. Hypomania induced by herbal and pharmaceutical psychotropic medicines following mild traumatic brain injury. *Brain Injury* 2002; 16(4): 359.

66. Wonnemann M, Singer A, Siebert B and Muller WE. Evaluation of synaptosomal uptake inhibition of most relevant constituents of St. John's wort. *PharmacoPsych* 2001; 34 Suppl 1: S148–S151.

67. Nathan PJ. *Hypericum perforatum* (St. John's Wort): a non-selective reuptake inhibitor? A review of the recent advances in its pharmacology. *J Psychopharmacol* 2001; 15(1): 47.

68. Galluzzi S, Zanetti O, Binetti G, Trabucchi M and Frisoni GB. Coma in a patient with Alzheimer's disease taking low dose trazodone and gingko biloba. *J Neurol Neurosurg Psych* 2000; 68(5): 679–680.

69. Hu Z, Yang X, Ho PC, Chan SY, Heng PW, Chan E, Duan W, Koh HL, Zhou S. Herb-drug interactions: a literature review. *Drugs* 2005; 65(9): 1239–1282.

70. Sasaki K, Hatta S, Haga M and Ohshika H. Effects of bilobalide on gamma-aminobutyric acid levels and glutamic acid decarboxylase in mouse brain. *Eur J Pharmacol* 1999; 367(2-3): 165–173.

71. Shinozuka K, Umegaki K, Kubota Y, Tanaka N, Mizuno H, Yamauchi J, Nakamura K, Kunitomo M. Feeding of Ginkgo biloba extract (GBE) enhances gene expression of hepatic cytochrome P-450 and attenuates the hypotensive effect of nicardipine in rats. *Life Sci* 2002; 70(23): 2783–2792.

72. Sala F, Mulet J, Choi S, Jung SY, Nah SY, Rhim H, Valor LM, Criado M, Sala S. Effects of ginsenoside Rg2 on human neuronal nicotinic acetylcholine receptors. *J Pharmacol Exp Ther* 2002; 301(3): 1052–1059.

73. Kim S, Ahn K, Oh TH, Nah SY and Rhim H. Inhibitory effect of ginsenosides on NMDA receptor-mediated signals in rat hippocampal neurons. *Biochem Biophys Res Commun* 2002; 296(2): 247–254.

74. Demers RG, McDonagh PH and Moore RJ. Pyridoxine deficiency with phenelzine. *South Med J* 1984; 77(5): 641–642.

75. Stewart JW, Harrison W, Quitkin F and Liebowitz MR. Phenelzine-induced pyridoxine deficiency. *J Clin Psychopharmacol* 1984; 4(4): 225–226.

76. Malcolm DE, Yu PH, Bowen RC, O'Donovan C, Hawkes J and Hussein M. Phenelzine reduces plasma vitamin B_6. *J Psychiatr Neurosci* 1994; 19(5): 332–334.

77. Lydiard RB, Laraia MT, Howell EF and Fossey MD. Phenelzine treatment of panic disorder: lack of effect on pyridoxal phosphate levels. *J Clin Psychopharmacol* 1989; 9(6): 428–431.

78. Brown C, Taniguchi G and Yip K. The monoamine oxidase inhibitor-tyramine interaction. *J Clin Pharmacol* 1989; 29(6): 529–532.

79. Gardner DM, Shulman KI, Walker SE and Tailor SA. The making of a user-friendly MAOI diet. *J Clin Psych* 1996; 57(3): 99–104.

80. Shulman KI, Walker SE. Refining the MAOI diet: tyramine content of pizzas and soy products. *J Clin Psych* 1999; 60(3): 191–193.

81. Tanskanen A, Hibbeln JR, Tuomilehto J, Uutela A, Haukkala A, Viinamaki H, Lehtonen J, Vartiainen E. Fish consumption and depressive symptoms in the general population in Finland. *Psychiatr Serv* 2001; 52(4): 529–531.

82. Maes M, Christophe A, Delanghe J, Altamura C, Neels H and Meltzer HY. Lowered omega-3 polyunsaturated fatty acids in serum phospholipids and cholesteryl esters of depressed patients. *Psych Res* 1999; 85(3): 275–291.

83. Peet M, Horrobin DF. A dose-ranging study of the effects of ethyl-eicosapen-taenoate in patients with ongoing depression despite apparently adequate treatment with standard drugs. *Arch Gen Psych* 2002; 59(10): 913–920.

84. Nemets B, Stahl Z and Belmaker RH. Addition of omega-3 fatty acid to mainte-nance medication treatment for recurrent unipolar depressive disorder. *Am J Psych* 2002; 159(3): 477–479.

85. Sontrop J, Campbell MK. Omega-3 polyunsaturated fatty acids and depression: a review of the evidence and a methodological critique. *Prev Med* 2005; 42(1): 4–13.

86. Horrobin DF, Bennett CN. Depression and bipolar disorder: relationships to impaired fatty acid and phospholipid metabolism and to diabetes, cardiovascular disease, immunological abnormalities, cancer, ageing and osteoporosis. Possible candidate genes. *Prostaglandins Leukot Essent Fatty Acids* 1999; 60(4): 217–234.

87. Kodas E, Galineau L, Bodard S, Vancassel S, Guilloteau D, Besnard JC, Chalon S. Serotoninergic neurotransmission is affected by n-3 polyunsaturated fatty acids in the rat. *J Neurochem* 2004; 89(3): 695–702.

88. Maes M, Smith RS. Fatty acids, cytokines, and major depression. *Biol Psych* 1998; 43(5): 313–314.

7 Supplements and Anesthesiology

Alan D. Kaye, Amir Baluch, and Jason M. Hoover

CONTENTS

7.1 INTRODUCTION

The use of supplements such as minerals, vitamins, and herbal products has increased dramatically in recent years. Reasons for such an increase in prevalence include anecdotal reports on efficacy, impressive advertisement, lower cost of products compared to prescription medications, and ease of attainment of the supplements. Regardless of the reasons, it is important that physicians, particularly the anesthesiologist, be cognizant of the effects of these agents, whether beneficial or harmful.

7.2 MINERALS

7.2.1 CALCIUM

It may be reasonable for patients to supplement their diet with calcium, as calcium deficiency is a common problem.[1] Many women supplement with calcium to improve symptoms associated with premenstrual syndrome.[2]

Calcium may interfere with a host of commonly used drugs. The anesthesiologist must be aware of patients with cardiac problems that may be taking calcium channel blockers or beta-blockers. The effects of calcium channel blockers may be affected by calcium supplementation, as calcium has been shown to antagonize the effects of verapamil.[3] In fact, calcium has recently been used in the successful management of calcium channel blocker overdose.[4] Calcium supplementation may also decrease levels of beta-blockers, leading to a greater chronotropic and inotropic presentation than one would expect.[5]

Thiazide diuretics have been shown to increase serum calcium concentrations, possibly leading to hypercalcemia due to increased reabsorption of calcium in the kidneys. Dysrhythmias may occur in patients taking digitalis and calcium together. The antibiotic effect of tetracyclines and quinolone, and pharmacological blood levels of bisphosphonates and levothyroxine may be decreased with calcium supplementation; these medications should not be taken within 2 hours of calcium intake.[6,7]

Calcium supplementation may also affect the choice of anesthesia used in operative procedures. Elevated levels of calcium may complicate cardiopulmonary bypass procedures by worsening mechanical injury to erythrocytes. Recent data suggest that the use of propofol may have a protective effect on erythrocytes in patients with elevated levels of calcium.[8] Documenting the use of calcium by patients preoperatively may prevent many of these drug interactions.

7.2.2 CHROMIUM

Chromium is an essential nutrient involved in metabolism of carbohydrates and lipids. Recently, chromium has received attention from consumers in the belief that it may improve glucose tolerance in diabetics, reduce body fat, and reduce atherosclerotic formation. These purported effects stem from chromium's effect on insulin resistance. However, the evidence regarding its use for insulin resistance and mildly impaired glucose tolerance is inconclusive.[9-12]

A double blind trial with 180 patients concluded that high doses of chromium supplementation (1000 mg) could have beneficial effects on hemoglobin A1c, insulin, cholesterol, and overall glucose control in type 2 diabetics.[13] The anesthesiologist should consider asking any diabetics if they supplement with chromium in an attempt to attain these effects. Because of chromium's effects on insulin resistance and impaired glucose control, some patients will supplement with this mineral to prevent risk of cardiovascular disease. Human studies have shown decreased levels of cholesterol and triglycerides in elderly patients taking 200 µg twice a day.[14]

Chromium is generally well tolerated; however, some patients may experience nervous system symptoms, such as perceptual, cognitive, and motor dysfunction with doses as low as 200 to 400 µg.[15] In addition, toxicity has been reported with chromium consumption. In one case, a woman developed anemia, thrombocytopenia, hemolysis, weight loss, and liver and renal toxicity when attempting weight loss with 1200 to 2400 µg of chromium picolinate. These problems resolved after discontinuation of chromium ingestion.[16] A lower dose of only 600 µg was demonstrated to have resulted in interstitial nephritis in another female patient.[17]

7.2.3 MAGNESIUM

Magnesium plays many important roles in structure, function, and metabolism and is involved in numerous essential physiologic reactions in the human body. The supplementing of magnesium has been used extensively by patients with cardiovascular disease, diabetes, osteoporosis, asthma, and migraines, although most individuals consume adequate levels in their diet.[18] Patients with a history of these illnesses may be supplementing with magnesium and, therefore, should be questioned.

The most obvious anesthetic consideration in treating a patient taking magnesium supplementation has to do with its effect on muscle relaxants. The mineral can potentiate the effects of nondepolarizing skeletal muscle relaxants, such as tubocurarine. Therefore, it may be advisable to ask patients about their magnesium usage preoperatively to avoid complications.[6]

Anesthesiologists caring for obstetrical patients must be aware of the effects of magnesium sulfate in the patient undergoing caesarean section. Literature suggests that the duration of action of relaxant anesthetics, such as mivacuronium, may be affected by subtherapeutic serum magnesium levels.[19] Magnesium may also interfere with the absorption of antibiotics, such as tetracyclines, flurorquinolones, nitrofurantoins, penicillamine, ACE inhibitors, phenytoin, and H2 blockers. Absorption problems can be ameliorated by not taking doses of magnesium within 2 hours from these other medications.[20-23] The mineral may also make oral hypoglycemics, specifically sulfonylureas, more effective when used, thus increasing the risk of hypoglycemic episodes.[24]

7.2.4 IRON

In both developed and underdeveloped countries, iron deficiency is the most common nutrient deficiency. Worldwide, at least 700 million individuals have iron-deficiency anemia.[25] More than just a constituent of hemoglobin and myoglobin, iron is a key component in nearly every living organism and, in humans, is associated with hundreds of enzymes and other proteins structures. People have supplemented with iron in order to treat iron deficiency anemia, alleviate poor cognitive function in children, increase athletic performance, and suppress restless legs syndrome (RLS).

High concentrations of iron in the blood may worsen neuronal injury secondary to cerebral ischemia.[26] Increased iron levels during pregnancy may lead to preterm delivery and neonatal asphyxia.[27] These complications may occur even with normal iron intake if the patient also takes vitamin C, as high doses of the vitamin can increase iron absorption.[28]

Iron may inhibit absorption of many drugs including levodopa, methyldopa, carbidopa, penicillamine, thyroid hormone, captopril, and antibiotics in the quinolone and tetracycline family.[29–33] Some medications may decrease iron absorption and lead to decreased therapeutic levels of the mineral. This includes antacids, histamine (H2) receptor antagonists, proton pump inhibitors, and cholestyramine resin.[6,7] Iron should not be given orally within 2 hours of other pharmaceuticals to avoid alterations in drug or mineral absorption.

7.2.5 SELENIUM

Selenium, an essential trace element, functions in a variety of enzyme-dependent pathways, especially those utilizing selenoproteins. Much of its supplemental efficacy is due to its antioxidant properties. Glutathione peroxidase incorporates this mineral at its active site and, as dietary selenium intake decreases, glutathione levels drop.[34]

Patients supplement with selenium for a variety of reasons, most notably a supposed improvement in immune status. Elderly patients may be inclined to supplement with selenium for this reason. Toxicity with selenium supplementation begins at intake greater than 750 μg/day and may manifest as garlic-like breath, loss of hair and fingernails, gastrointestinal distress, or central nervous system changes.[35,36] Few interactions with other pharmacological agents have been found.[6]

7.2.6 ZINC

Zinc deficiency was first described in 1961, when it was found to be associated with "adolescent nutritional dwarfism" in the Middle East.[37] Deficiency is this mineral is thought to be quite common in infants, adolescents, women, and the elderly.[38–41] The most well-known use for zinc supplementation is in treatment of the common cold, caused principally by the rhinovirus.

Patients self-medicating with zinc supplements may inadvertently overmedicate themselves. Signs of zinc toxicity include anemia, neutropenia, cardiac abnormalities, unfavorable lipid profiles, impaired immune function, acute pancreatitis, and copper deficiency.[42,43] Zinc supplements may interfere with the absorption of antibiotics, such as tetracyclines, flurorquinolones, and penicillamine.[42] Zinc should not be ingested within 2 hours of antibiotics.[7]

7.3 VITAMINS

7.3.1 VITAMIN A

The term "vitamin A" refers to a large number of related compounds: preformed retinol (an alcohol) and retinal (an aldehyde). Vitamin A deficiency is common in teenagers, lower socioeconomic groups, and in developing countries.[44] Furthermore, some studies indicate that diabetic patients are at an increased risk for vitamin A deficiency.[45] This deficiency may manifest as night blindness, immune deterioration, birth defects, or decreased red blood cell production.[46] Purported therapeutic uses for vitamin A include diseases of the skin, acute promyelotic leukemia, and viral infections.

Retinoids (a class of chemical compounds that are related chemically to vitamin A) have been used as pharmacologic agents to treat disorders of the skin. Psoriasis, acne, and rosacea have been treated with natural or synthetic retinoids. Moreover, retinoids are effective in treating symptoms associated with congenital keratinization disorder syndromes. Therapeutic effects stem from its antineoplastic activity.[47] Patients suffering from these illnesses may be supplementing with vitamin A and their dosages should be explored.

Vitamin A may increase anticoagulant effects of warfarin.[48] This interaction could increase the risk of bleeding complications in surgical patients, which can be avoided by informing the patient of this effect preoperatively

Excess vitamin A intake during pregnancy, as well as deficiency, may lead to birth defects. For this reason, pregnant woman who are not vitamin A deficient should not consume more than 2600 IU/day of supplemental retinol.[49] Patients using isotretinoin and pregnant women taking valproic acid, likewise, are at increased risk for vitamin A toxicity.[46,50] Finally, alcohol consumption decreases the liver toxicity threshold for vitamin A, thereby narrowing its therapeutic window in alcoholics.[51]

7.3.2 VITAMIN B$_{12}$

Vitamin B$_{12}$, the largest and most complex of all vitamins, is unique in that it contains cobalt, a metal ion. B$_{12}$ deficiency may affect up to 10 to 15% of people over the age of 60.[52] B$_{12}$ deficiency manifests as pernicious anemia. This syndrome includes a megaloblastic anemia as well as neurologic symptoms. The neurologic manifestations result from degeneration of the lateral and posterior spinal columns and include symmetrical paresthesis with loss of proprioception and vibratory sensation, especially involving the lower extremities.[46]

The most documented use of vitamin B_{12} is in the treatment of pernicious anemia. Many of the neurological, cutaneous, and thrombotic clinical manifestations have been successfully treated with oral or intramuscular cyanocobalamin.[53] A commonly used anesthetic, nitrous oxide, inhibits both vitamin B_{12}-dependent enzymes and may produce clinical features of deficiency, such as megaloblastic anemia and neuropathy. Some experts believe that vitamin B_{12} deficiency should be ruled out before the use of nitrous oxide, since many elderly surgical patients have this deficiency.[52,54]

The drugs colchicines, metformin, phenformin, and zidovudine (AZT) may decrease the levels of vitamin B_{12} in a patient.[55-58] Histamine2 (H2) receptor blockers and proton pump inhibitors may decrease absorption of vitamin B_{12} from food, but not absorption from dietary supplements.[59-61]

7.3.3 VITAMIN C

Ascorbic acid, also known as vitamin C, is an essential water-soluble vitamin. The symptoms of scurvy, which include bleeding and easy bruising, can be prevented with as little as 10 mg of vitamin C due to its association with collagen, but it can also be used to prevent a host of other disease processes.[62]

Numerous people moderately supplement their diet with vitamin C in order to prevent infection from viruses responsible for the common cold, yet research reviews over the past 20 years conclude that there is no significant impact on the incidence of infection.[63] However, there are a few studies that show that certain groups of people who are susceptible to low dietary intake of vitamin C, such as marathon runners, may be less susceptible when supplementation is used. Furthermore, vitamin C may decrease the duration or severity of colds via an antihistamine effect when taken in large doses.[64]

There is some evidence that patients taking vitamin C supplements may have a reduced anticoagulant effect from warfarin or heparin. Increased doses of these anticoagulants might be advised to achieve therapeutic levels.[65,66] It is recommended that patients on anticoagulation therapy should limit vitamin C intake to 1 g/day. As always, the precise dosage regimen must be monitored by the appropriate lab studies. Since high doses may also interfere with certain laboratory tests, such as serum bilirubin, creatinine, and stool guaiac assay, it is crucial to inquire about any over-the-counter supplementation with the vitamin.[6] There is evidence that vitamin C may increase the inotropic effect of dobutamine in patients with abnormal left ventricular function. Infusion of vitamin C into individuals with normal heart function was shown to increase contractility of the left ventricle.[67] High doses of vitamin C may increase acetaminophen levels, while aspirin and oral contraceptives may lower serum levels of vitamin C.[68-70]

7.3.4 Vitamin D

Vitamin D deficiency does occur in the elderly and shows increased incidence in people that live in Northern latitudes.[71,72] The main function of this vitamin is in calcium homeostasis. Individuals with osteoporosis frequently have a deficiency in vitamin D.[73] With increasing age, vitamin D and calcium metabolism increase the risk of deficiency. Studies show a clear benefit of vitamin D and calcium supplementation in older postmenopausal women. Supplementation results in increased bone density, decreased bone turnover, and decreased nonvertebral fractures, as well as decreases in fall risk and body sway.[74]

Hypervitaminosis D can occur with high doses of the vitamin. Symptoms include nausea, vomiting, loss of appetite, polydipsia, polyuria, itching, muscular weakness, joint pain, and, in some cases, can lead to coma and death.[46] In order to prevent the syndrome, the Food and Nutrition Board has set an upper limit of supplementation at 2000 IU/day for adults.[75]

The cardiac patient taking calcium channel blockers may present for surgery while concurrently taking supplemental vitamin D and calcium. The combination of vitamin D and calcium may interfere with calcium channel blockers by antagonizing its effect. Hypercalcemia exacerbates arrhythmias in patients taking digitalis. A state of hypercalcemia may be induced by the concomitant use of thiazide diuretics with vitamin D, which may lead to these complications. Conversely, anticonvulsants, cholesterol-lowering medications, and the fat substitute olestra may decrease the absorption of vitamin D.[76]

7.3.5 Vitamin E

Antioxidant properties define the primary function of vitamin E. Dietary deficiency is quite prevalent even in the developed world; therefore, supplementation is reasonable.[77] The anesthesiologist must be keenly aware of vitamin E supplementation, as it may increase the effects of anticoagulant and antiplatelet drugs. Concomitant use of vitamin E with these drugs may increase the risk of hemorrhage.[78] Further, preliminary evidence suggests that type 2 diabetics may have an increased risk of hypoglycemia since vitamin E may enhance insulin sensitivity and, therefore, adjustment of oral hypoglycemics would be advisable.[79,80] Cholestyramine, colestipol, isoniazid, mineral oil, orlistat, sucralfate, and the fat substitute olestra may possibly decrease the absorption of vitamin E, leading to decreased levels in the serum.[6]

7.3.6 Folate

Folic acid and folate have been used interchangeably, although the most stable form that is used by the human body is folic acid. This water-soluble, B-complex vitamin occurs naturally in foods and in metabolically active forms.[81] Since 1998, the fortification of cereal with folate has significantly decreased the prevalence of folate deficiency.[82]

Excess folate intake has not been associated with any significant adverse effects. Patients taking large amounts of nonsteroidal antiinflammatory drugs (NSAIDs), such as aspirin or ibuprofen, experience interference in folate metabolism, although regular use shows no significant changes. Patients suffering from seizures who use phenytoin for therapy may report decrease in seizure threshold when taking folate supplements.[83] The body's ability to absorb or utilize folate may be decreased if taking nitrous oxide, antacids, bile acid sequestrants, H2 blockers, certain anticonvulsants, and high-dose triamterene. Supplementation of folic acid may also correct for megaloblastic anemia due to B_{12} deficiency, but the neurological damage will not be prevented. In these cases, one must be careful to pinpoint the true cause of the anemia to prevent neurological complications.[43]

7.4 HERBALS

7.4.1 SAW PALMETTO

Saw palmetto is used mainly for treatment of benign prostatic hyperplasia with free fatty acids and sterols being the main components.[84] Despite an uncertain mechanism, the literature does demonstrate antagonism at the androgen receptor for dihydrotestosterone and 5α-reductase enzyme.[84] Though prostate size and prostate-specific antigen level are not decreased by saw palmetto, biopsies have demonstrated decreases in transitional zone epithelia in prostates of men treated with this agent compared to a placebo.[84] When compared with finasteride, a 5α-reductase inhibitor, saw palmetto use resulted in fewer side effects and increased urine flow.[84] However, a study of patients with prostatitis/chronic pelvic pain syndrome that evaluated the safety and efficacy of saw palmetto compared to finasteride reported that at the end of the investigation, more patients opted to continue finasteride treatment rather than the saw palmetto treatment. The researchers found that in patients with the studied condition, saw palmetto had no appreciable long-term improvement and, with the exception of voiding, patients on finasteride experienced significant improvement in all other analyzed parameters.[85]

Adverse reactions to saw palmetto are rare, but there are reports of mild gastrointestinal symptoms and headaches.[84] Results of a recent investigation indicated that recommended doses of saw palmetto are not likely to alter the pharmacokinetics of co-administered medications dependent on the cytochrome P-450 isoenzymes CYP2D6 or CYP3A4, such as dextromethorphan and alprazolam.[86] Further, there are few herbal–drug interactions in the literature regarding saw palmetto, but, as always, care and responsibility should be exercised when taking this agent.[84]

7.4.2 ST. JOHN'S WORT

St. John's wort is used to treat anxiety, mild-to-moderate depression, and sleep-related disorders.[84,87] Other uses have included treatment of cancer, fibrositis, headache, obsessive-compulsive disorder, and sciatica.[88] Active compounds in the agent include the naphthodihydrodianthrones, hypericin and pseudohypericin, the flavonoids, quercitrin, rutin, and hyperin, and the xanthones.[84,89]

It is thought that extracts of St. John's wort, such as WS 5570, are widely used to treat mild-to-moderate depression.[90,91] Such extracts are standardized based on their hypericin content and have demonstrated an effectiveness superior to placebo and potentially as great as selective serotonin reuptake inhibitors and low-dose tricyclic antidepressants.[88]

The exact mechanism of action of St. John's wort remains controversial. This herbal substance demonstrates irreversible inhibition of monoamine oxidase *in vitro*, but such inhibition has yet to be observed *in vivo*.[92] In the feline lung vasculature, St. John's wort exhibited a vasodepressor effect that was mediated or modulated by both a gamma-aminobutyric acid (GABA) receptor and an L-type calcium channel sensitive mechanism.[93] Studies performed *in vitro* have demonstrated GABA receptor inhibition by hypericum perforatum. This finding may indicate that a GABA inhibitory mechanism is responsible for the antidepressant effect.[94,95] However, other theorized pathways include inhibition of serotonin, dopamine, and norepinephrine reuptake in the central nervous system, thus making its mechanism of action somewhat similar to traditionally used antidepressant medications.[84]

Regarding side effects, St. John's wort is typically well tolerated.[84] Associated side effects may include photosensitivity, restlessness, dry mouth, dizziness, fatigue, constipation, and nausea[84,87] (Table 7.1). Other noteworthy side effects of St. John's wort include its induction of the cytochrome P-450 system (CYP 34A), thus affecting serum levels of cyclosporine in patients after organ transplantation, and the potential threat of serotonergic syndrome in patients concurrently taking prescription antidepressants.[84] The serotonergic syndrome is characterized by hypertonicity, myoclonus, autonomic dysfunction, hallucinosis, tremors, hyperthermia, and potentially death.[96,97] Specifically, use of St. John's wort is not recommended with photosensitization drugs such as tetracyclines, antidepressants such as monoamine oxidase inhibitors and selective serotonin reuptake inhibitors, and β-sympathomimetics such as ephedra and pseudoephedrine hydrochloride. Finally, there is little to no data regarding the potential anesthetic–St. John's wort interactions.

7.4.3 ECHINACEA

Echinacea is part of the daisy family found throughout North America. There are nine species of echinacea in total and the medicinal preparations are derived from three of these: *Echinacea purpurea* (purple coneflower), *Echinacea pallida* (pale purple coneflower), and *Echinacea angustifolia* (narrow-leaved coneflower).[96,98,99] Echinacea is recommended as a prophylactic and treatment substance for upper respiratory infections. However, data are insufficient at present to support the former.[84] It has alkylamide and polysaccharide substances that possess significant

TABLE 7.1
Herbal Agents, Potential Side Effects, and Anesthesia Considerations

Herbal Agents	Potential Side Effects	Anesthesia Considerations
Echinacea	Unpleasant taste, tachyphylaxis, affects cytochrome P-450 enzyme, hetatotoxicity	Can potentiate barbiturate toxicity
Ephedra (Ma Huang)	Hypertension, tachycardia, cardiomyopathy, stroke, cardiac arrythmias	Can interact with anesthetics, i.e., halothane, and cause cardiac dysrhythmias
Feverfew	Aphthous ulcers, gastrointestinal irritability, headache	Can increase risk of intraoperative hemodynamic instability
Garlic	Halitosis, increases in bleeding time, hypotension, affects cytochrome P-450 enzyme	Can increase risk of intraoperative hemodynamic instability
Ginger	Increases in bleeding time	Can increase risk of intraoperative hemodynamic instability
Gingko biloba	Platelet dysfunction	Can increase perioperative bleeding tendencies and decrease effectiveness of intravenous barbiturates
Ginseng	Hypertension, increases in bleeding time, hypoglycemia, insomnia, vomiting, epistaxis	Can increase risk of intraoperative hemodynamic instability
Kava kava	Dermopathy, affects cytochrome P-450 enzyme, hepatotoxicity	Can potentiate the effect of barbiturates/benzodiazepines resulting in excessive sedation
St. John's wort	Dry mouth, dizziness, affects cytochrome P-450 enzyme, constipation, nausea, serotonergic syndrome	Pseudoephedrine, MAOIs, SSRIs should be avoided

Note: MAOIs = monoamine oxidase inhibitors, SSRIs = selective serotonin reuptake inhibitors

Source: Modified from Kaye AD, Clarke RC, Sabar R, et al. Herbal medicines: current trends in anesthesiology practice — a hospital survey. *J Clin Anest* 12: 468–471, 2000.

in vitro and *in vivo* immunostimulation properties due to enhanced phagocytosis and nonspecific T-cell stimulation.[100]

The consumption of echinacea at the onset of symptoms has been clinically shown to decrease both the severity and duration of the cold and flu. Employing quantitative polymerase chain reaction (PCR) to identify *in vivo* alterations in the expression of immunomodulatory genes in response to echinacea has been performed.[101] Investigations conducted on *in vivo* gene expression within peripheral leukocytes were evaluated in six healthy nonsmoking subjects. Blood samples were obtained at baseline and on subsequent days following consumption of a commercially blended echinacea product. The overall gene expression pattern between 48 hours and 12 days after taking echinacea was consistent with an antiinflammatory response. The expression of interleukin-1beta, intracellular adhesion molecule, tumor necrosis factor-alpha, and interleukin-8 was modestly depressed up through day 5, and returned to baseline by day 12. Further, the expression of interferon-alpha consistently increased through day 12, thus indicating an antiviral response. Therefore, initial data yielded a gene expression response pattern consistent with the ability of echinacea to decrease both the intensity and duration of cold and flu symptoms.[101]

Aside from the effects of echinacea on innate immunity, few studies are available that have examined the ability for enhancement of humoral immunity. Although a study using female Swiss mice as the model found support for the use of *Echinacea purpurea*, as suggested by anecdotal reports, and demonstrated potential enhancement of humoral immune responses, in addition to innate immune responses.[102] However, it is important to note that the use of *Echinacea purpurea*, as dosed in one study, was not effective in treating upper respiratory tract infections and related symptoms in pediatric patients, aged 2 to 11. Further, the consumption of *Echinacea purpurea* was associated with an increased risk of rash.[103]

Regarding side effects, echinacea is often well tolerated with the most common side effect being its unpleasant taste.[84,104] Extended use of echinacea for more than 2 months may lead to tachyphylaxis.[105] Anaphylaxis has also been reported with a single dose of this herbal agent.[96] Further, echinacea use has been associated with hepatatoxicity if taken with hepatotoxic agents, including anabolic steroids, amiodarone, ketoconazole, and methotrexate.[106] Further, flavinoids from *Echinacea purpurea* can affect the hepatic cytochrome P-450 and sulfotransferase systems.[107,108] For example, one investigation found that echinacea decreased the oral clearance of substrates of the cytochrome P-450 1A2 system, but not the oral clearance of substrates of the 2C9 and 2D6 isoenzymes *in vivo*. The herbal also selectively modulates the activity of the cytochrome P-450 P3A isoenzyme at both hepatic and intestinal sites. The researchers, therefore, urged caution when echinacea is combined with medications dependent upon the cytochrome P-450 3A or 1A2 systems for elimination.[109] Drug levels may become elevated with concomitant use of echinacea. Some drugs that are metabolized by the cytochrome P-450 3A enzyme include lovastatin, clarithromycin, cyclosporine, diltiazem, estrogens, indinavir, triazolam, and numerous others. Taking midazolam and echinacea together seems to increase levels of the sedative.[109] Finally, echinacea use should exceed 4 weeks and it should not be used in patients with systemic or autoimmune disorders, patients who are pregnant, or patients who are immunocompromised.[84]

The immunostimulatory effects of echinacea may antagonize the immunosuppressive actions of corticosteroids and cyclosporine.[110] Echinacea may also lead to inhibition of the hepatic microsomal enzyme system and, as such, its use with drugs, such as phenobarbital, phenytoin, and rifampin, which are metabolized by these enzymes, should be avoided as toxicity may result.

7.4.4 FEVERFEW

Feverfew is used to treat headache, fever, menstrual abnormalities, and prevent migraines.[111] The name is derived from the Latin word *febrifugia*, which means "fever reducer."[112] Although feverfew is commonly used for migraine headaches, the literature is inconclusive regarding its efficacy.[113,114] In a study reviewing evidence from double-blind, randomized controlled trials of the clinical efficacy of feverfew vs. placebo for migraine prophylaxis, investigators found insufficient evidence to suggest a benefit of feverfew over placebo for the prevention of migraines.[115] As with most herbal compounds, analyses of feverfew-based products have yielded significant variations in the parthenolide contents, which are believed to be the active ingredients.[116]

Regarding the effects of the antiinflammatory lactone parthenolide, a German study indicated that parthenolide may support T-cell survival by downregulating the CD95 system. The CD95 system is a critical component of the apoptotic, or programmed cell death pathway of activated T-cells. Further, the authors reported that pathenolide can have therapeutic potential as an antiapoptotic substance blocking the activation-induced cell death of T-cells.[117]

Feverfew also has demonstrated inhibition of serotonin release from aggregating platelets. This mechanism may be related to the inhibition of arachidonic acid release via a phosholipase pathway.[118–120] It has also been found that feverfew has decreased approximately 86 to 88% of prostaglandin production without exhibiting inhibition of the cyclooxygenase enzyme.[121]

Adverse reactions to feverfew include apthous ulcers, abdominal pain, nausea, and vomiting. A rebound headache may occur with abrupt cessation of this herbal.[111–112] Better tolerance to feverfew has been suggested when compared to conventional migraine medications because in studies feverfew use resulted in no alteration in heart rate, blood pressure, body weight, or blood chemistry like conventional migraine medications.[111] A condition known as "post-feverfew syndrome" can occur in long-term users, which manifests as fatigue, anxiety, headaches, insomnia, arthralgias, and muscle and joint stiffness.[111,122]

Feverfew may inhibit platelet action; therefore, it is reasonable to avoid the concomitant use of this herb in patients taking medications, such as heparin, warfarin, NSAIDs, aspirin, and vitamin E.[123,124] Furthermore, herbs, like feverfew, can interact with iron preparations, thereby reducing the bioavailability of that substance.[106]

7.4.5 EPHEDRA

Since the U.S. government's ban on ephedra-based products, there has been an obvious decline in its prevalent use in this country. However, patients may still present for perioperative assessment with a history of use of ephedra. Ma huang, an ephedra-based alkaloid, is similar in structure to amphetamines and is traditionally indicated for the treatment of various respiratory disorders, such as the flu, the common cold, allergies, and bronchitis. Additionally, it is commonly used as an appetite suppressant.[84] Ma huang, or ephedra, acts as a sympathomimetic agent and exhibits potent positive ionotropic and chronotropic responses. In addition to its antitussive actions, ephedra may also possess bacteriostatic properties.[112] As a cardiovascular and respiratory sympathomimetic, it utilizes an α- or β-adrenergic sensitive pathway.[125] Recent laboratory data using the cat lung vascular bed indicate that ephedra-mediated pulmonary hypertension is dependent upon $\alpha(1)$-adrenoreceptor-sensitive mechanisms.[126]

The appetite suppressant and metabolic enhancer effects of ma huang made it a potent ingredient of various over-the-counter weight loss compounds. However, even prior to the U.S.'s federal ban on ma huang, many herbal manufacturers were already promoting their ephedra-free supplements due to the numerous reported adverse effects of ephedra.

Dangerous side effects of ma huang administration include hypertension, tachycardia, cardiomyopathy, cardiac dysrrhythmias, myocardial infarction, stroke, seizures, psychosis, and death.[84] Many of these complications have been attributed to a lack of standardization in its formulation.[127,128] Before the U.S. ban of ma huang, approximately 16,000 cases of adverse events, including 164 deaths, had been reported to the U.S. Food and Drug Administration from 1994.[129] Further, the Bureau of Food and Drug Safety of the Texas Department of Health reported eight ephedra associated fatalities during a 21-month period between 1993 and 1995; seven of the fatalities were due to myocardial infarction or stroke.[89] Patients at highest risk of side effects include those who are pregnant, have hypertension, coronary vascular disease, seizures, glaucoma, anxiety, or mania.[84]

The use of ma huang is highly relevant to the perioperative period. The possibility of hypertension causing myocardial ischemia or stroke needs to be considered. Further, ephedra can potentially interact with general anesthetic agents, such as halothane, isoflurane, desflurane, or cardiac glycosides, like digitalis, to cause cardiac dysrrhythmias. Patients taking ephedra for prolonged periods of time can also deplete their peripheral catecholamine stores. Therefore, under general anesthesia, these patients can potentially experience profound intraoperative hypotension, which can be controlled with a direct vasoconstrictor (e.g., phenylephrine) instead of ephedrine. Finally, use of ephedra with phenelzine or other monoamine oxidase inhibitors may result in insomnia, headache, and tremulousness, and concurrent use with the obstetric drug oxytocin has resulted in hypertension.[130]

7.4.6 GINGER

Ginger has been used for the treatment of nausea, vomiting, motion sickness, and vertigo.[87] A study of the effects of ginger on subjects with vertigo found that no subjects experienced nausea after caloric stimulation of the vestibular system, in contrast to those treated with a placebo.[131] It is postulated that ginger may be superior to dimenhydrinate in decreasing motion sickness.[132] For vomiting episodes, this herbal has also been effective in decreasing symptoms associated with hyperemesis gravidarum.[133]

The effect of ginger on the clotting pathway has also been investigated. Ginger has exhibited potent inhibition of thromboxane synthetase and this results in an increased bleeding time.[134] The ability of ginger constituents and related substances to inhibit arachidonic acid-induced platelet activation in human whole blood has also been investigated. The data from that study revealed ginger compounds and derivatives are more potent antiplatelet agents than aspirin under conditions employed in the study. [8]-Paradol, a constituent of ginger, was identified the most potent antiplatelet aggregation agent and cyclooxygenase 1 inhibitor.[135] In another study, administration of ginger has also resulted in decreases in blood pressure, serum cholesterol, and serum triglycerides in diabetic rats.[136] Thus, further investigation into these effects in this disease is warranted.

Adverse effects of ginger include bleeding dysfunction and its use is contraindicated in patients with coagulation abnormalities or those on anticoagulant medications such as NSAIDs, aspirin, warfarin, and heparin.[87] Ginger may increase bleeding risk, enhance barbiturate effects, and, as a result of an inotropic effect, interfere with cardiac medications. Large quantities of ginger may also cause cardiac arrhythmias and central nervous system depression.[137]

7.4.7 GARLIC

Garlic's use is prevalent and is available in powdered, dried, and fresh forms.[84] Allicin, the main active ingredient in garlic, contains sulfur, and crushing the clove activates the enzyme allinase, thus facilitating the conversion of alliin to allicin.[96]

Recommended uses for garlic have focused on treating hypercholesterolemia, hypertension, and cardiovascular disease and studies have targeted its hypocholesterolemic and vasodilatory activity.[84,138–142] Investigations have found that garlic may lead to inhibition of the HMG-CoA reductase and 14α-demethylase enzyme systems, thereby exerting a lipid-reducing effect.[84] Garlic may also be used for its antiplatelet, antioxidant, and fibrinolytic actions.[140,143,144] There is minimal data present to support the use of garlic for hypertension, as its depressor effects on systolic and diastolic blood pressure appear to range from minimal to modest.[84,96]

Chronic oral use of garlic has been reported to augment the endogenous antioxidants of the heart.[146] A recent study hypothesized that garlic-induced cardiac antioxidants may provide protection against acute adriamycin-induced cardiotoxicity. Using the rat model, researchers discovered an increase in oxidative stress as evidenced by a significant increase in myocardial thiobarbituric acid reactive substances (TBARS) and a decrease in myocardial superoxide dismutase (SOD), catalase, and glutathione peroxidase activity in the adriamycin group. However, in the garlic treated rats, the increase in myocardial TBARS and a decrease in endogenous antioxidants by adriamycin was significantly attenuated. Therefore, one may conclude garlic administration may help prevent this form of drug-induced cardiotoxicity.[145] The effects of allicin in the feline and rat lung vasculature have also been studied. Allicin has shown significant vasodepressor activity in the pulmonary vascular bed of the rat and cat.[146] Although allicin has been found to lower blood pressure, insulin, and triglycerides levels in fructose-fed rats, it has also been considered important to investigate its effect on the weight of animals.

Recent data indicate garlic may be an effective treatment against methicillin-resistant *Staphylococcus aureus* (MRSA) infection. In a study using mice, investigators demonstrated that the garlic extracts, diallyl sulphide and diallyl disulphide, showed protective qualities against MRSA infection. Such conclusions, coupled with further investigation, may result in the use of such extracts in MRSA infection treatment.[147]

Side effects of garlic are minimal, with odor and gastrointestinal discomfort being the most commonly reported.[84] Induction of the cytochrome P-450 system may occur as evidenced by reduction of serum levels of one medication.[84] Anesthesiologists must be aware that garlic may augment the effects of warfarin, heparin, aspirin, and may result in an abnormal bleeding time. This effect can result in increased risk of peri-operative hemorrhage.[148] Thus, monitoring of cardiovascular function in this period is crucial.

7.4.8 Gingko Biloba

There are many active components present in gingko, including the flavinoid glycosides and terpenoids. The flavinoids have demonstrated antioxidant activity while the terpenoids have shown antagonism to platelet action.[84] Gingko has been used to treat intermittent claudication, vertigo, and enhance memory.[89] Subjects using this herbal have reported decreased pain in the affected lower extremities and increased symptom-free distance in ambulation. In addition to inhibiting the platelet-activating factor, gingko may also mediate nitric oxide release and decrease inflammation.[84,149-154]

To evaluate the efficacy of gingko on dementia, a double-blind and placebo-controlled randomized trial using the extract EGB761 was performed. It was found that EGB761 had the potential to stabilize and modestly improve cognitive performance and social functioning.[84,155] In addition, the improvement in cognition was comparable to the effect of donazepil on dementia.[84] This effect on cognition function and memory may be related to activation of cholinergic neurotransmitters. It is important to note, however, that data are inconclusive regarding the ability of this herbal to improve memory in subjects without dementia.[84]

Although the pathogenesis of acute pancreatitis is not well understood, there are numerous data that suggest a role for oxygen free radicals in the progression and complications of pancreatitis. The effects of EGB761 have shown a positive effect on acute pancreatitis and this effect may be linked to a free radical scavenger effect by gingko.[156]

Gingko is generally well tolerated in healthy adults for about 6 months.[84] However, aside from the mild gastrointestinal distress, the potential of gingko on antiplatelet activating factor has resulted in gingko biloba-induced spontaneous hyphema (bleeding from the iris, the anterior chamber of the eye), spontaneous bilateral subdural hematomas, and subarachnoid hemorrhage.[84,87,157–160] Therefore, the use of anticoagulants and gingko should be strictly monitored and possibly avoided.[84]

Regarding the effects of gingko on pharmacokinetics, an open-labeled and randomized crossover trial was conducted on healthy human volunteers to determine if ginkgo alters the pharmacokinetics of digoxin. The investigators found the concurrent use of orally administered gingko and digoxin did not seem to have a significant effect on the pharmacokinetics of digoxin in healthy volunteers.[161] Therefore, one may conclude that concurrent use of gingko biloba with aspirin, NSAIDs, warfarin, and heparin is not recommended as gingko may increase the potential for bleeding in these patients. It is also advisable to avoid use of gingko with anticonvulsant drugs, such as carbamazapine, phenytoin, and phenobarbital, as the herbal may decrease the effectiveness of these medications.[106] Concurrent use of gingko and tricyclic antidepressants also is not advised because of the potential to lower the seizure threshold in these patients.[106]

7.4.9 KAVA KAVA

Kava kava, an extract of the Piper methysticum plant, is employed for its proposed anxiolytic, antiepileptic, antidepressant, antipsychotic, and sedative properties.[162–164] Some of the active ingredients of kava kava include the lactones or pyrones, kawain, methysticin, dihydrokawain, dihydromethysticin.[165,166] Kava extracts available commercially are usually found to contain approximately 30 to 70% kava lactones.[165]

The extract WS 1490 has been investigated to determine its effectiveness in the treatment of anxiety.[166] WS 1490 has been shown effective in anxiety disorders as a treatment alternative to benzodiazepines and tricyclic antidepressants, and reported not to have the problems associated with those two classes of drugs.[166] However, therapeutic effect may take up to 4 weeks and data have indicated treatment for 1 to 8 weeks to obtain significant improvement.[165,167]

Although the exact mechanism of kava kava's effects on the central nervous system is largely unknown, the pyrones have demonstrated competitive inhibition of the monoamine oxidase B enzyme.[165] Inhibition of this enzyme may result in the psychotropic effects related to kava kava use, as this enzyme is responsible for the breakdown of amines that play a role in psychoses.[168]

Regarding adverse effects, patients that experience hepatic adverse reactions are known as "poor metabolizers." Typically, these patients have a deficiency in the cytochrome P-450 2D6 isozyme.[165] Therefore, it is recommended that patients who use kava kava receive routine liver function tests to monitor for the development of hepatotoxicity.[165] Furthermore, there have been 24 documented cases of hepatotoxicity following the use of kava kava and, in some cases, death or liver transplant occurred after 1 to 3 months of use.[165] In countries, such as Germany and Australia, kava kava use longer than 3 months is not recommended.[167] Other side effects of kava kava use include visual changes, a pellagra-like syndrome with characteristic ichthyosiform dermopathy, and hallucinations.[165,169,170]

Regarding drug interactions, kava kava may react adversely with the benzodiazepine alprazolam, other central nervous system depressants, statins, alcohol, and levodopa, consequently resulting in excessive sedation, among other side effects; therefore, the supplement should be avoided in those patients with endogenous depression.[165,171–173] Finally, kava kava may also affect platelets in an antithrombotic fashion by inhibiting cyclooxygenase and, thus, attenuating thromboxane production.[165] Pain relief mechanisms utilized by the herbal may be similar to local anesthetic responses and could be dependent on a nonopiate sensitive pathway.[174,175]

7.4.10 GINSENG

There are three main groups of ginseng that are classified based on their geographic origin.[84] These are Asian ginseng, American ginseng, and Siberian ginseng, with the pharmacologically active ingredient in ginseng being ginsenosides.[84,89,112] Asian and American ginsengs have been used to increase resistance to environmental stress, promote diuresis, stimulate the immune system, and aid digestion.[176,177] Further, while Asian ginseng has shown promise in improving cognition when combined with the herbal agent gingko, American ginseng has been studied for its potential to stimulate human tumor necrosis factor alpha (TNF-alpha) production in cultured human white blood cells.[177,178] American ginseng may also possess hypoglycemic activity.[179,180] Such effects have been observed in both normal and diabetic subjects and may be attributed to ginseng's components, specifically ginsenoside Rb2 and panaxans I, J, K, and L.[181–185]

Typically ginseng is well tolerated, but side effects, such as bleeding abnormalities secondary to antiplatelet effects, headache, vomiting, Stevens-Johnson syndrome, epistaxis, and hypertension have been reported.[186–192] Drug interactions between Asian ginseng and calcium channel blockers, warfarin, phenelzine, and digoxin have also been noted.[84] It may be advisable for patients on anticoagulant medications, such as warfarin, heparin, aspirin, and NSAIDs, to avoid ginseng. Further, because of ginseng's association with hypertension and the deleterious outcomes linked to chronic hypertension, the anesthesiologist should be aware of whom and for how long patients may have been taking this herbal product. Since many anesthetic agents can cause generalized vasodilation, hemodynamic lability may be seen.

Regarding ginseng's interaction with antidepressants, such as monoamine oxidase inhibitors, concurrent use of ginseng with phenelzine sulphate should be avoided as manic episodes have been reported with routine use of both.[193,194] Finally, as a result of ginseng's potential to cause decreased blood glucose levels, it should be used cautiously in diabetic patients on insulin or other oral hypoglycemic agents, and blood glucose levels should be monitored.

7.5 CONCLUSION

The growing use of supplements, such as minerals, vitamins, and herbals, in the world warrants a more comprehensive understanding of these agents by the medical community. It is important for the anesthesiologist to recognize certain facts regarding these supplements. For example, there are about 1300 g of calcium in a 70 kg adult and the mineral magnesium activates approximately 300 enzyme systems in the human body; most of these systems are involved in energy metabolism.[195] Aside from these, the anesthesiologist must regulate the patient's physiological functions and appreciate the effect of these supplements on such functions during various operative procedures. As demonstrated in this chapter, the use of these compounds may prove beneficial for some patients, but result in alterations in normal physiologic functions in others, thus potentially resulting in deleterious consequences. These agents, in addition to all other medications taken by the patient, should be screened by medical practitioners, in particular anesthesiologists, as some of these compounds may interact with chosen anesthetics during the stages of anesthesia. Furthermore, education of patients regarding the serious potential drug-supplement interactions should be an integral component of the preoperative assessment. Specifically, the American Society of Anesthesiologists (ASA) recommends that all herbal medications be discontinued 2 to 3 weeks prior to elective surgery.

Due to current lax regulations in some countries, some of these agents are poorly categorized and standardized, thus resulting in a high risk of adverse effects when used by an uninformed or misinformed public. Within the past few decades, hundreds of deaths have been linked to the use of these agents, specifically the herbals. Data also suggest that less than 1% of adverse effects associated with herbals are reported. In general, whether the patient is taking minerals, vitamins, and/or herbals, one thing is for certain, an open line of communication between medical practitioner and patient should exist regarding all of these agents. This communication is essential to ensure quality patient treatment, a stable and secure rapport, and a properly informed and educated general public.

REFERENCES

1. McCarron DA, Hatton D. Dietary calcium and lower blood pressure: we can all benefit. *JAMA* 1996; 275: 1128–1129.
2. Thys-Jacobs S, Starkey P, Bernstein D, et al. Calcium carbonate and the premenstrual syndrome: effects on premenstrual and menstrual symptoms. Premenstrual Syndrome Study Group. *Am J Obstet Gynecol* 1998; 179: 444–452.
3. Bar-Or D, Gasiel Y. Calcium and calciferol antagonize effect of verapamil in atrial fibrillatin. *Br Med J* (Clin Res Ed) 1981; 282: 1585–1586.
4. Durward A. Guerguerian AM. Lefebvre M. Shemie SD. Massive diltiazem overdose treated with extracorporeal membrane oxygenation. [Case Reports. Journal Article] *Ped Crit Care Med* 2003; 4(3): 372–376.

5. Kirch W, Schafer-Korting M, Axthelm T, et al. Interaction of atenolol with furosemide and calcium and aluminum salts. *Clin Pharmacol Ther* 1981; 30: 429–435.

6. Hendler SS, Rorvik DR, Eds. *PDR for Nutritional Supplements*. Montvale, NJ: Medical Exonomics, Inc., 2001.

7. Minerals. *Drug Facts and Comparisons*. St. Louis, MO: Facts and Comparisons, 27–30.

8. Zhang S, Yao S. The protective effect of propofol on erythrocytes during cardiopulmonary bypass. *J Tongji Med Univer* 2001; 21(1): 65–67.

9. Anderson RA, Polansky MM, Bryden NA, et al. Supplemental-chromium effects on glucose, insulin, glucagons, and urinary chromium losses in subjects consuming controlled low-chromium diets. *Am J Clin Nutr* 1991; 54: 909–916.

10. Uusitupa MI, Mykkanen L, Siitonen O, et al. Chromium supplementation in impaired glucose tolerance of elderly: effects on blood glucose, plasma insulin, C-peptide and lipid levels. *Br J Nutr* 1992; 68: 209–216.

11. Bahijri SM. Effect of chromium supplementation on glucose tolerance and lipid profile. *Ausdi Med J* 2000; 21: 45–50.

12. Shinde Urmila A, Sharma G, Xu Yan J, et al. Anti-diabetic activity and mechanism of action of chromium chloride. *Exp Clin Endocrinol Diabetes*. 2004; 112(5): 248–252.

13. Anderson RA, Cheng N, Bryden NA, et al. Elevated intakes of supplemental chromium improve glucose and insulin variables in individuals with type 2 diabetes. *Diabetes* 1997; 46: 1786–1791.

14. Rabinovitz H, Friedensohn A, Leibovitz A, et al. Effect of chromium supplementation on blood glucose and lipid levels in type 2 diabetes mellitus elderly patients. *Int J Vitam Nutr Res* 2004; 74(3): 178–182.

15. Fox GN, Sabovic Z. Chromium picolinate supplementation for diabetes mellitus. *J Fam Pract* 1998; 46(1): 83–86.

16. Cerulli J, Grabe DW, Gauthier I, et al. Chromium picolinate toxicity. *Ann Pharmacother*. 1998; 32: 428–431.

17. Wasser WG, Feldman NS, D'Agati VD. Chronic renal failure after ingestion of over-the-counter chromium picolinate [letter]. *Ann Intern Med* 1997; 126 :410.

18. Institute of Medicine. *Dietary Reference Intakes for Calcium, Phosphorus, Magnesium, Vitamin D and Fluoride*. Washington, D.C.: National Academy Press, 2001.

19. Hodgson RE, Rout CC, Rocke DA, Louw NJ. Mivacurium for caesarean section in hypertensive parturients receiving magnesium sulphate therapy. *Int J Obstet Anesth* 1998; 7(1): 12–17.

20. Tatro D, Ed. *A to Z Drug Facts*. St. Louis: Facts and Comparisons, 1999.

21. Shiba K, Sakamoto M, Nakazawa Y, et al. Effects of antacid on absorption and excretin of new quinolones. *Drugs* 1995; 49(suppl 2): 360–361.

22. Naggar VF, Khalil SA. Effect of magnesium trisilicate on nitrofurantoin absorption. *Clin PHarmacol Ther* 1979; 25: 857–863.

23. Osman MA, Patel RB, Schuna A, et al. Reduction in oral penicillamine absorption by food, antacid and ferrous sulfate. *Clin Pharmacol Ther* 1983; 33: 465–470.

24. Kivisto KT, Neuvonen PJ. Effect of magnesium hydroxide on the absorption and efficacy of tolbutamide and chlorpropamide. *Eur J Clin Pharmacol*. 1992; 42: 675–679.

25. Shils ME, Olson JA, Shike M, Eds. *Modern Nutrition in Health and Disease*. 9th ed. Baltimore: Williams and Wilkins, 1999: 210, 860, 1422, 1424, 1772.

26. Davolos A, Castillo J, Marrugat J, et al. Body iron stores and early neurologic deterioration in acute cerebral infarction. *Neurology* 2000; 54: 1568–1574.

27. Lao TT, Tam K, Chan LY. Third trimester iron status and pregnancy outcome in non-anemic women; pregnancy unfavourably affected by maternal iron excess. *Hum Reprod* 2000; 15: 1843–1848.

28. Siegenberg D, Baynes RD, Bothwell TH, et al. Ascorbic acid prevents the dose-dependent inhibitory effects of polyphenols and phytates on nonheme-iron absorption. *Am J Clin Nutr* 1991; 53: 537–541.

29. Lehto P, Kivisto KT, Neuvonen PJ. The effect of ferrous sulphate on the absorption of norfloxacin, ciprofloxacin and ofloxacin. *Br J Clin Pharmacol* 1994; 37: 82–85.

30. Campbell NR, Hasinoff BB. Iron supplements: a common cause of drug interactions. *Br J Clin Pharmacol* 1991; 31: 251–255.

31. Heinrich HC, Oppitz KH, Gabbe EE. Inhibition of iron absorption in man by tetracycline [German]. *Klin Wochenschr.* 1974; 52: 493–498.

32. Osman MA, Patel RB, Schuna A, et al. Reduction in oral penicillamine absorption by food, antacid, and ferrous sulfate. *Clin Pharmacol Ther* 1983; 33: 465–470.

33. Campbell NR, Hasinoff BB, Stalts H, et al. Ferrous sulfate reduces thyroxine efficacy in patients with hypothyroidism. *Ann Intern Med* 1992; 117: 1010–1013.

34. Ursini F, Heim S, Kiess M, et al. Dual function of the selenoprotein PHGPx during sperm maturation. *Science* 1999; 285(5432): 1393–1396.

35. Patterson BH, Levander OA. Naturally occurring selenium compounds in cancer chemoprevention trials: a workship summary. *Cancer Epidemiol Biomarkers Prev* 1997; 6: 63–69.

36. Fan AM, Kizer KW. Selenium: nutritional, toxicologic, and clinical aspects, *West J Med* 1990; 153: 160–167.

37. Prasad AS, Halsted JA, Nadimi M. Syndrome of iron deficiency anemia, hepatosplenomegaly, hypogonadism, dwarfism, and geophagia. *Am J Med* 1961; 31: 532–546.

38. Sandstead HH. Is zinc deficiency a public health problem? *Nutrition* 1995; 11: 87–92.

39. Goldenberg RL, Tamura T, Neggers Y, et al. The effect of zinc supplementation on pregnancy outcome. *JAMA* 1995; 274: 463–468.

40. Ma J, Betts NM. Zinc and copper intakes and their major food sources for older adults in the 1994-96 continuing survey of food intakes by individuals (CSFII). *J Nutr* 2000; 130: 2838–2843.

41. Prasad AS. Zinc deficiency in women, infants, and children. *J Am Coll Nutr* 1996; 15: 113–120.

42. Bratman S, Girman AM. *Handbook of Herbs and Supplements and their Therapeutic Uses.* St. Louis: Mosby, Inc., 2003.

43. Mikszewski JS, Saunders HM, Hess RS. Zinc-associated acute pancreatitis in a dog. *J Small Anim Pract* 2003; 44(4): 177–180.

44. Combs GF. *The Vitamins: Fundamental Aspects in Nutrition and Health.* 2nd ed. San Diego: Academic Press, 1998: 5–6.

45. Queiroz E, Ramalho A, Saunders C, et al. Vitamin A status in diabetic children. *Diabetes Nutr Metab.* 2000; 13(5): 298–299.

46. Higdon, J. *An Evidence-Based Approach to Vitamins and Minerals.* New York: Thieme Medical Publishers, Inc., 2003: 148–-156.

47. Brzezinska-Wcislo L, Pierzchala E, Kaminska-Budzinska G, et al. [The use of retinoids in dermatology] [Polish]. *Wiad Lek* 2004; 57(1-2): 63–69.

48. Harris JE. Interaction of dietary factors with oral anticoagulants: review and applications. *J Am Diet Assoc* 1995; 95: 580–584.
49. Binkley N, Krueger D. Hypervitaminosis A and bone. *Nutr Rev* 2000; 58(5): 138–144.
50. Nau H, Tzimas G, Mondry M, et al. Antiepileptic drugs alter endogenous retinoid concentrations: a possible mechanism of teratogenesis of anticonvulsant therapy. *Life Sci* 1995; 57: 53–60.
51. Leo MA, Lieber CS. Alcohol, vitamin A, and beta-carotene: adverse interactins, including hepatotoxicity and carcinogenicity. *Am J Clin Nutr* 1999; 69(6): 1071–1085.
52. Baik HW, Russel RM. Vitamin B12 deficiency in the elderly. *Annu Rev Nutr* 1999; 19: 357–377.
53. Loikili NG, Noel E. Blaison G, et al. Update of pernicious anemia. A retrospective study of 49 cases. [French] *Rev Med Interne* 2004; 25(8): 556–561.
54. Weimann J. Toxicity of nitrous oxide. *Best Pract Res Clin Anaesthesiol* 2003; 17(1): 47–61.
55. Webb DI, Chodos RB, Mahar CQ, et al. Mechanism of vitamin B12 malabsorption in patients receiving colchicines. *N Engl J Med* 1968; 279: 845–850.
56. Adams JF, Clark JS, Ireland JT, et al. Malabsorption of vitamin B12 and intrinsic factor secretion during biguanide therapy. *Diabetologia* 1983; 24: 16–18.
57. Flippo TS, Holder WD Jr. Neurologic degeneration associated with nitrous oxide anesthesia in patients with vitamin B12 deficiency. *Arch Surg* 1993; 128: 1391–1395.
58. Baum MK, Javier JJ, Mantero-Atienza E, et al. Zidovudine-associated adverse reactions in a longitudinal study of asymptomatic HIV-1-infected homosexual males. *J Acquir Immune Defic Syndr* 1991; 4: 1218–1226.
59. Marcuard SP, Albernaz L, Khazanie PG. Omeprazole therapy causes malabsorption of cyanocobalamin (vitamin B12). *Ann Intern Med* 1994; 120: 211–215.
60. Streeter AM, Goulston KJ, Bathur FA, et al. Cimetidine and malabsorption of cobalamin. *Dig Dis Sci* 1982; 27: 13–16.
61. Aymard JP, Aymard B, Netter P, et al. Haematological adverse effects of histamine H2-receptor antagonists. *Med Toxicol Adverse Drug Exp* 1988; 3: 430–448.
62. Sauberlich HE. A history of scurvy and vitamin C. In Packer L, Fuchs J, Ed. *Vitamin C in Health and Disease*. New York: Marcel Decker, 1997: 1–24.
63. Hemila H. Vitamin C intake and susceptibility to the common cold. *Br J Nutr* 1997; 77(1): 59–72.
64. Johnston CS, Martin LJ, Cai X. Antihistamine effect of supplemental ascorbic acid and neutrophil chemotaxis. *J Am Coll Nutr* 1992; 11(2): 172–176.
65. Rosenthal G. Interaction of ascorbic acid and warfarin [letter]. *JAMA* 1971; 215: 1671.
66. Harris JE. Interaction of dietary factors with oral anticoagulants: review and applications. *J Am Diet Assoc* 1995; 95: 580–584.
67. Mak S, Newton GE. Vitamin C augments the inotropic response to dobutamine in humans with normal left ventricular function. *Circulation* 2001; 103: 826–830.
68. Houston JB, Levy G. Drug biotransformation interactions in man. VI. Acetaminophen and ascorbic acid. *J Pharm Sci* 1976; 65 :1218–1221.
69. Molloy TP, Wilson CW. Protein-binding of ascorbic acid. 2. Interaction with acetyl-salicylic acid. *Int J Vitam Nutr Res* 1980; 50: 387–392.

70. Rivers JM, Devine MM. Plasma ascorbic acid concentrations and oral contraceptives. *Am J Clin Nutr* 1972; 25: 684–689.

71. Utiger R. The need for more vitamin D. *N Engl J Med* 1998; 338: 828–829.

72. Semba RD, Garrett E, Johnson BA, et al. Vitamin D deficiency among older women with and without disability. *Am J Clin Nutr* 2000; 72: 1529–1534.

73. Mezquita-Raya P, Munoz-Torres M, De Dios Luna J, et al. Relation between vitamin D insufficiency, bone density, and bone metabolism in healthy postmenopausal women. *J Bone Miner Res* 2001; 16: 1408–1415.

74. Malabanan AO, Holick MF. Vitamin D and bone health in postmenopausal women. *J Womens Health* (Larchmt) 2003; 12(2): 151–156.

75. Food and Nutrition Board, Institute of Medicine. *Vitamin D. Dietary Reference Intakes: Calcium, Phosphorus, Magnesium, Vitamin D, and Fluoride.* Washington, D.C.: National Academy Press, 1997: 250–287.

76. Vitamins. *Drug Facts and Comparisons.* St. Louis: Facts and Comparisons, 6–33.

77. Ford ES, Sowell A. Serum alpha-tocopherol status in the United States population: findings from the Third National Health and Nutrition Examination Survey. *Am J Epidemiol* 1999; 150: 290–300.

78. Liede KE, Haukka JK, Saxen LM, et al. Increased tendency towards gingival bleeding caused by joint effect of alpha-tocopherol supplementation and acetylsalicylic acid. *Ann Med* 1998; 30: 542–546.

79. Paolisso G, D'Amore A, Galzerano D, et al. Daily vitamin E supplements improve metabolic control but not insulin secretion in elderly type II diabetic patients. *Diabetes Care* 1993; 16: 1433–1437.

80. Paolisso G, D'Amore A, Giugliano D, et al. Pharmacologic doses of vitamin E improve insulin action in healthy subjects and non-insulin-dependent diabetic patients. *Am J Clin Nutr* 1993; 57: 650–656.

81. Food and Nutrition Board, Institute of Medicine. *Folic acid. Dietary Reference Intakes: Thiamin, Riboflavin, Niacin, Vitamin B-6, Vitamin B-12, Pantothenic Acid, Biotin, and Choline.* Washington, D.C.: National Academy Press, 1998: 193–305.

82. Cembrowski GS, Zhang MM, Prosser CI, et al. Folate is not what it is cracked up to be. *Arch Intern Med* 1999; 159: 2747–2748.

83. Lewis DP, Van Dyke DC, Willhite LA, et al. Phenytoin-folic acid interaction. *Ann Pharmacother* 1995; 29: 726–735.

84. Hughes EF, Jacobs BP, Berman BM. Complementary and alternative medicine. In Tierney Jr. LM, McPhee SJ, Papadakis MA, Eds. *Current Medical Diagnosis and Treatment.* New York: Lange Medical Books/McGraw-Hill, 2004: 1681–1703.

85. Kaplan SA, Volpe MA, Te AE. Prospective, 1-year trial using saw palmetto versus finasteride in the treatment of category III prostatitis/chronic pelvic pain syndrome. *J Urol* 2004; 171: 284–288.

86. Markowitz JS, Donovan JL, Devane CL, et al. Multiple doses of saw palmetto (serenoa repens) did not alter cytochrome P450 2D6 and 3A4 activity in normal volunteers. *Clin Pharmacol Ther* 2003; 74: 536–542.

87. Kaye AD, Sabar R, Vig S, et al. Neutraceuticals-current concepts and the role of the anesthesiologist. *Am J Anesthesiol* 2000; 27: 405–407.

88. Jellin JM, Gregory PJ, Batz F, et al, Eds. *St. John's Wort. Natural Medicines: Comprehensive Database.* 4th ed. Stockton, CA: Therapeutic Research Faculty, 2002; 1180–1184.

89. Leak JA. Herbal medicine: is it an alternative or an unknown? A brief review of popular herbals used by patients in a pain and symptom management practice setting. *Cur Rev Pain* 1999; 3: 226–236.

90. Hostanska K, Reichling J, Bommer S, et al. Aqueous ethanolic extract of St. John's wort (*Hypericum perforatum* l) induces growth inhibition and apoptosis in human malignant cells *in vitro*. *Pharmazie* 2002; 57: 323–331.

91. Lecrubier Y, Clerc G, Didi R, et al. Efficacy of St. John's wort extract WS 5570 in major depression: a double-blind, placebo-controlled trial. *Am J Psychiatry* 2002; 159: 1361–1366.

92. Staffeldt B, Kerb R, Brockmoller J, et al. Pharmacokinetics of hypericin and pseudohypericin after local intake of the hypericum perforatum extract LI160 in healthy volunteers. *J Geriatr Psych Neurol* 1994; 7: S47–S53.

93. Hoover JM, Kaye AD, Ibrahim IN, et al. Analysis of responses to St. John's wort in the feline pulmonary vascular bed. *J Herb Pharmacother* 2004; 4(3): 47–62.

94. Cott JM. *In vitro* receptor binding and enzyme inhibition by *Hypericum perforatum* extract. *Pharmacopsychiatry* 1997; 30: 108–112.

95. Cott JM, Misra R. Medicinal plants: a potential source of new psychotherapeutic drugs. In Kanba S, Richelson SE, Eds. *New Drug Development from Herbal Medicines in Neuropharmacology*, vol 5. New York: Brunner/Mazel, 1998.

96. Ness J, Sherman FT, Pan CX. Alternative medicine: what the data say about common herbal therapies. *Geriatrics* 1999; 54: 33–43.

97. Czekalla J, Gastpar M, Hubner WD, et al. The effect of hypericum extract on cardiac conduction as seen in the electrocardiogram compared to that of imipramine. *Pharmacopsychiatry* 1997; 30: 86–88.

98. Bauer R, Khan IA. Structure and stereochemistry of new sesquiterpene esters from *E. purpurea*. *Helv Chim Acta* 1985; 68: 2355–2358.

99. Melchart D, Walther E, Linde K, et al. Echinacea root extracts for the prevention of upper respiratory tract infections: a double-blind, placebo-controlled, randomized trial. *Arch Fam Med* 1998; 7: 541–545.

100. Grimm W, Muller HH. A randomized controlled trial of the effect of fluid extract of *Echinacea purpurea* on the incidence and severity of colds and respiratory infections. *Am J Med* 1999; 106: 138–143.

101. Randolph RK, Gellenbeck K, Stonebrook K, et al. Regulation of human immune gene expression as influenced by a commercial blended echinacea product: preliminary studies. *Exp Biol Med* (Maywood) 2003; 228: 1051–1056.

102. Freier DO, Wright K, Klein K, et al. Enhancement of the humoral immune response by *Echinacea purpurea* in female Swiss mice. *Immunopharmacol Immunotoxicol* 2003; 25: 551–560.

103. Taylor JA, Weber W, Standish L, et al. Efficacy and safety of echinacea in treating upper respiratory tract infections in children: a randomized controlled trial. *JAMA* 2003; 290: 2824–2830.

104. Parnham MJ. Benefit-risk assessment of the squeezed sap of the purple coneflower (*E. purpurea*) for long-term oral immunostimulation. *Phytomedicine* 1996; 3: 95–102.

105. Blumenthal M, Gruenwald J, Hall T, et al, Eds. *German Commission E Monographs: Therapeutic Monographs on MedicinalPplants for Human Use*. Austin, TX: American Botanical Council, 1998.

106. Miller LG. Herbal medicinals. *Arch Intern Med* 1998; 158: 2200–2211.

107. Eaton EA, Walle UK, Lewis AJ, et al. Flavinoids, potent inhibitors of the human form of phenolsulfotransferase: potential role in drug metabolism and chemoprevention. *Drug Met Disp* 1996; 24: 232–237.

108. Schubert W, Eriksson U, Edgar B, et al. Flavinoids in grapefruit juice inhibit the *in vitro* hepatic metabolism of 17 beta-estradiol. *Eur J Drug Metab Pharmacokinet* 1995; 20: 219–224.

109. Gorski JC, Huang SM, Pinto A, et al. The effect of echinacea (*Echinacea purpurea* root) on cytochrome P450 activity *in vivo*. *Clin Pharmacol Ther* 2004; 75: 89–100.

110. Chavez ML, Chavez PI. Echinacea. *Hosp Pharm* 1998; 33: 180–188.

111. Jellin JM, Gregory PJ, Batz F, et al, Eds. Feverfew. *Natural Medicines: Comprehensive Database*, 5th ed. Stockton: Therapeutic Research Faculty, 2003: 541–543.

112. Kaye AD, Sabar R, Vig S, et al. Neutraceuticals-current concepts and the role of the anesthesiologist. *Am J Anesthesiol* 2000; 27: 467–471.

113. Murphy J, Heptinstall S, Mitchell JR, et al. Randomized double-blind, placebo-controlled trial of feverfew in migrane prevention. *Lancet* 1988; 2: 189–192.

114. De Weerdt C, Bootsma H, Hendricks H. Herbal medicines in migrane prevention: randomized double-blind, placebo-controlled crossover trial of a feverfew preparation. *Physomed* 1996; 3: 225–230.

115. Pittler M, Ernst E. Feverfew for preventing migraine. Cochrane Database Syst Rev 1: CD002286, 2004.

116. Nelson MH, Cobb SE, Shelton J. Variations in parthenolide content and daily dose of feverfew products. *Am J Health Syst Pharm* 2002; 59: 1527–1531.

117. Li-Weber M, Giaisi M, Baumann S, et al. The anti-inflammatory sesquiterpene lactone parthenolide suppresses CD95-mediated activation-induced-cell-death in T-cells. *Cell Death Differ* 2002; 9: 1256–1265.

118. Marles RJ, Kaminski J, Arnason JT, et al. A bioassay of inhibition of serotonin release from bovine platelets. *J Nat Prod* 1992; 55: 1044–1056.

119. Fozard JR. 5-Hydroxytryptamine in the pathophysiology of migrane. In Bevan JA, Ed. *Vascular Neuroeffector Mechanisms*. Amsterdam: Elsevier, 1985: 321–328.

120. Makheja AN, Bailey JM. A platelet phospholipase inhibitor from the medicinal herb feverfew (*Tanacatum parthenium*). Proostaglandins Leukot Med 1982; 8: 653–660.

121. Collier HO, Butt NM, McDonald-Gibson WJ, et al. Extract of feverfew inhibits prostaglandins biosynthesis. *Lancet* 1980; 2: 922–923.

122. Baldwin CA, Anderson LA, Phillipson JD, et al. What pharmacists should know about feverfew. *J Pharm Pharmacol* 1987; 239: 237–238.

123. Heptinstall S, Groenwegen WA, Spangenberg P, et al. Extracts of feverfew may inhibit platelet behavior neutralization of sulphydryl groups. *J Pharm Pharmacol* 1987; 39: 459–465.

124. Makheja AN, Bailey J. The active principle in feverfew [letter]. *Lancet* 1981; 2: 1054.

125. Tinkleman DG, Avner SE. Ephedrine therapy in asthmatic children. Clinical tolerance and absence of side effects. *JAMA* 1977; 237: 553–557.

126. Fields AM, Kaye AD, Richards TA, et al. Pulmonary vascular responses to ma huang extract. *J Altern Complement Med* 2003; 9: 727–733.

127. Gurley BJ, Gardner SF, White LM, et al. Ephedrine pharmacokinetics after ingestion of nutritional supplements containing ephedra sinica (ma huang). *Ther Drug Monit* 1998; 20: 439–445.

128. Centers for Disease Control and Prevention (CDC). Adverse events associated with ephedrine-containing products — Texas, December 1993–September 1995. *MMWR Morb Mortal Wkly Rep* 1996, August 16; 45: 689–693.

129. Jurgensen K, Stevens C, Eds. Finally, a Ban on Ephedra. *USA Today* Newspaper, p. 22A, April 13, 2004.

130. Gruenwald J, Brendler T, Jaenicke C, et al. *PDR for Herbal Medicines*, Ed. 1. Montvale: Medical Economics Company, 1998: 826-827.

131. Grontved A, Hentzer E. Vertigo-reducing effect of ginger root. *J Otolaryngol* 1986; 48: 282–286.

132. Holtmann S, Clarke AH, Scherer H, et al. The anti-motion sickness mechanism of ginger. *Acta Otolaryngol* (Stockh) 1989; 108: 168–174.

133. Fischer-Rasmussen W, Kjaer SK, Dahl C, et al. Ginger treatment of hyperemesis gravidarum. *Eur J Obstet Gyn Rep Biol* 1990; 38 :19–24.

134. Backon J. Ginger: inhibition of thromboxane synthetase and stimulation of prostacyclin: relevance for medicine and psychiatry. *Med Hypoth* 1986; 20: 271–278.

135. Nurtjahja-Tjendraputra E, Ammit AJ, Roufogalis BD, et al. Effective anti-platelet and COX-1 enzyme inhibitors from pungent constituents of ginger. *Thromb Res* 2003; 111: 259–265.

136. Akhani SP, Vishwakarma SL, Goyal RK. Anti-diabetic activity of *Zingiber officinale* in streptozotocin-induced type I diabetic rats. *J Pharm Pharmacol* 2004; 56: 101–105.

137. Jellin JM, Batz F, Hitchens K, et al, Eds. *Ginger. Natural Medicines: Comprehensive Database*, 2nd ed. Stockton: Therapeutic Research Faculty, 1999: 416–418.

138. Jain AK, Vargas R, Gotzowsky S, et al. Can garlic reduce levels of serum lipids? A controlled clinical study. *Am J Med* 1993; 94: 632–635.

139. Silagy CA, Neil HAW. A meta-analysis of the effect of garlic on blood pressure. *J Hyperten* 1994; 12: 463–468.

140. Neil HAW, Silagy CA, Lancaster T, et al. Garlic powder in the treatment of moderate hyperlipidemia: a controlled trial and meta-analysis. *J R Coll Physician* 1996; 30: 329–334.

141. Berthold HK, Sudhop T, von Bergmann K. Effect of a garlic oil preparation on serum lipoproteins and cholesterol metabolism: a randomized controlled trial. *JAMA* 1998; 279: 1900–1902.

142. Cooperative group for essential oil of garlic: the effect of essential oil of garlic on hyperlipidemia and platelet aggregation: an analysis of 308 cases. *J Trad Chin Med* 1986; 6: 117–120.

143. Reuter HD. Allium sativum and allium ursinum, part 2: pharmacology and medicinal applications. *Phytomedicine* 1995; 2: 73–91.

144. Beaglehole R. Garlic for flavor, not cardioprotection. *Lancet* 1996; 348: 1186–1187.

145. Mukherjee S, Banerjee SK, Maulik M, et al. Protection against acute adriamycin-induced cardiotoxicity by garlic: role of endogenous antioxidants and inhibition of TNF-alpha expression. *BMC Pharmacol.* 2003; 3: 16.

146. Kaye AD, Nossaman BD, Ibrahim IN, et al. Analysis of responses of allicin, a compound from garlic, in the pulmonary vascular bed of the cat and in the rat. *Eur J Pharmacol* 1995; 276: 21–26.

147. Tsao SM, Hsu CC, Yin MC. Garlic extract and two diallyl sulphides inhibit methicillin-resistant *Staphylococcus aureus* infection in BALB/cA mice. *J Antimicrob Chemother* 2003; 52: 974–980.

148. Bordia A. Effect of garlic on human platelet aggregation *in vitro*. *Atherosclerosis* 1978; 30: 355–360.

149. Bauer U. Six-month double-blind randomized clinical trial of gingko biloba extract versus placebo in two parallel groups in patients suffering from peripheral arterial insufficiency. *Arz-neimittelforschung* 1984; 34: 716–720.

150. Peters H, Kieser M, Holscher U. Demonstration of the efficacy of Gingko biloba special extract EGB 761 on intermittent claudication — a placebo controlled, double-blind multicenter trial. *Vasa* 1998; 27: 106–110.

151. Braquet P. BN 52021 and related compounds: a new series of highly specific PAF-acether receptor antagonists isolated from gingko biloba. *Blood Vessels* 1985; 16: 559–572.

152. Braquet P, Bourgain RH. Anti-anaphylactic properties of BN 52021: a potent platelet activating factor antagonist. *Adv Exp Med Biol* 1987; 215: 215–233.

153. Marcocci L. The nitric oxide scavenging properties of gingko biloba extract Egb761: inhibitory effect on nitric oxide production in the macrophage cell line RAW 264.7. *Biochem Pharmacol* 1997; 53: 897–903.

154. Kobuchi H, Ldroy-Lefaix MT, Christen Y, et al. Gingko biloba extract (Egb 761): inhibitory effect on nitric oxide production in macrophage cell line RAW 264.7. *Biochem Pharmacol* 1997; 53: 897–903.

155. LeBars PL, Katz MM, Berman N, et al. A placebo controlled, double-blind, randomized trial of an extract of gingko biloba for dementia. *JAMA* 1997; 278: 1327–1332.

156. Zeybek N, Gorgulu S, Yagci G, et al. The effects of gingko biloba extract (EGb 761) on experimental acute pancreatitis. *J Surg Res* 2003; 115: 286–293.

157. Rosenblatt M, Mindel J. Spontaneous hyphema associated with ingestion of gingko biloba extract [letter]. *NEJM* 1997; 336: 1108.

158. Rowin J, Lewis SL. Spontaneous bilateral subdural hematomas associated with chronic gingko biloba ingestion have also occurred. *Neurology* 1996; 46: 1775–1776.

159. Gilbert GJ. Gingko biloba [commentary]. *Neurology* 1997; 48: 1137.

160. Vale S. Subarachanoid hemorrhage associated with Gingko biloba [letter]. *Lancet* 1998; 352: 36.

161. Mauro VF, Mauro LS, Kleshinski JF, et al. Impact of ginkgo biloba on the pharmacokinetics of digoxin. *Am J Ther* 2003; 10: 247–251.

162. Nowakowska E, Ostrowicz A, Chodera A. Kava-kava preparations-alternative anxiolytics. *Pol Merkuriusz Lek* 1998; 4: 179–180a.

163. Skidmore-Roth L. *Kava. Mosby's Handbook of Herbs and Natural Supplements*. St. Louis: Mosby-Harcourt Health Sciences, 2001: 486–490.

164. Uebelhack R, Franke L, Schewe HJ. Inhibition of platelet MAO-B by kava pyrone-enriched extract from Piper methysticum Forster (kava-kava). *Pharmacopsychiatry* 1998; 31: 187–192.

165. Jellin JM, Gregory PJ, Batz F, et al, Eds. *Kava. Natural Medicines: Comprehensive Database*, 4th ed. Stockton: Therapeutic Research Faculty, 2002: 759–761.

166. Volz HP, Kieser M. Kava-kava extract WS 1490 versus placebo in anxiety disorders a randomized placebo-controlled 25-week outpatient trial. *Pharmacopsychiatry* 1997; 30: 1–5.
167. Forget L, Goldrosen J, Hart JA, et al, Eds. *Herbal Companion to AHFS DI.* Bethesda, MD: American Society of Health-System Pharmacists, Inc., 2000.
168. Seitz U, Schule A, Gleitz J. [3H]-monoamine uptake inhibition properties of kava pyrones. *Planta Med* 1997; 63: 548–549.
169. Winslow LC, Kroll DJ. Herbs as medicines. *Arch Intern Med* 1998; 158: 2192–2199.
170. Garner LF, Klinger JD. Some visual effects caused by the beverage kava. *J Ethnopharm* 1985; 13: 307–311.
171. Jellin JM, Gregory PJ, Batz F, et al, Eds. *Kava. Natural Medicines: Comprehensive Database*, 5th ed. Stockton: Therapeutic Research Faculty, 2003: 788–791.
172. Jamieson DD, Duffield PH. Positive interaction of ethanol and kava resin in mice. *Clin Exp Pharm Physiol* 1990; 17: 509–514.
173. Gruenwald J, Brendler T, Jaenicke C, et al. *PDR for Herbal Medicines*, 1st ed. Montvale: Medical Economics Company, 1998: 1043–1045.
174. Jamieson DD, Duffield PH. The antinociceptive actions of kava components in mice. *Clin Exp Pharm Physio* 1990; 17: 495–507.
175. Singh YN. Effects of kava on neuromuscular transmission and muscular contractility. *J Ethnopharm* 1983; 7: 267–276.
176. Ng TB, Li WW, Yeung HW. Effects of ginsenosides, lectins and Momordica charantia insulin-like peptide on corticosterone production by isolated rat adrenal cells. *J Ethnopharm* 1987; 21: 21–29.
177. Jellin JM, Gregory PJ, Batz F, et al, Eds. *Ginseng, American, Ginseng, Panax. Natural Medicines: Comprehensive Database*, 5th ed. Stockton: Therapeutic Research Faculty, 2003: 614–619.
178. Zhou DL, Kitts DD. Peripheral blood mononuclear cell production of TNF-alpha in response to North American ginseng stimulation. *Can J Physiol Pharmacol* 2002; 80: 1030–1033.
179. Jie YH, Cammisuli S, Baggiolini M, et al. Immunomodulatory effects of panax ginseng: CA Meyer in the mouse. *Agents Actions Suppl* 1984; 15: 386–391.
180. Sotaniemi EA, Haapakkoski E, Rautio A, et al. Ginseng therapy in non-insulin dependent diabetic patients. *Diabetes Care* 1995; 18: 1373–1375.
181. Yokozawa T, Kobayashi T, Oura H, et al. Studies on the mechanism of hypoglycemic activity of ginsenoside-Rb2 in streptozotocin-diabetic rats. *Chem Pharm Bull* 1985; 33: 869–872.
182. Oshima Y, Kkonno C, Hikono H. Isolation and hypoglycemic activity of panaxans I, J, K and L, glycans of panax ginseng roots. *J Ethnopharm* 1985; 14: 255–259.
183. Konno C, Murakami M, Oshima Y, et al. Isolation and hypoglycemic activity of panaxans Q, R, S, T and U, glycans of panax ginseng roots. *J Ethnopharm* 1985; 14: 69–74.
184. Konno C, Sugiyama K, Oshima Y, et al. Isolation and hypoglycemic activity of panaxans A, B, C, D and E glycans of panax ginseng roots. *Planta Med* 1984; 50: 436–438.
185. Tokmoda M, Shimada K, Konno M, et al. Partial structure of panax A: a hypoglycemic glycan of panax ginseng roots. *Planta Med* 1984; 50: 436–438.
186. Baldwin CA. What pharmacists should know about ginseng. *Pharm J* 1986; 237: 583–586.

187. Hammond TG, Whitworth JA. Adverse reactions to ginseng [letter]. *Med J Aust* 1981; 1: 492.

188. Dega H, Laporte J, Frances C, et al. Ginseng a cause of Steven-Johnson syndrome? [letter] *Lancet* 1996; 347: 1344.

189. Greenspan EM. Ginseng and vaginal bleeding [letter]. *JAMA* 1983; 249: 2018.

190. Hopkins MP, Androff L, Benninghoff AS, et al. Ginseng face cream and unexpected vaginal bleeding. *Am J Obs Gyn* 1988; 159: 1121–1122.

191. Palmer BV, Montgomery AC, Monterio JC, et al. Ginseng and mastalgia. *BMJ* 1978; 1: 1284.

192. Kuo SC, Teng CM, Lee JG, et al. Antiplatelet components in panax ginseng. *Planta Med* 1990; 56: 164–167.

193. Shader RI, Greenblatt DJ. Phenelzine and the dream machine-ramblings and reflections [edit.] *J Clin Psychopharmacol* 1985; 5: 65.

194. Jones BD, Runikis AM. Interactions of ginseng with phenelzine. *J Clin Psychopharm* 1987; 7: 201–202.

195. Kaye AD, Grogono AW. Fluid and electrolyte physiology. In Miller RD, Cucchiara RF, Miller ED Jr, et al, Eds. *Anesthesia* vol. 1, 5th ed. Philadelphia: Churchill Livingstone, 2000: 1586–1612.

8 Nutrient- and Drug-Responsive Polymorphic Genes as Nutrigenomic Tools for Prevention of Cardiovascular Disease and Cancer

Kevin Wood and Marica Bakovic

CONTENTS

8.1   INTRODUCTION

Nutrigenomics is an integrative science combining biotechnology, molecular medicine, and pharmacogenomics, which is revolutionizing how nutrition and diet are viewed.[1] A working definition of this new branch of genomics, by Kaput and Rodriguez, is that "it seeks to provide a genetic understanding for how dietary chemicals can affect the balance between health and disease by altering the expression of an individual's genetic makeup."[2] In an attempt to clarify the term, they have proposed the following five tenets:

1. Common dietary compounds act on the human genome, directly or indirectly, to alter gene expression or structure.
2. In some individuals under certain circumstances, diet can be a serious risk factor for a number of diseases.
3. Some diet-regulated genes (and their normal, common variants) are susceptibility genes and likely to play a role in the onset, incidence, progression, and/or severity of chronic diseases.
4. The degree to which diet influences the balance between healthy and disease states depends on an individual's genetic makeup.
5. Dietary interventions based on knowledge of nutritional requirement, nutrition status, and genotype (i.e., "individualized nutrition") can be used to prevent, mitigate, or cure chronic disease.

The possible applications of nutrigenomics could be numerous. Genomic information could be used to understand the basis of individual differences in response to dietary patterns.[1] Nutrigenomic data could be gathered to provide a sound basis for the development of safe and effective diet therapies for individuals or subgroups in specific populations. Therefore, the main goal of nutrigenomics is to understand each individual's responses to micro- and macronutrients via genetic screening in order to create safe and effective dietary treatments for them. Nutrigenomics can establish more flexible, long-term dietary strategies for early prevention of chronic diseases, based on genetic predispositions and the knowledge of specific dietary requirements of individuals and particular (ethnic) groups, relying less on the entire population.[3]

In particular, single nucleotide polymorphisms (SNPs) will be very important in identifying individual variations in responses to nutrients. SNPs are changeable sites within a genome, occurring once every 1000 to 2000 nucleotides,[4] where the rarer nucleotide is present at a frequency of greater than 1% in a population.[5] SNPs are different than sporadic mutations, which are germline polymorphisms occurring with a frequency of less than 1%.[5] These genetic variations alter protein structure and function when the nucleotide base substitution occurs in a gene's coding region.[6] Alternatively, a polymorphism may have no effect on the protein product because the base substitution occurs in a DNA region that is not involved in gene transcription or translation; however, it could be a part of regulatory promoters.

Molecular techniques for detecting SNPs (polymerase chain reaction, restriction enzyme detection) have been used extensively in pharmaceutical, toxicological, and clinical research disciplines, but not so much in nutritional sciences.[4] The recent development of extensive genomic databases and high throughput genetic screening made it possible for the study of the interactions of interindividual variation and nutrition. The greatest potential for benefit from those studies will be for health maintenance by preventing or slowing the early stages of diet-related diseases. Nutrigenomics could also provide the means to develop better molecular biomarkers of early changes between health maintenance and disease progression.

The most common diseases, such as cardiovascular disease (CVD) and cancer, are known to be polygenic, meaning that the incidence of the disease is attributable to polymorphisms of multiple interacting genes.[6,7] These multifactorial diseases involve the interaction of many genes as well as gene–environment and gene–diet interactions. Complex interactions of multiple internal and external factors determine the probability of developing these multifactorial diseases. Since the interactions can make it increasingly difficult to identify and characterize what combinations of genetic variants are relevant to CVD and cancer, the study of gene–diet interactions can help to establish the strongest relationships between gene variations and phenotypes in healthy individuals in order to relate their specific genotype to biomarkers of disease risk.[5] Defining these pathophysiologic mechanisms in each individual can aid in identifying individuals at risk for disease and to apply diet and lifestyle changes to modify disease risk factors.[6] This chapter focuses on certain polymorphisms where the intake of a specific nutrient related to that polymorphism affects the pathogenesis of CVD and/or cancer.

8.2 GENETIC POLYMORPHISMS AND CVD

Our health is maintained through the integration of numerous complex homeostatic physiological processes operating at the cellular, tissue, and organ level.[8] Genes encode the proper amount of functional proteins and enzymes necessary for these processes and, hence, a disease such as CVD may be thought of as a result of failure of adequate homeostasis within a physiological system. This failure may result from failure at the genetic level or from environmental exposure or from an imbalance of the two. CVD most often does not result from a single mutation in one gene, but since it is polygenic, it is more likely that CVD risk is a result of many interacting mutations in several different genes (except for single autosomal dominant inheritance, such as familial hypercholesterolemia). A single polymorphism in a single gene likely plays a small role in CVD, but it is the combination of several polymorphic genes that determines susceptibility to CVD. Even though pharmaceutical agents can successfully normalize plasma lipid concentrations, dietary modification is currently the cornerstone of primary CVD prevention.[9] The success of this approach is known to vary and depend on individual responses to recommended dietary changes, which is determined by gene–nutrient interactions. Hence, exposure to the same level of a dietary factor can decrease the risk in one person, but not in another, depending on specific gene variants. There are many genes involved in CVD pathogenesis that have been documented; however, they are either not affected by diet or are still not well established as risk factors.

8.2.1 APOLIPOPROTEIN E AND CVD

Apolipoprotein E (APOE), a constituent of triglyceride-rich chylomicrons, very low-density lipoprotein (VLDL) particles, and their remnants,[10] is a protein associated with the metabolism of triacylglycerol-rich lipoproteins and high-density lipoprotein (HDL).[11] It also serves as a ligand for low-density lipoprotein (LDL) receptors and LDL-receptor related proteins and, therefore, mediates chylomicron and VLDL clearance from plasma.[11,12] The APOE gene, located on human chromosome 19, is 3.7kb in length and contains four exons. Genetic variation at the APOE gene locus is an important determinant of serum LDL-cholesterol concentrations.[13]

Three common alleles of the APOE gene have been described: *E2*, *E3*, and *E4*, which produce three isoforms of the protein E2, E3, and E4. These isoforms differ in amino acid sequence at positions 112 and 158.[14] E3 has a cysteine at 112 and an arginine at 158. E2 has a cysteine at both positions and E4 has an arginine at both positions. Population studies have shown that plasma total cholesterol and LDL cholesterol (LDL-C) concentrations are lowest in subjects with the *E2* allele, intermediate in those with the *E3* allele, and highest in those with the *E4* allele.[11] APOE allele frequencies vary, with the major allele in all populations being *E3* (gene frequency of 0.49 to 0.91), followed by *E4* (gene frequency 0.06 to 0.37) and *E2* (gene frequency 0 to 0.15).[12] The *E4* variant has been associated with increased cholesterol absorption, increased LDL production from VLDL, and decreased bile acid synthesis and LDL clearance from plasma. The *E4* allele is also associated with a greater risk of coronary artery disease in both men and women.

8.2.2 APOE GENOTYPE AND SATURATED FAT INTAKE

In Western societies, where diets are high in saturated fat and cholesterol, studies have shown that the *E4* allele is associated with higher LDL-C and triglyceride and lower HDL cholesterol (HDL-C) concentrations.[12] In 2001, Campos et al. studied how the genetic variants of APOE would interact with habitual saturated fat intake to affect the plasma lipid profile. Higher saturated fat intake was associated with higher VLDL cholesterol, lower HDL-C, and smaller LDL particles in *E2* carriers, and the opposite or no effect was observed in the *E4* and *E3* carriers. This suggests that carriers of the E2 variant allele may actually be particularly susceptible to coronary disease when exposed to high saturated fat diets. It was found that the E2 allele has a more detrimental influence on the lipoprotein profile in individuals eating a high saturated fat diet compared to low saturated fat, and the mechanism for this response may be due to the effect of the E2 allele on receptor-mediated VLDL clearance. Compared to E3, E2 binds poorly to lipoprotein receptors leading to delayed clearance and increased accumulation of chylomicron and VLDL remnants.[11]

8.2.3 APOE GENOTYPE AND SUCROSE INTAKE

Erkkila et al.[11] conducted a cross-sectional study to investigate the interaction between APOE genotype and dietary intake of fat and carbohydrate (sucrose), on serum cholesterol and triacylglycerol concentrations in patients with coronary artery disease. The allele frequencies for *E2*, *E3*, and *E4* were 0.039, 0.757 and 0.204, respectively. Patients had to complete 4-day food records and all amounts and qualities of foods in the records were checked by a clinical nutritionist for completion. Results showed that LDL-C and total cholesterol were lower in patients with the *E2* allele than in patients with the *E3* and *E4* allele, while serum triacylglycerol levels tended to be higher in *E2* carriers. In addition, a high intake of sucrose was associated with high serum triacylglycerol only in patients with the *E2* allele, while high triacylglycerol content was more observed in *E4* carriers with a low sucrose intake. The investigators concluded that coronary artery disease patients with the *E2* allele will likely have a greater triacylglycerol response to high dietary sucrose intake than will patients with the *E3* or *E4* allele.

8.2.4 METHYLENETETRAHYDROFOLATE REDUCTASE AND CVD

The enzyme methylenetetrahydrofolate reductase (MTHFR), a 70 kDA flavoprotein is a member of the MTHFR family.[15] MTHFR catalyzes the conversion of 5,10-methylenetetrahydrofolate to 5-methyltetrahydrofolate (Figure 8.1), which is a methyl donor group in the methylation of homocysteine to methionine.[4–6,16,17] The human MTHFR gene is located on chromosome 1p36.3 and has a coding region length of 1.980 bp.[16] A common polymorphism of the MTHFR gene has been associated with CVD risk and is well documented.[18] The polymorphism, which consists of a C→T change at nucleotide 677, results in an amino acid substitution of alanine in place of valine.[19] This amino acid substitution produces an enzyme with decreased activity (approximately 35% of the value in individuals without the mutation) and decreased thermal stability. The TT genotype is predictive of increased plasma homocysteine and an increased risk for CVD.[20] Elevated plasma homocysteine has also been identified as a risk factor for cardiovascular-related diseases of the coronary, cerebral and peripheral arteries, and venous thrombosis.[21] Although there have been some studies to show the contrary,

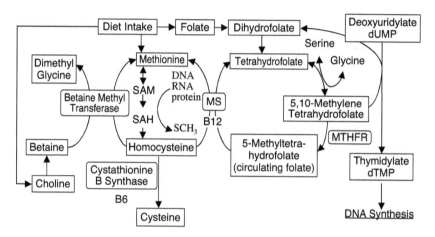

FIGURE 8.1 Schematic representation of folate/homocysteine/methionine metabolism in DNA methylation and DNA synthesis. (Adapted from Steenge et al. (2003) Betaine supplementation lowers plasma homocysteine in healthy men and women. *J Nutr* 133: 1291–1295; and Ma et al. (1999) A polymorphism of the methionine synthase gene: association with plasma folate, vitamin B_{12}, homocysteine, and colorectal cancer risk. *Canc Epidemiol Biomark Prev* 8: 825-829.) Abbreviations: MS = methionine synthase, SAM = S-adenosyl methionine, SAH = S-adenosyl homocysteine, MTHFR = methylene-tetrahydrofolate reductase, dUMP = deoxyuridine 5′-monophosphate, dTMP = deoxythymidine 5′-monophosphate.

total homocysteine does seem to be a predictor of CVD, particularly in high-risk populations, but is only weakly associated with risk in otherwise healthy subjects.[16] Homocysteine concentrations can be modulated by genetic and physiological factors, diet, folate supplementation, riboflavin, choline, and vitamins B_6 and B_{12}.[17]

8.2.5 MTHFR 677 C→T Polymorphism, Folate Intake, and CVD

Observational studies have shown that when folate status is less than adequate, individuals with the MTHFR 677 TT genotype have lower blood folate and higher plasma homocysteine concentrations than those with the MTHFR 677 CC genotype.[22–26] One of the most recent studies in this area, by Shelnutt et al.,[27] recruited only 677 CC and TT, nonpregnant healthy women, aged 20 to 30 years old and placed them on folate deficient and folate rich diets. The folate depletion diet provided approximately 115 μg dietary folate equivalents (DFE) per day for 7 weeks, and the folate repletion diet consisted of a combination of the depletion diet, plus 400 μg DFE/d for 7 weeks. Serum folate concentrations did not differ between the two genotypes at baseline. Results showed that TT individuals were less capable of maintaining normal blood folate concentration during the depletion phase than CC individuals.[27] Mean plasma homocysteine concentration was

~3 μmol/l higher in TT subjects with low folate status postdepletion than in CC subjects. Seven weeks of folate repletion was also insufficient to decrease the mean plasma homocysteine concentration in women with the TT genotype. Hence, this study, in which nutrient intake was controlled, supports the conclusion that folate deficiency alone is sufficient to negatively affect plasma homocysteine concentration in TT individuals.[27]

Studies by Ashfield-Watt et al.[28] and de Bree et al.[24] have both shown similar results for men and women. Ashfield-Watt et al. placed subjects on three different diets, each for 4 months. The "exclusion diet" was a usual diet, but folate-fortified foods were replaced with unfortified foods, and a placebo tablet taken daily. The "folate-rich diet" was a usual diet plus additional folate-fortified foods and naturally folate-rich foods to reach a total of at least 400 μg/d. The "supplement diet" was the exclusion diet plus a 400 μg folate supplement daily instead of the placebo. The folate supplement did have a significantly greater effect on plasma folate than the folate-rich diet did, but the supplement had minimal additional homocysteine-lowering capacity compared with diet alone.[28] The folate-rich and supplement interventions significantly increased plasma folate in TT individuals above the baseline concentrations observed in those with the CC genotype. The TT genotypes showed a greater homocysteine-lowering response to active folate interventions than subjects with the other genotypes.

The study by de Bree et al. also supports this result. They showed that at any folate intake, TT subjects have lower plasma folate than CT and CC subjects, yet at high plasma folate concentrations, the homocysteine concentrations in TT subjects are as low as those in CT and CC subjects. Overall, findings show TT homozygotes have a greater requirement for folate to achieve homocysteine concentrations comparable with the prevalent concentrations seen in CT and CC individuals.[28] These studies provide very useful data on folic acid fortification for public health reasons and of supplementation, which is relevant for CVD prevention.

8.2.6 Hepatic Lipase and CVD

Hepatic lipase (HL), a lipolytic enzyme synthesized primarily in hepatocytes, located on human chromosome 15q21, plays a critical role in lipid metabolism, particularly in HDL metabolism.[29–32] HL attaches to the sinusoidal endothelial surface after being secreted from hepatocytes and hydrolyzes triglycerides and phospholipids in plasma lipoproteins.[30,31,33] HL has been implicated in regulating HDL cholesterol levels, although the precise mechanism by which HL modulates lipoprotein metabolism has yet to be characterized.[34] It is thought that increased HL activity is linked with generating small LDLs and contributes to its association with low HDL because HL can also increase the hepatic uptake of HDL lipids.[35] There have been several polymorphisms identified in the HL gene, including some causing a rare HL deficiency condition.[36,37] Recent studies have also shown that polymorphisms in the HL gene promoter region are related to variations in plasma HDL concentrations and that there are associations between HL gene promoter polymorphisms and HL activity.[38–41] A polymorphism in the HL gene, which causes a C→T substitution at nucleotide 514, is favorable.[38,39] The T allele is associated with decreased HL activity, therefore, increasing HDL concentrations.[38,39] Hence, there is a good deal of research supporting the fact that rare alleles of common promoter polymorphisms, such as the nucleotide 514 C→T substitution, are associated with a significant decrease in plasma HL activity and increased HDL levels.[33,39,42]

8.2.7 HL-514 C→T POLYMORPHISM AND CVD

Using a multiethnic population in Singapore and subjecting them to a highly Westernized lifestyle, Tai et al.[9] investigated the possible gene–nutrient interactions between the −514 C→T polymorphism and dietary fat on HDL metabolism. When there was no stratification by fat intake considered, the T allele was associated with higher plasma HDL concentrations, higher triglyceride (TG) concentrations and higher HDL/TG ratios. The TT subjects showed higher TG levels only when fat intake was greater than 30% of total energy. An earlier study by Ordovas et al.[43] supports the results of Tai et al. using subjects from the Framingham Study. They were also able to show that the T allele was associated with significantly greater HDL concentrations only in those subjects consuming less than 30% of energy from fat. When the total intake of fat was greater than 30% of energy, the mean HDL concentrations were lowest among those individuals with the TT genotype, and no differences were observed between CT and CC individuals.[43] Overall, both studies indicate that the TT genotype is associated with a more atherogenic lipid profile when subjects consume diets with a fat content of at least 30% of total energy.[9,43]

8.2.8 STATINS, NIACIN, AND POLYMORPHISMS RELATED TO THE LOWERING OF CHOLESTEROL

For individuals with lipoprotein abnormalities, lowering LDL-C continues to be the primary target of cholesterol-lowering therapy. Lifestyle modification is the first means of lowering LDL-C and drug therapy is reserved for those where lifestyle modification is ineffective.[44] The most commonly used hypocholesterolemic drugs are hydroxyl methylglutaryl coenzyme-A (HMG CoA) reductase inhibitors, known as statins. The use of statins has become popular since the 1990s due to their high efficacy and low secondary effects.[45] Their principal action is to lower plasma lipids via a considerable decrease in plasma LDL-C as well as a slight decrease in triglycerides and a modest increase in HDL-C.[46–48] However, hypolipidemic agents show considerable individual variation in their effects. The differences may be attributable to the interaction of environmental and genetic factors.[44,45] Among the genetic factors that may be responsible for this individual variation, the APOE locus has been the most widely studied.[44,49,50] There is a significant difference in response to statins associated with the APOE locus. Subjects carrying the *E2* allele have a significantly higher response to LDL-C lowering and those carrying the *E4* allele have a significantly lower response.[51] Plasma total cholesterol, LCL-C, and triglyceride responses were significantly greater for E2 subjects as compared to E3 and E4 subjects when taking atorvastatin, one of the most effective statins available.

Other polymorphisms involved in the individual response to statins are the *Pvu*II and *Ava*II polymorphisms of the LDL-receptor gene. These polymorphisms have been shown to influence the levels of LDL-C in both normo- and hypercholesterolemic subjects and may influence the response to treatment with statins.[52] There has been minimal work done on these polymorphisms with conflicting results. Studies have reported that subjects with the P2 allele of the *Pvu*II polymorphism have a better response than those homozygous for the P1 allele, but this has yet to be reproduced.[45,53] Lahoz has shown a significant trend in the *Ava*II polymorphism showing that those homozygous for the (−) allele responded less than heterozygotes, who in turn responded less than homozygotes for the (+) allele. Clinical importance for these polymorphisms is currently unknown and requires further studies to determine an effect.

The −514C/T hepatic lipase and apolipoprotein A-1 promoter polymorphisms can also influence the effectiveness of statin therapy. Individuals who are homozygous for the C allele had scarce modification of HDL-C with pravastatin treatment while in carriers of the T allele, the increase in HDL-C was almost 7%.[54] However, it has been reported that those with the CC genotype may benefit more from statins since they appear to have greater improvement in coronary lesions than CT and TT genotypes. Carriers of the A allele for the apoA-1 polymorphism showed HDL-C concentrations significantly higher than G allele carriers with pravastatin treatment. The mechanisms by which the G/A polymorphism influences HDL-C levels and its response to pravastatin are not known. This is the case for many of the above-mentioned polymorphisms interacting with statins. The value of determining genetic polymorphisms in order to predict the effects of statin treatment is still unclear, but will improve with further research.

Niacin (nicotinic acid) has been used as a lipid lowering agent to treat dyslipidemia since 1954.[55–57] Niacin is one of the most effective agents available for raising HDL-C and lowering triglycerides and, hence, adding niacin to statin therapy may be desirable. There has been reluctance to take immediate-release niacin due to possible side effects of flushing and skin rash, but extended-release niacin is both better tolerated and safer.[58] Many studies suggest that combination niacin–statin therapy leads to improved lipoprotein profiles and clinical outcomes over monotherapy using either niacin or a statin.[59,60] The addition of 2000 mg/d of extended-release niacin to patients on statin therapy can decrease total cholesterol an additional 21%, LDL-C by 31%, triglycerides by 27%, and increase HDL-C by an additional 27%. Therefore, drug–nutrient interactions need to be considered for each individual and these drug therapies could be more effective if they are tailored better to individual needs.

8.3 GENETIC POLYMORPHISMS AND CANCER

There has been a wealth of evidence from epidemiological, clinical, and laboratory studies to suggest that nutrition and dietary factors can influence the risk for the development of cancer, prognosis after diagnosis, as well as the quality of life during treatment.[61] It is estimated that many of the cancers in the U.S. are related to nutritional and dietary factors.[61,62] The molecular pathologies of cancer are known to involve many steps involving the culmination of genetic changes resulting from the interaction between genetics and the environment.[61,63,64] The great challenge has been to show the actual causative relationships and underlying mechanisms that link dietary constituents to cancer risk.[61] Although it has been difficult to define relationships between nutritional factors and disease due to the limitations of methodologies for assessing exposure to these factors, complexity of dietary patterns, as well as the trouble in untangling the influence of dietary constituents, it has been recognized that not all persons exposed to the same risk factors will develop the associated disease.[61,63,65,66] This is why it is now clear that differential genetic susceptibility may explain the variation in response seen among those with apparently similar diets or exposure to nutritional factors.

There are many genetic factors that can increase the risk for cancer, but the most well-known are the highly penetrant, dominant mutations that epidemiological studies show to have very high relative risks. However, in contrast with the highly penetrant dominant mutations are the genetic mutations, which are not sufficient to cause disease, but may affect cancer susceptibility or the response to environmental exposure. These mutations can actually have a much greater effect on a population, despite posing lower individual risk.[64] The most studied of these mutations are gene variants that influence metabolic activation, detoxification, or elimination of carcinogens. Some of these gene variants/polymorphisms can be relatively common in the general population (up to 53%) and are known to play a role in the ability of an individual to withstand exposure to carcinogens or to inhibit the initiation, promotion, or proliferation in carcinogenesis.[67,68] With much speed, nutrition and cancer research is transitioning from an observational approach to more of a molecular approach as the knowledge of genomics and new technologies grows.[69] Not only will nutritional genomics determine which nutrient-related genetic and epigenetic changes cause phenotypic changes that influence cancer risk, but it will also establish which interactions are the most important under certain circumstances.[68] Although this area is receiving more and more attention, it is still not entirely clear as to how genetic polymorphisms are related to the impact of diet on the cancer process, but it is plausible that polymorphic differences have been a contributing factor in the inconsistencies surrounding diet and health.[70] This section focuses on certain genes and nutrients that are known to play a role in mitigating cancer based on specific variations in diet–gene interactions and gene functions.

8.3.1 VITAMIN D AND THE VITAMIN D RECEPTOR

Vitamin D is an essential nutrient that is mainly produced in the skin as a photoproduct of 7-dehyrocholesterol, or obtained through the diet via such foods as dairy products (milk, cheese, butter) and seafood (fish, oysters).[71,72] Other sources of vitamin D include fortified milk products, breakfast cereals, and vitamin D-containing multivitamins and supplements. Vitamin D is a prohormone necessary for the regulation of serum calcium and phosphorous. One of the active hormonal forms, 1,25-hydroxycholecalciferol [1,25(OH)$_2$D] produced in the kidney, enhances calcium absorption from the small intestine and is tightly regulated to ensure calcium homeostasis. Vitamin D does undergo several hydroxylations to become biologically active.[73] The first hydroxylation occurs in the liver, at carbon 25, to yield 25-hydroxyvitamin D [25(OH)$_2$D]. Since this reaction is not tightly regulated, 25(OH)D levels reflect exposure to sunlight and dietary intake and, hence, plasma 25(OH)D is the best indicator of nutritional vitamin D status.[72–74]

1,25(OH)$_2$D is a specific ligand for the nuclear vitamin D receptor (VDR), which is expressed in different tissues, especially in the intestine, bone, pancreas, breast, prostate, pituitary, gonads, mononuclear cells, activated T lymphocytes, and skin.[73] Once 1,25(OH)$_2$D binds with VDR, the resulting complex translocates to the nucleus and interacts with respective vitamin D-responsive elements (VDRE) within regulatory (promoter) regions; hence, initiating or repressing transcription of various target genes. When VDR is bound to the 1,25(OH)$_2$D form, it transactivates genes that inhibit proliferation,[75] promote differentiation,[76,77] or induce apoptosis.[78,79] Vitamin D and its various forms have been investigated as dietary anticarcinogens, and observational and cohort studies have supported an inverse relationship between vitamin D and prostate, colorectal, and breast cancers.[65,72]

Biological activity of circulating 1,25(OH)$_2$D is modulated through variants in the VDR gene, which was found to be polymorphic at multiple sites.[80] These polymorphisms include FokI (FF, Ff, ff), BsMI (BB, Bb, bb), TaqI (TT, Tt, tt), and a 3'-untranslated region poly-A site (SS, Ss, ss) of the VDR gene.[68,71,73,81] Except for FokI, all polymorphisms are in strong linkage disequilibrium with each other and may potentially influence the expression or function of the VDR protein. The FokI polymorphism influences the development of colorectal adenomas.[81] The BsMI B polymorphism and short poly-A polymorphisms have been associated with increased breast cancer risk.[68,80] BsMI has also been associated with decreased risk of prostate cancer and benign prostatic hyperplasia.[68,81] The TaqI polymorphism may reduce the risk of lymph node metastasis, inhibit tumor progression, and increase survival among ER (+), tamoxifen-treated women. TaqI has also shown reductions in prostate cancer risk.[71,83]

8.3.2 VDR POLYMORPHISMS, VITAMIN D INTAKE, AND COLORECTAL CANCER

Vitamin D had first been implicated as protective against cancer by ecological studies linking colorectal cancer mortality to latitude, which correlates with sunlight exposure.[81,84] The ecological studies were then followed by analytic epidemiologic studies of vitamin D and cancer, most of which found weak inverse relationships between vitamin D status and colorectal cancer risk.[81,85,86] It has been suggested that vitamin D reduces epithelial cell proliferation and promotes differentiation in various cell cultures.[87,88] Other studies have also shown that vitamin D induces apoptosis in colorectal tumor cell lines and premalignant adenoma cells.[89] Clinical evidence has shown that a high level of VDR expression is associated with a favorable prognosis of colorectal cancer.[90]

Ingles et al.[81] examined whether the 5′ start codon FokI polymorphism and the 3′ UTR BsMI VDR polymorphism are associated with risk of colorectal adenoma in a multiethnic population of men and women aged 50 to 74 with no history of invasive cancer or inflammatory bowel disease. Cases had a first-time diagnosis of one or more colorectal adenomas, confirmed by histology, and controls had no past adenoma and were matched to cases by gender, age, and date of sigmoidoscopy. The frequency of the FokI F allele was highest in African Americans (74%) and the frequency of the BsMI B allele was highest in Caucasians (42%). Only large, not small, adenomas were associated with the FokI genotype, suggesting that this genotype may influence the progression of adenomas to a more malignant phenotype. No association between the BsMI genotype and the risk of large adenoma was seen.[81]

A study by Peters et al.[85] investigated the association of a VDR polymorphism with colorectal adenomas and the interactions with vitamin D and calcium in subjects between the ages of 18 and 74. Detailed information about sun exposure, use of vitamin and mineral supplements, medical history, physical activity, and alcohol and tobacco consumption was collected from each subject, along with blood samples for measuring serum 25(OH)D levels and for FokI genotyping. The results showed no evidence for an overall effect of the FokI polymorphism and colorectal adenoma nor interaction with either serum vitamin D or calcium intake; however, an inverse association of serum vitamin D with colorectal adenoma was found. A similarly designed study by Slattery et al.[91] also found no evidence for an inverse association with the FokI polymorphism and colon cancer, but did find inverse associations for the SS poly-A, BsMI and TaqI polymorphisms, and colon cancer. Wong et al.[84] have reported that the FokI variant actually increases the risk of colorectal cancer in a Singapore Chinese population. Compared to those individuals carrying the FF genotype, those with the Ff genotype had a 51% increase in risk and those with the ff genotype had an 84% increase in risk.

There are studies, though, that show a decrease in colon cancer risk based on vitamin D-VDR interaction. Slattery et al.[92] found the greatest reduced risk for colon cancer was observed for individuals with a high intake of calcium, vitamin D, and low-fat dairy products, and with the SS poly-A or BB BsMI genotypes. Also, calcium, vitamin D, and low-fat dairy products were inversely associated with rectal cancer in women, but not in men. These results are supported by Kim et al.[93] who showed that those with the BB BsMI genotype and the lowest calcium and vitamin D intake were at a reduced risk of colorectal adenomas relative to those with the bb BsMI genotype and the highest levels of intake, although this interaction wasn't statistically significant.[92] It has been proposed that the antineoplastic activity of the BB and SS alleles is due to the increased $1,25(OH)_2D$ levels associated with those alleles.[92] It may also be possible that different VDR genotypes interact differently with VDREs, which could lead to altered ability to transcriptionally regulate target genes.

8.3.3 METHYLENETETRAHYDROFOLATE REDUCTASE, FOLATE STATUS, AND CANCER

As mentioned earlier, MTHFR irreversibly converts 5,10- methylenetetrahydrofolate to 5-methyl tetrahydrofolate, which is the major form of circulating folate in plasma[71] (see Figure 8.1). Besides being the major circulating form of intracellular folate, 5,10-methylenetetrahydrofolate is also the cofactor for methylating deoxyuridylate to produce thymidylate, the rate-limiting nucleotide in DNA synthesis (see Figure 8.1). Decreasing the availability of MTHFR increases the availability of methylenetetrahydrofolate and, therefore, reduces the chances of insufficient thymidylate and misincorporation of uracil into DNA.[71] The reduced incorporation of uracil into DNA leads to less chromosome breaking, and possibly a lower cancer risk.[94,95]

There are many common genetic polymorphisms that appear to modulate cancer risk through their influence on folate metabolism. Two polymorphisms in the MTHFR gene, one consisting of a C to T substitution at nucleotide 677 (alanine to valine), and another consisting of an A to G substitution at nucleotide 1298 (glutamate to alanine) both result in a reduction in MTHFR activity. Methionine synthase (MS) catalyzes the transfer of a methyl group from 5-methyl tetrahydrofolate to homocysteine, producing methionine and tetrahydrofolate (see Figure 8.1), which is necessary for maintaining an adequate level of intracellular methionine, the precursor of the methyl donor S-adenosyl methionine (SAM).[71,96] SAM is an important methyl group donor that is involved in over 100 methylation reactions that includes DNA methylation. A polymorphism of the methionine synthase gene (MTR), consisting of an A to G substitution at nucleotide 2756, results in a conversion of aspartate to glycine and reduces MS activity. A lack of sufficient SAM can lead to DNA hypomethylation and modify cancer risk.[96] These polymorphisms can have different effects on cancer pathogenesis depending on individual folate status.

8.3.4 MTHFR 677 C→T POLYMORPHISM, FOLATE INTAKE, AND COLORECTAL CANCER

Because colorectal carcinomas are derived from rapidly proliferating tissues, they have a great requirement for DNA synthesis and are affected by the metabolic fate of folic acid. Epidemiological studies have shown that colorectal cancer was reduced (~50%) in individuals with the MTHFR 677 TT genotype when folate intake was adequate, compared to those with the MTHFR 677 CC genotype.[71] Slattery and Potter[96] analyzed a mixed-ethnicity population of individuals aged 30 to 79 who were diagnosed with first primary colon cancer matched with control subjects. Dietary food frequency questionnaires were distributed. After genotyping for the MTHFR 677 C→T polymorphism, frequencies of the CC, CT, and TT genotypes among all cases were 45.9%, 44.7%, and 9.5%, respectively, and were very similar for the controls. High intakes of folate were associated with a 30 to 40% risk reduction in colon cancer among those with the TT genotype relative to those with low folate intake who were CC genotypes.[97] Shannon et al.[98] provided further support by showing that the MTHFR TT genotype conferred an increased risk of colorectal cancer in subjects older but not younger than 70 years of age. Hence, the variant TT form of the MTHFR gene appears to be slightly inversely associated with colon cancer, while the heterozygote CT and wild-type CC genotypes appear to have similar associations with colon cancer.[97]

8.3.5 MTHFR 677 C→T AND 1298 A→C POLYMORPHISMS AND ACUTE LEUKEMIA

The etiology of most types of leukemia is still unknown, but it is unlikely to be caused by a single genetic defect, and is most likely a result of adverse gene-environment interactions, with susceptibility being related to polymorphisms in multiple genes.[95] Skibola et al. have hypothesized that there may be a correlation between functional polymorphisms in the MTHFR gene and leukemogenesis due to the association between folate status and susceptibility to genetic damage in dividing cells. Since leukemias, like colorectal carcinomas, are also derived from rapidly proliferating tissues, they have a great requirement for DNA synthesis and are likely to be affected similarly by the metabolic fate of folic acid. These investigators designed their study to evaluate what role, either individually or combined, the 677 C→T and 1298 A→C MTHFR polymorphisms play in leukemia susceptibility. They hypothesized that the carriers of the variant alleles may have a protective advantage against leukemia. Case individuals consisted of those diagnosed with acute leukemia and were matched with controls. After genotyping, the MTHFR 677 CC, CT, and TT genotype frequencies for cases and controls were 57.9%, 32.5%, and 9.6%, and 53.2%, 35.0%, and 11.8%, respectively. The MTHFR 1298 AA, AC, and CC genotype frequencies for cases and controls were 49.8%, 41.9%, and 8.3%, and 45.0%, 44.3%, and 10.7%, respectively. Results demonstrated that individuals with at least one MTHFR mutation at 677 or 1298 were less likely to develop acute lymphocytic leukemia.

When examining joint effects between the two polymorphisms, it was found that the double heterozygotes (677 CT/1298 AC) were approximately five times less likely than 677 CC/1298 AA individuals to develop acute lymphocytic leukemia.[95]

8.3.6 MTR 2756 A→G POLYMORPHISM AND CANCER

The MTR 2756 GG genotype has been reported to be associated with a reduced risk of adenomas in colorectal cancer, up to a 41% lower risk than in MTR 2756A.[71,96,99] The most recent study, by Ulvik et al., genotyped 2179 subjects with colorectal cancer matched with controls for age and gender. In this Norwegian population, the MTR variant form GG was associated with a significant risk reduction of more than 25%, and the same was seen for the variant MTFHR 677 TT genotype. Specifically for the MTR AG genotype, the risk was considered intermediate. A similar study by Ma et al.[96] found that the MTR GG genotype was associated with a 40% decreased risk of colorectal cancer, but was not associated with plasma levels of folate or total homocysteine. A possible explanation for this lack of association is that homocysteine may be remethylated to methionine through an alternative pathway by betaine methyltransferase[96] (see Figure 8.1). This pathway adds yet another nutrient, choline, to the equation, which could have a role in modulating the processes involved with folate deficiency, DNA methylation, and cancer. This study, however, took into account alcohol intake since ethanol can interfere with folate and methyl group metabolism as well as MS activity. Colorectal cancer risk conferred by high alcohol intake may overcome the protective effect of these polymorphisms. Out of 10 cases and 21 controls that had the MTR GG genotype, the risk was 10-fold higher in those men who drank one or more drinks per day than those who drank less.[96]

8.4 CONCLUSIONS

In this new millennium, research in nutrition and disease prevention must now prioritize in understanding the molecular basis by which nutrients affect the disease process.[68,100,101] A well-coordinated, multidisciplinary effort must be made amongst all types of scientists — nutritional scientists, molecular biologists, geneticists, statisticians, and clinical cancer researchers — in order to move this research forward. There are many more genes related to the pathogenesis of cancer and CVD that have not been included in this paper because there hasn't yet been information for those genes showing relevance for dietary interventions. For each gene there may be one or more polymorphisms associated with it, hence, creating even more possible interactions between genetic polymorphisms and diet. This creates an ongoing challenge in trying to solve multifactorial, polygenic diseases. The individualization of treatments has been one of the strongest therapeutic tools, yet also one of the biggest challenges of the pregenomic era. However, now, with the availability of comprehensive genetic and molecular profiles and with improved molecular techniques, it will be possible to respond to diseases with individual strategies based on genetic profiles.[16] Nutrigenomics has a powerful message — food and nutrients have the potential to affect the balance between health and disease by affecting gene expression and function.[102]

Exploring the role that functional gene polymorphisms play in determining risk and in determining the levels of intermediate phenotypes is important to our understanding of the key metabolic pathways and physiology in both the disease and disease-free states.[7] More research in this area is still required, as there are many more genetic polymorphisms and nutrient interactions that are related to cancer and CVD. As was seen for the added benefit of including niacin with statins for treating hypercholesterolemia, there is great potential to improve treatment by adding a simple nutrient to drug therapy. These benefits will vary according to each individual's genotype. Yet, also, there is the potential for adverse effects with adding a nutrient to a drug therapy, which can also vary depending on one's genotype; hence, caution is required as well. It seems that only the surface has been scratched in the pursuit of solving the genetic–nutrient–drug mechanisms of CVD and cancer, but a great deal of research will undoubtedly follow. The key now is for researchers to always think of nutrient, drug, and gene interactions when designing experiments because the three are no longer solely independent of each other, but inevitably linked.

REFERENCES

1. Fogg-Johnson, N. and Merolli, A. (2000) Nutrigenomics: The next wave in nutrition research. *Nutraceuticals World* March 2000: 86–95.
2. Kaput, J. and Rodriguez, R. L. (2004) Nutritional genomics: the next frontier in the postgenomic era. *Physiol Genomics* 16(2): 166–177.
3. Bakovic, M. (2005) An Introduction to Nutrigenomics: What Consumers Need to Know. *FAQ's and Facts Sheet; Dietitians of Canada* (Available online: http://www.dietitians.ca)
4. Elliott, R. and Ong, T. J. (2002) Science, medicine, and the future. Nutritional genomics. *BM J* 324: 1438–1442.
5. Kirk, B. W., Feinsod, M., Favis, R., Kilman, R. M., and Barany, F. (2002) Single nucleotide polymorphism seeking long-term association with complex disease. *Nucleic Acids Res* 30: 3295–3311.
6. Iannuzzi, M. C., Maliarik, M., and Rybicki, B. (2002) Genetic polymorphism in lung disease: bandwagon or breakthrough? *Respir Res* 3: 15.
7. Loktionov, A. (2003) Common gene polymorphisms and nutrition: emerging links with pathogenesis of multifactorial chronic diseases (Review). *J Nutr Biochem* 14: 426–451.
8. Stephens, J. W. and Humphries, S. E. (2003) The molecular genetics of cardiovascular disease: clinical implications. *J Intern Med* 253: 120–127.
9. Tai, E. S., Corella, D., Deurenberg-Yap, M., Cutter, J., Chew, S. K., Tan, C. E., and Ordovas, J. M. (2003) Dietary fat interacts with the −514 CT polymorphism in the hepatic lipase gene promoter on plasma lipid profiles in a multiethnic Asian population: the 1998 Singapore national health survey. *J Nutr* 133: 3399–3408.

10. Hagberg, J. M., Wilund, K. R., and Ferrell, R. E. (2000) APOE gene and gene-environment effects on plasma lipoprotein-lipid levels. *Physiol Genomics* 4: 101–108.
11. Erkkila, A. T., Sarkkinen, E. S., Lindi, V., Lehto, S., Laakso, M., and Uusitupa, M. I. (2001) APOE polymorphism and the hypertryglyceridimic effect of dietary sucrose. *Am J Clin Nutr* 73: 746–752.
12. Campos, H., D'Agostino, M., and Ordovas, J. M. (2001) Gene–diet interactions and plasma lipoproteins: role of apolipoprotein E and habitual saturated fat intake. *Genet Epidemiol* 20: 117–128.
13. Corella, D., Tucker, K., Lahoz, C., Coltell, O., Cupples, L. A., Wilson, P., Schaefer, E. J., and Ordovas, J. M. (2001) Alcohol drinking determines the effect of the APOE locus on LDL-cholesterol concentrations in men: the Framingham Offspring Study. *Am J Clin Nutr* 73: 736–745.
14. Eichner, J. E., Dunn, S. T., Perveen, G., Thompson, D. M., Stewart, K. E., and Stroehla, B. C. (2002) Apolipoprotein E polymorphism and cardiovascular disease: a HuGE review. *Am J Epidemiol* 155(6): 487–495.
15. Jimenez-Sanchez, G., Childs, B., and Valle, D. (2001) Human disease genes. *Nature* 409: 853–855.
16. Gerling, I. C., Solomen, S. S., and Bryer-Ash, M. (2003) Genomes, transcriptomes, and proteomes. *Arch Intern Med* 163: 190–198.
17. Fodinger, M., Horl, W. H., and Sunder-Plassmann, G. (2000). Molecular biology of 5,10-methylenetetrahydrofolate reductase. *J Nephrol* 13: 20–33.
18. Frosst, P., Blom, H. J., Milos, R., Gryette, P., Sheppard, C. A., Matthews, R. G., Boers, G. J. H., Heijer, M., Kluijtmans, L. A. J., Heuval, L. P., and Rozen, R. (1995) A candidate genetic risk factor for vascular disease: a common mutation in methylenetetrahydrofolate reductase. *Nat Genet* 10: 111–113.
19. Ueland, P. M., Hustad, S., Schneede, J., Refsum, H., and Vollset, S. E. (2001) Biological and clinical implications of the MTHFR C677T polymorphism. *Trend Pharmacol Sci* 22: 195–201.
20. Kang, S. S., Passen, E. L., Ruggie, N., Wond, P. W., and Sora, H. (1993) Thermolabile defect of methylenetetrahydrofolate reductase in coronary artery disease. *Circulation* 88: 1463–1469.
21. Refsum, H., Ueland, P. M., Nygard, O., and Vollset, S. E. (1998) Homocysteine and cardiovascular disease. *Annu Rev Med* 49: 31–62.
22. Molloy, A. M., Daly, S., Mills, J. L., Kirke, P. N., Whitehead, A. S., Ramsbottom, D., Conley, M. R., Weir, D. G., and Scott, J. M. (1997) Thermolabile variant of 5,10-methylenetetrahydrofolate reductase associated with low red-cell folates: implications for folate intake recommendations. *Lancet* 349: 1591–1593.
23. de Bree, A., Verschuren, W. M., Bjorke-Monsen, A. L., van der Put, N. M., Heil, S. G, Trijbels, F. J., and Blom, H. J. (2003) Effect of the methylenetetrahydrofolate reductase 677 CT mutation on the relations among folate intake and plasma folate and homocysteine concentrations in a general population sample. *Am J Clin Nutr* 77: 687–693.
24. Brattstrom, L., Wilcken, D. E., Ohrvik, J. and Brudin, L. (1998) Common methylenetetrahydrofolate reductase gene mutation leads to hyperhomocysteinemia but not to vascular disease: the result of a meta-analysis. *Circulation* 98: 2520–2526.

25. Zittoun, J., Tonetti, C., Bories, D., Pignon, J. M., and Tulliez, M. (1998) Plasma homocysteine levels related to interactions between folate status and methylene-tetrahydrofolate reductase: a study in 52 healthy subjects. *Metabolism* 47: 1413–1418.

26. Lievers, K. J., Boers, G. H., Verhoef, P., den Heijer, M., Kluijtmans, L. A., van der Put, N. M., Trijbels, F. J. and Blom, H. J. (2001) A second common variant in the methylenetetrahydrofolate reductase (MTHFR) gene and its relationship to MTHFR enzyme activity, homocysteine, and cardiovascular disease risk. *J Mol Med* 79: 522–528.

27. Shelnutt, K. P., Kauwell, G. P., Chapman, C. M., Gregory III, J. F, Maneval, D. R., Browdy, A. A., Theriaque, D. W., and Bailey, L. B. (2003) Folate status response to controlled folate intake is affected by the methylenetetrahydrofolate reductase 677 CT polymorphism in young women. *J Nutr* 133: 4107–4111.

28. Ashfield-Watt, P. A., Pullin, C. H., Whiting, J. M., Clark, Z. E., Moat, S. J., Newcombe, R. G., Burr, M. L., Lewis, M. J., Powers, H. J., and McDowell, I. F. Methylenetetrahydrofolate reductase 677 CT genotype modulates homocysteine responses to a folate-rich diet or a low-dose folic acid supplement: a randomized controlled trial. *Am J Clin Nutr* 76: 180–186.

29. van't Hooft, F. M., Lundahl, B., Ragogna, F., Karpe, F., Olivecrona, G., and Hamsten, A. (2000) Functional characterization of 4 polymorphisms in promoter region of hepatic lipase gene. *Arterioscler Thromb Vasc Biol* 20: 1335–1339.

30. Connelly P. W. (1999) The role of hepatic lipase in lipoprotein metabolism. *Clin Chim Acta* 286: 243–245.

31. Galan, X., Robert, M. Q., Llobera, M., and Ramirez, I. (2000) Secretion of hepatic lipase by perfused liver and isolated hepatocytes. *Lipids* 35: 1017–1026.

32. Campos, H., Dreon, D. M., and Krauss, R. M. (1995) Associations of hepatic and lipoprotein lipase activities with changes in dietary composition and low-density lipoproteins subclasses. *J Lipid Res* 36: 462–472.

33. Deeb, S. S. and Peng, R. (2000) The C-514T polymorphism in the human hepatic lipase gene promoter diminishes its activity. *J Lipid Res* 41: 155–158.

34. Kuusi, T., Saarinen, P., and Nikkila, E. A. (1980) Evidence for the role of hepatic endothelial lipase in the metabolism of plasma high-density lipoprotein2 in man. *Atherosclerosis* 36B: 589–593.

35. Grundy, S. M., Vega, G. L., Otvos, J. D., Rainwater, D. L., and Cohen, J. C. (1999) Hepatic lipase activity influences high density lipoprotein subclass distribution in normotriglyceridaemic men: genetic and pharmacological evidence. *J Lipid Res* 40: 229–234.

36. Hegele, R.A, Tu, L., and Connelly, P. W. (1992) Human hepatic lipase mutations and polymorphisms. *Hum Mutat* 1: 320–324.

37. Hegele, R. A., Little, J. A., Vezina, C., Maguire, G. F., Tu, L., Wolever, T. S., Jenkins, D. A., and Connelly, P. W. (1993) Hepatic lipase deficiency: clinical, biochemical, and molecular genetic characteristics. *Arterioscler Throm* 13: 720–728.

38. Pihlajamaki, J., Karjalainen, L., Karhapaa, P. Vauhkonen, I., Taskinen, M. R., Deeb, S. S., and Laakso, M. (2000) G-250A substitution in promoter of hepatic lipase gene is associated with dyslipidemia and insulin resistance in healthy control subjects and in members of families with familial combined hyperlipidemia. *Arteriosclerosis* 20: 1789–1795.

39. Couture, P., Otvos, J. D., Cupples, L. A., Lahoz, C., Wilson, P. W., Schaefer, E. J., and Ordovas, J. M. (2000) Association of the C-514T polymorphism in the hepatic lipase gene with variations in lipoprotein subclass profiles: The Framingham Offspring Study. *Arterioscler Thromb Vasc Biol* 20: 815–822.

40. Guerra, R., Wang, J., Grundy, S. M., and Cohen, J. C. (1997) A hepatic lipase (LIPC) allele associated with high plasma concentration of high density lipoprotein cholesterol. *Proc Natl, Acad Sci USA* 94: 4532–4537.

41. Zambon, A., Deeb, S. S., Hokanson, J. E., Brown, B. G., and Brunzell, J. D. (1998) Common variants in the promoter of the hepatic lipase gene are associated with lower levels of hepatic lipase activity, buoyant LDL, and higher HDL2 cholesterol. *Arterioscler Thromb Vasc Biol* 18: 1723–1729.

42. Shohet, R. V., Vega, G. L., Anwar, A. Cigarroa, J. E., Grundy, S. M., and Cohen, J. C. (1999) Hepatic lipase (LIPC) promoter polymorphism in men with coronary artery disease. Allele frequency and effects on hepatic lipase activity and plasma HDL-C concentrations. *Arterioslcer Thromb Vasc Biol* 19: 1975–1978.

43. Ordovas, J. M., Corella, D., Demissie, S., Cupples L. A., Couture, P., Coltell, O., Wilson, P. W., Schaefer, E. J., and Tucker, K. L. (2002) Dietary fat intake determines the effect of a common polymorphism in the hepatic lipase gene promoter on high-density lipoprotein metabolism. *Circulation* 106: 2315–2321.

44. Pedro-Botet, J., Schaefer, E. J., Bakker-Arkema, R. G., Black, D. M., Stein, E. M., Corella, D., and Ordovas, J. M. (2001) Apolipoprotein E genotype affects plasma lipid response to atorvastatin in a gender specific manner. *Atherosclerosis* 158: 183–193.

45. Lahoz, C., Pena, R., Mostaza, J. M., Laguna, F., Garcia-Iglesias, M. F., Taboada, M., and Pinto, X. (2005) Baseline levels of low-density lipoprotein cholesterol and lipoprotein (a) and the *Ava*II polymorphism of the low-density lipoprotein receptor gene influence the response of low-density lipoprotein cholesterol to pravastatin treatment. *Metab Clin Exper* 54: 741–747.

46. Shepherd, J., Cobbe, S. M., Ford, I., Isles, C. G., Lorimer, A. R., MacFarlane, P. W., McKillop, J. H., and Packard, C. J. (2004) Prevention of coronary heart disease with pravastatin in men with hypercholesterolemia. *Atherscler Supples* 5: 91–97.

47. Downs, J. R., Clearfeld, M., Weis, S., Whitney, E., Shapiro, D. R., Beere, P. A., Langendorfer, A., Stein, E. A., Kruyer, W., and Gotto Jr, A. M. (1998) Primary prevention of acute coronary events with lovastatin in men and women with average cholesterol levels: results of AFCAPS/TexCAPS. Air Force/Texas Coronary Athersclerosis Prevention Study *JAMA* 279: 1615–1622.

48. Sacks, R. M., Pfeffer, M. A., Moye, L. A., Rouleau, J. L., Rutherford, J. D., Cole, T. G., Brown, L., Warnica, J. W., Arnold, J. M., Wun, C. C., Davis, B. R., and Braunwald, E. (1996) The effect of pravastatin on coronary events after myocardial infarction in patients with average cholesterol levels. Cholesterol and Recurrent Events Trial investigators. *N Engl J Med* 335: 1001–1009.

49. Nestel, P., Simons, L., Barter, P., Clifton, P., Colquhoun, D., Hamilton-Craig, I., Sikaris, K., and Sullivan, D. (1997) A comparative study of the efficacy of simvastatin and gemfibrozil in combined hyperlipoproteinemia: prediction of response by baseline lipids, apoE genotype, lipoprotein(a) and insulin. *Athersclerosis* 129: 231–239.

50. Sanllehy, C., Casals, E., Rodriguez-Villar, C., Zambon, D., Ojuel, J., Ballesta, A. M., and Ros, E. (1998) Lack of interaction of apolipoprotein E phenotype with the lipoprotein response to lovastatin or gemfibrozil in patients with primary hypercholesterolemia. *Metabolism* 47: 560–565.

51. Ordovas, J. M., Lopez-Miranda, J., Perez-Jimenez, F., Rodriguez, C., Park, J. S., Cole, T., and Schaefer, E. J. (1995) Effect of apolipoprotein E and A-IV phenotypes on the low-density lipoprotein response to HMG CoA reductase inhibitor therapy. *Atherosclerosis* 113: 157–166.

52. Salazar, L. A., Hirata, M. H., Giannini, S. D., Forti, N., Diament, J., Issa, J. S., and Hirata, R. D. (1999) Effects of *Ava*II and *Hinc*II polymorphisms at the LDL receptor gene on serum lipid levels of Brazilian individuals with high risk for coronary heart disease. *J Clin Lab Anal* 13: 251–258.

53. Salazar, L. A., Hirata, M. H., Quintao, E. C., and Hirata, R. D. (2000) Lipid-lowering response of the HMG-CoA reductase inhibitor fluvastatin is influenced by polymorphisms in the low-density lipoprotein receptor gene in Brazilian patients with primary hypercholesterolemia. *J Clin Lab Anal* 14: 125–131.

54. Lahoz, C., Pena, R., Mostaza, J. M., Laguna, F., Garcia-Iglesias, M. F., Taboada, M., and Pinto, X. (2005) The -514C/T polymorphism of the hepatic lipase gene significantly modulates the HDL-cholesterol response to statin treatment. *Atherosclerosis* 182: 129–134.

55. Kashyap, M. L., McGovern, M. E., Berra, K., Guyton, J. R., Kwiterovich, P. O., Harper, W. L., Toth, P. D., Favrot, L. K., Kerzner, B., Nash, S. D., Bays, H. E., and Simmons, P. D. (2002) Long-term safety and efficacy of a once-daily niacin/lovastatin formulation for patients with dyslipidemia. *Am J Cardiol* 89: 672–678.

56. Birjmohun, R. S., Hutten, B. A., Kastelein, J. J. P., and Stroes, E. S. G. (2004) Increasing HDL cholesterol with extended-release nicotinic acid: from promise to practice. *Neth J Med* 62: 229–234.

57. Ganji, S. H., Kamanna, V. S., and Kashyap, M. L. (2003) Niacin and cholesterol: role in cardiovascular disease (review). *J Nutr Biochem* 14: 298–305.

58. Wolfe, M. L., Vartanian, S. F., Ross, J. L., Bansavich, L., Mohler, E. R., Meagher, E, Friedrich, C. A., and Rader, D. J. (2001) Safety and effectiveness of niaspan when added sequentially to a statin for treatment of dyslipidemia. *Am J Cardiol* 87: 476–479.

59. Ito, M. K. (2003) Advances in the understanding and management of dyslipidemia: using niacin-based therapies. *Am J Health-Syst Pharm* 60: S15–S21.

60. Rosenson, R. S. (2003) Antiatherothrombotic effects of nicotinic acid. *Atherosclerosis* 171: 87–96.

61. Rock, C. L., Lampe, J. W., and Patterson, R. E. (2000) Nutrition, genetics, and risks of cancer. *Annu Rev Public Health* 21: 47–64.

62. Greenwald, P. (1996) The potential of dietary modification to prevent cancer. *Prev Med* 25: 41–43.

63. Lai, C. and Shields, P. G. (1999) The role of interindividual variation in human carcinogenesis. *J Nutr* 129: 552S–555S.

64. Perera, F. P. (1997) Environment and cancer: who are susceptible? *Science* 278: 1067–1073.

65. Steinmetz, K. A. and Potter, J. D. (1996) Vegetables, fruit, and cancer prevention: a review. *J Am Diet Assoc* 96 (10): 1027–1039.

66. Mathers, J. C. (2003) Nutrition and cancer prevention: diet-gene interactions. *Proc Nutr Soc* 62: 605–610.

67. Patterson, R. E, Eaton, D. L. and Potter, J. D. (1999) The genetic revolution: change and challenge for the dietetics profession. *J Am Diet Assoc* 99 (11): 1412–1420.

68. Milner, J. A. (2002) Strategies for cancer prevention: the role of diet. *Br J Nutr* 87: S265–S272.

69. Greenwald, P., Milner, J. A. and Clifford, C. K. (2000) Creating a new paradigm in nutrition research within the national cancer institute. *J Nutr* 130: 3103–3105.

70. Cotton, S. C., Sharp, L., Little, J., and Brockton, N. (2000) Glutathione *S*-transferase polymorphisms and colorectal cancer: a HuGE review. *Am J Epidemiol* 151(1): 7–32.

71. Milner, J. A., McDonald, S. S., Anderson, D. E., and Greenwald, P. (2001) Molecular targets for nutrients involved with cancer prevention. *Nutr Cancer* 41(1&2): 1–16.

72. Platz, E. A., Leitzmann, M. F., Hollis, B. W., Willett, W. C., and Giovannucci, E. (2004) Plasma 1,25-dihydroxy- and 25-hydroxyvitamin D and subsequent risk of prostate cancer. *Canc Causes Cont* 15: 255–265.

73. Giovannucci, E. (1998) Dietary influences of 1,25(OH)$_2$ vitamin D in relation to prostate cancer: a hypothesis. *Canc Causes Cont* 9: 657–582.

74. Platz, E. A., Hankinson, S. E., Hollis, B. W., Colditz, G. A., Hunter, D. J., Speizer, F. E., and Giovannucci, E. (2000) Plasma 1,25-dihydroxy- and 25-hydroxyvitamin D and adenomatous polyps of the distal colorectum. *Canc Epidemiol Biomark Prev* 9: 1059–1065.

75. Kallay, E., Pietschmann, P., Toyokuni, S., Bajna, E., Hahn, P., Mazzucco, K., Bieglmayer, C., Kato, S., and Cross, H. S. (2001) Characterization of a vitamin D receptor knockout mouse as a model of colorectal hyperproliferation and DNA damage. *Carcinogenesis* 22: 1429–1435.

76. Liu, M., Lee, M. H., Cohen, M., Bommakanti, M., and Freedman, L. P. (1996) Transcriptional activation of the Cdk inhibitor p21 by vitamin D3 leads to the induced differentiation of the myelomonocytic cell line U937. *Genes Dev* 10: 142–153.

77. Palmer, H. G., Gonzalez-Sancho, J. M., and Espada, J. (2001) Vitamin D(3) promotes the differentiation of colon carcinoma cells by the induction of E-cadherin and the inhibition of beta-catenin signaling. *J Cell Biol* 154: 369–387.

78. Mathiasen, I. S., Lademann, U. and Jaattela, M. (1999) Apoptosis induced by vitamin D compounds in breast cancer cells is inhibited by Bcl-2 but does not involve known caspases or p53. *Canc Res* 59: 4848–4856.

79. Donohue, M. M. and Demay, M. B. (2002) Rickets in VDR null mice is secondary to decreased apoptosis of hypertrophic chondrocytes. *Endocrinology* 143: 3691–3694.

80. Morrison, N. A., Qi, J. C., Tokita, A., Kelly, P. J., Crofts, L., Nguyen, T. V., Sambrook, P. N., and Eisman, J. A. (1994) Prediction of bone density from vitamin D receptor alleles. *Nature* 367: 284–287.

81. Ingles, S. A., Wang, J., Coetzee, G. A., Lee, E. R., Frank, H. D., and Haile, R. W. (2001) Vitamin D receptor polymorphisms and risk of colorectal adenomas. *Canc Causes Cont* 12: 607–614.

82. Habuchi, T., Suzuki, T., Sasaki, R., Wang, L., Sato, K., Satoh, S., Akao, T., Tsuchiya, N., Shimoda, N., Wada, Y., Koizumi, A., Chihara, J., Ogawa, O., and Kato, T. (2000) Association of vitamin D receptor gene polymorphism with prostate cancer and benign prostatic hyperplasia in a Japanese population. *Canc Res* 60: 305–308.

83. Sinha, R. and Caporaso, N. (1999) Diet, genetic susceptibility and human cancer etiology. *J Nutr* 129: 556S–559S.

84. Wong, H-L., Seow, A., Arakawa, K., Lee, H-P., Yu, M. C., and Ingles, S. A. (2003) Vitamin D receptor start codon polymorphism and colorectal risk: effect modification by dietary calcium and fat in Singapore Chinese. *Carcinogenesis* 24: 1091–1095.

85. Peters, U., McGlynn, K. A., Chatterjee, N., Gunter, E., Garcia-Closas, M, Rothman, N., and Sinha, R. (2001) Vitamin D, calcium, and vitamin D receptor polymorphism in colorectal adenomas. *Canc Epidemiol Biomark Prev* 10: 1267–1274.

86. Niv, Y., Sperber, A. D., Figer, A., Igael, D., Shany, S., Fraser, G., and Schwartz, B. (1999) In colorectal carcinoma patients, serum vitamin D levels vary according to the stage of carcinoma. *Cancer* 86: 391–397.

87. Xue, L., Lipkin, M, Newmark, H., and Wang, J. (1999) Influence of dietary calcium and vitamin D on diet-induced epithelial cell hyperproliferation in mice. *J Natl Canc Inst* 91: 176–181.

88. Tong, W. M., Kallay, E., Hofer, H., Hulla, W., Manhardt, T., Peterlik, M., and Cross, H. S. (1999) Growth regulation of human colon cancer cells by epidermal growth factor and 1,25-dihydroxyvitamin D_3 is mediated by mutual modulation of receptor expression. *Eur J Canc* 34: 2119–2125.

89. Diaz, G. D., Paraskeva, C., Thomas, M. G., Binderup, L., and Hague, A. (2000) Apoptosis is induced by the active metabolite of vitamin D_3 and its analogue, EB1089 in colorectal adenoma and carcinoma cells: possible implications for prevention and therapy. *Canc Res* 60: 2304–2312.

90. Evans, S. R., Nolla, J., Hanfelt, J., Shabahang, M., Nauta, R. J., and Shchepotin, I. B. (1998) Vitamin D receptor expression as a predictive marker of biological behavior in human colorectal cancer. *Clin Canc Res* 4: 1591–1595.

91. Slattery, M. L., Yakumo, K., Hoffman, M., and Newhausen, S. (2001) Variants of the VDR gene and risk of colon cancer. *Canc Causes Cont* 12: 359–364.

92. Slattery, M. L., Newhausen, S. L., Hoffman, M., Caan, B., Curtin, K., Ma, K., and Samowitz, W. (2004) Dietary calcium, vitamin D, VDR genotypes and colorectal cancer. *Int J Canc* 111: 750–756.

93. Kim, H. S., Newcomb, P. A., Ulrich, C. M., Keener, C. L., Bigler, J., and Farin, F. M. (2001) Vitamin D receptor polymorphism and the risk of colorectal adenomas: evidence of interaction with dietary vitamin D and calcium. *Canc Epidemiol Biomark Prev* 10: 869–874.

94. Bailey, L. B. and Gregory III, J. F. (1999) Polymorphisms of methylenetetrahydrofolate reductase and other enzymes: metabolic significance, risks and impact on folate requirement. *J Nutr* 129: 919–922.

95. Skibola, C. F., Smith, M. T., Kane, E., Roman, E., Rollinson, S., Cartwright, R. A., and Morgan, G. (1999) Polymorphisms in the methylenetetrahydrofolate reductase gene are associated with susceptibility to acute leukemia in adults. *PNAS* 96: 12810–12815.

96. Ma, J., Stampfer, M. J., Christensen, B., Giovannucci, E., Hunter, D. J., Chen, J., Willett, W. C., Selhub, J., Hennekens, C. H., Gravel, R., and Rozen, R. (1999) A polymorphism of the methionine synthase gene: association with plasma folate, vitamin B_{12}, homocysteine, and colorectal cancer risk. *Canc Epidemiol Biomark Prev* 8: 825–829.

97. Slattery, M. L., Potter, J. D., Samowitz, W., Schaffer, D., and Leppert, M. (1999) Methylenetetrahydrofolate reductase, diet, and risk of colon cancer. *Canc Epidemiol Biomark Prev* 8: 513–518.

98. Shannon, B., Gnanasampanthan, S., Beilby, J. and Lacopetta, B. (2002) A polymorphism in the methylenetetrahydrofolate reductase gene predisposes to colorectal cancers with microsatellite instability. *Gut* 50: 520–524.

99. Ulvik, A., Vollset, S. E., Hansen, S., Gislefoss, R., Jellum, E., and Ueland, P. M. Colorectal cancer and the methylenetetrahydrofolate reductase 677C→T and methionine synthase 2756A→G polymorphisms: a study of 2168 case-control pairs from the JANUS cohort. *Canc Epidemiol Biomark Prev* 13: 2175–2180.

100. Rankinen, T. and Tiwari, H. (2004) Genome scans for human nutritional traits: what have we learned? *Nutr* 20: 9–13.

101. Kaput, J. (2004) Diet-disease gene interactions. *Nutrition* 20(1): 26–31.

102. Bakovic, M. (2005) Nutrigenomics: balancing diet to gene function proposes a new-age recipe for better health *Resource Information; Dietitians of Canada* Available online: http://www.dietitians.ca

9 Nutrigenomics and Pharmacogenomics of Human Cancer: On the Road from Nutrigenetics and Pharmacogenetics

Alexandre Loktionov

CONTENTS

9.1 INTRODUCTION

Recent rapid progress in the determination of the human genome sequence has strongly stimulated the development of genomic approaches to the investigation of a broad spectrum of medical problems.[1,2] Functional genomics is now expanding into several bioscientific domains, which previously had little relation to genetic research. Emerging amalgamation of functional genomics with nutritional sciences has recently been called nutrigenomics; however this new discipline is just entering its embryonal state, being mainly discussed in numerous reviews devoted to future opportunities rather than existing reality.[3–6] This dream-like state of the subject has brought about a very vague concept of suggested boundaries of nutrigenomics, which often tend to incorporate transcriptomics, proteomics, and, eventually, metabolomics. However, the integrative ideas, more appropriately attributable to the systems biology, still have little impact on our knowledge regarding the relationship between human genome, nutritional factors, and genesis of major human chronic diseases, such as cardiovascular disease and cancer.

Cancer remained one of the most enigmatic conditions still challenging scientists and physicians at the beginning of the new millennium. Although it is generally accepted that genetic component plays a leading role in the pathogenesis of neoplastic disorders, only a minor fraction of all human cancers (i.e., hereditary cancer syndromes accounting for 5 to 10% of all cancer cases) inevitably results from specific deteriorating mutations transmitted through germ line.[7,8] In contrast, the development of sporadic tumors is regarded as a complex pathogenetic process involving interactions of multiple contributing factors, both internal (intrinsic host factors) and external.[9] In this context, diet obviously constitutes an omnipresent combination of external influences potentially important for all malignancies at different stages of neoplastic growth. Furthermore, dietary factors can interact with anticancer drugs used at later stages of the disease, thus affecting chemotherapy outcome.

Although it would be extremely tempting to have a chance to look at cancer pathogenesis and medicamentous treatment through the prism of genome-governed network of interactions between nutrition, chemotherapeutic agents, and biological systems in all their complexity, the existing knowledge is obviously insufficient to allow any fact-based analysis of this type. In the context of this chapter, it appears to be justified to use a limited meaning of the term "nutrigenomics," analogous to "pharmacogenomics," which is often defined as a field aiming to investigate the genetic basis for interindividual differences in drug response using genome-wide approaches.[10] It is, however, clear that the effects of drugs, which are administered as pure compounds in precise doses, are much easier to assess than combined and interfering effects of numerous food constituents.[4] Nevertheless, this chapter is an attempt to analyze the present state of nutrigenomic and pharmacogenomic research in relation to human cancer.

9.2 DIET, GENETIC BACKGROUND, AND CANCER RISK

It is generally accepted that diet can affect cancer risk in humans. The relationship had been well demonstrated by epidemiological studies; however, precise biological mechanisms involved in these interactions remain obscure since simultaneous determination of various biological effects exerted by thousands of food components ingested daily is a formidable problem.[11–13] At this level of complexity, application of the traditional reductionist approach attempting to separately analyze effects of individual diet-derived bioactive substances could easily lead to flawed conclusions. Persistent lack of clear understanding of the cancer pathogenesis further aggravates the situation.

Figure 9.1 roughly illustrates the present state of general scientific knowledge regarding the relationship between diet and neoplastic growth (the scheme also includes the main therapeutic strategies presently applied in the management of cancer). It is transparent that the existing views on the diet–cancer relationship are mainly focused on the very beginning of the disease, i.e., cancer initiation, presuming that dietary composition shifts towards patterns corresponding to either "protection/prevention" or "high-risk/predisposition" can respectively reduce or increase diet-related risk of tumor development. This concentration of attention on the borderline separating physiological (normal) conditions from neoplasia has an obvious positive side, strongly stimulating research in the direction of dietary cancer prevention. At the same time, relatively little is known about effects of diet in cancer patients with the exception of some described interactions between dietary components and chemotherapeutic drugs, which are going to be considered from a nutrigenomic/pharmacogenomic point of view later in this chapter.

Identification of dietary components affecting cancer risk in humans has always been a difficult task. It was widely accepted for decades that excessive consumption of fat and red meat and insufficient intake of fruits, vegetables, and dietary fiber increase cancer risk.[11] However, discrepancies between positive results of earlier case-control studies (e.g., those indicating risk-increasing effect of dietary fat and protective action of fruits, vegetables, and dietary fiber) and failure to confirm these findings in recent large-scale prospective trials[11–15] create new uncertainties in the field. Among "traditional" dietary risk factors only relationship between consumption of red meat and increased risk of distal colon cancer has been clearly confirmed by several large-scale prospective studies.[16–18] Unexpected results of the prospective studies have already generated intense discussions with regard to the use of different methodologies of data collection in human nutrition studies.[19,20] In the meanwhile, new aspects of the problem emerge. Links between overeating/obesity and risk of cancer of several sites (colon, breast, esophagus, endometrium, kidney) have been repeatedly reported.[11,12,21–23] The latter area is especially important in view of the obesity "epidemic" rapidly spreading in the developed countries of Western Europe and North America.[24]

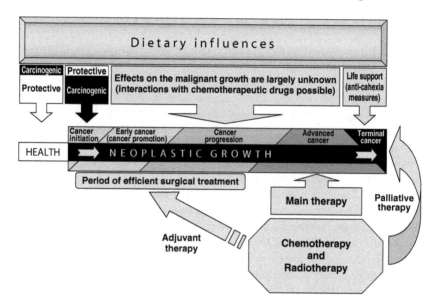

FIGURE 9.1 Schematic representation of neoplastic growth dynamics and influences of diet and anticancer treatments at its different stages.

The absence of complete clarity with regard to cancer-affecting dietary components makes application of systems biology approaches to nutritional science a challenging task for the future. The present knowledge in the field widely defined as nutrigenomics (see above) is limited by often patchy information on certain human genetic variants influencing (patho)physiological responses to the action of bioactive food components. Analysis of these (essentially nutrigenetic) observations is presented below.

9.2.1 Xenobiotic Metabolism-Controlling Pathways

The problem of associations between common gene polymorphisms, dietary influences, and cancer risk has attracted researchers since the early 1980s, when discovery of polymerase chain reaction made real analysis of human genetic variants possible. The prevailing idea of the field could be briefly summarized as the search for common gene variants responsible for deficient or altered metabolism of food-derived carcinogenic substances. Enzymatic pathways controlling metabolism of xenobiotics (including carcinogens) had been the main targets of these studies.[25] Special attention was paid to the genes encoding enzymes participating in Phase I and Phase II reactions. Reactions of Phase I, which often lead to procarcinogen activation, are mostly catalyzed by the cytochrome P450 (CYP) superfamily of enzymes providing catalytic hydroxylation of diverse compounds linked only by their lipophilic nature.[26,27] Numerous single nucleotide polymorphisms (SNPs) in the CYP genes (CYP1A1, CYP1A2, CYP1B1, CYP2A6 CYP2C9, CYP2C19, CYP2D6, CYP2E1, CYP3A4, and CYP3A5) have been studied in relation to cancer risk; however, no firm evidence in favor of this link has been produced.[28] It should be noted that the initial concept of the P450 family, regarding it mainly as a hepatic xenobiotic detoxification system, is now being expanded upon the discovery of multiple additional functions of these enzymes.[26,27] It also has become clear that some CYPs are closely involved in the metabolism of anticancer chemotherapeutic agents.[28] These interactions are going to be addressed later in this chapter.

Available information on interactions of dietary factors with polymorphic variants of the CYP genes is presented in the beginning of Table 9.1. Although the number of studies approaching gene–nutrient interactions as a factor in human cancer development is limited, it is obvious that polymorphic genes of the P450 family have been investigated mostly in the context of association between cooked red meat consumption and colorectal neoplasia. Several reports indicate possible risk-modulating effects of CYP gene variants (see Table 9.1), which might be in line with the idea of enhanced activation of meat processing-generated carcinogens, such as polycyclic aromatic hydrocarbons (PAH), heterocyclic amines (HCA), and N-nitroso compounds by some variant CYP enzymes.[70–72]

However, reported effects and interactions are usually weak and often difficult to reproduce. Moreover, the complexity of human diets and abundant presence of multiple bioactive dietary components makes investigation of isolated gene–nutrient interactions notoriously difficult. Furthermore, effects of different gene polymorphisms often overlap as several examples given in Table 9.1 show. For instance it is very difficult to separate influence of CYP family (especially CYP1A1 and CYP1A2) and N-acetyltransferase (NAT1 and NAT2) genes on colorectal cancer risk associated with cooked meat consumption. CYP family genes encode numerous xenobiotic-metabolizing enzymes, but CYP3A4, being the most abundant P450 enzyme in the human liver and gut[73–75] and a major factor in drug metabolism, deserves particular attention. Although over 70 SNPs are recently described in the corresponding gene,[75] knowledge of their physiological significance is still very scarce. Correlations between CYP3A4 gene polymorphisms and cancer risk only start to emerge,[75] and there is little doubt that further investigation of this gene can produce abundant information on carcinogenesis, responses to cancer treatment, and modulation of these processes by active components of diet (see also Chapter 2, Hypolipidemic Therapy: Drugs, Diet, and Interactive Effects).

Whereas polymorphic xenobiotic-metabolizing enzymes of Phase I are mostly responsible for a generation of active carcinogenic substances, Phase II metabolism is directed on detoxification of carcinogenic and mutagenic substances through conjugation reactions producing soluble and easily excretable products. Inherited deficiency of some Phase II enzymes, such as "Null" variants of glutathione S-transferases M1 (GSTM1) and T1 (GSTT1) caused by long deletions in the corresponding genes, has repeatedly been reported to be associated with increased risk of cancers of different sites.[76] GST family enzymes are strongly involved in the metabolism of PAH,[77] thus changes in their activity are likely to affect the probability of cancer initiation. Table 9.1 shows that

TABLE 9.1
Interactions between Common "Metabolic" Gene Variants and Dietary Factors in Cancer Risk Modulation

Gene	Tumor Site/Type	Dietary Factor(s)	Interactive Effects	Refs.
			Genes Encoding Phase I Metabolism Enzymes	
CYP1A1	Ovarian cancer	Caffeine	Elevated ovarian cancer risk related to increased caffeine intake was observed in individuals with the CYP1A1*2C allele.	(29)
	Colorectal cancer	White meat	No clear pattern of CYP1A1 polymorphism influence on colorectal cancer risk related to white meat consumption revealed.	(30)
CYP1A2	Colorectal cancer	Cooked red meat	Well-done red meat consumption was associated with an increased risk of colorectal cancer among ever-smokers with the CYP1A2 rapid phenotype (and NAT2 rapid).	(31)
			CYP1A2 rapid phenotype is associated with certain genetic variants, e.g., CYP1A2*F.	(32)
	Ovarian cancer	Caffeine	The associations of caffeine and coffee intake and ovarian cancer risk were stronger in women with CYP1A2 (high-rapid) genotype.	(33)
CYP2A6	Colorectal cancer	Cooked red meat	CYP2A6 high activity was associated with an increased risk of colorectal cancer, particularly among consumers of well-done meat (see also effect of GSTA1 genotype).	(34, 35)
			Information on the role CYP2A6 gene variants in the enzyme activity modulation is scarce; however, the effect appears to be likely.	(36)
CYP2E1	Colorectal cancer	Red meat and processed meat	Individuals with a 5' 96-bp promoter region insertion variant of the CYP2E1 gene had an increased rectal cancer risk associated with high red meat or processed meat consumption.	(37)

Gene	Cancer/phenotype	Dietary factor	Finding	Ref.
	Incomplete intestinal metaplasia (stomach cancer precursor)	Salted food (salted meat, dehydrated salted vegetables, salted raw fish)	Association between incomplete intestinal metaplasia and salted food intake was observed among subjects bearing homozygous c1/c1 CYP2E1 variant (defined by RsaI polymorphism in 5′ region). (See also effects of GSTM1 and GSTT1 genotypes.)	(38)
	Upper aerodigestive tract cancer	Alcohol	The highest risk of oral cavity/pharyngeal cancer was observed among the heaviest drinkers with either the CYP2E1 C (defined by DraI polymorphism in intron 6) or the CYP2E1 c2 (defined by RsaI polymorphism in 5′ region) allele.	(39)
Myeloperoxidase (MPO)	Breast cancer	Antioxidant-rich fruits and vegetables	The A-allele (G463A promoter region SNP) was associated with reduced breast cancer risk in women (especially premenopausal) who consumed higher amounts of fruits and vegetables.	(40)
Genes Encoding Enzymes with Dual (Predominantly Phase II, but Some Phase I Metabolism) Function				
N-acetyltransferase 1 (NAT1)	Breast cancer	Cooked red meat	Elevated breast cancer risk related to increased well-done red meat consumption was observed in women with putative rapid acetylation-associated NAT1*11 or NAT1*10 alleles.	(41, 42)
	Colorectal adenomas	Cooked red meat	Stronger association of well-done red meat consumption with colorectal adenoma development was observed in individuals with rapid acetylation-related NAT1 genotypes.	(43)
N-acetyltransferase 2 (NAT2)	Colorectal cancer	Cooked red meat	Well-done red meat consumption was associated with an increased risk of colorectal cancer among ever-smokers with NAT2 rapid phenotype (and CYP1A2 rapid phenotype).	(31)
	Colorectal adenoma	Cooked red meat	Frequent meat consumption combined with the NAT2 slow acetylation slightly increased colorectal adenoma risk.	(44)
	Breast cancer	Cooked red meat	Rapid/intermediate NAT2 genotype combined with consumption of well-done meat was associated with a nearly eight-fold increase of breast cancer risk.	(45)
			No NAT2 genotype or meat consumption effect on breast cancer risk found.	(46)

TABLE 9.1 (CONTINUED)
Interactions between Common "Metabolic" Gene Variants and Dietary Factors in Cancer Risk Modulation

Gene	Tumor Site/Type	Dietary Factor(s)	Interactive Effects	Refs.
	Hepatocellular cancer	Red meat	A trend of increased hepatocellular carcinoma risk with increasing red meat intake was observed in rapid acetylators (defined here as subjects homozygous for the wild type NAT2*4 allele).	(47)
Sulfotransferase 1A1 (SULT1A1)	Breast cancer	Red meat	The risk of breast cancer was elevated with increasing doneness of red meat intake among women with the Arg/Arg or Arg/His genotype, but not with the His/His homozygosity (lower enzyme activity-associated) at codon 213.	(48)
	Prostate cancer		An increased risk of prostate cancer was associated with the presence of the *1/*1 (His/His at 213) SULT1A1 genotype; however, there was no clear correlation among genotype, meat consumption, and cancer risk.	(49)
Microsomal epoxide hydrolase (EPHX1)	Colorectal adenomas	Cooked red meat	Elevated adenoma risk associated with meat consumption and high predicted EPHX1 activity (Tyr at codon 113 and Arg at codon 139).	(50)
			Increased adenoma risk was found to be associated with high meat intake and His 113 genotype.	(51)
	Lung cancer	Intake of protein, carbohydrates, animal fat, and dietary fiber	Among smokers with high animal fat and protein intake and low carbohydrate and fiber intake ("unhealthy" dietary pattern) individuals with His/His 113 homozygocity were at significantly lower lung cancer risk.	(52)
	Genes Encoding Phase II Metabolism Enzymes			
Glutathione S-transferase A1 (GSTA1)	Colorectal cancer	Well-done meat intake	GSTA1*B allele, which causes lower expression of the enzyme, was associated with an increased risk of colorectal cancer, especially among well-done meat consumers.	(34)

Gene	Cancer	Dietary factor	Finding	Ref.
Glutathione S-transferase M1 (GSTM1)	Lung cancer	Intake of isothiocyanate-rich cruciferous vegetables (esp. broccoli)	Increased intake of isothiocyanates was associated with cancer-protective effect in GSTM1-Null individuals.	(53–55)
	Colorectal cancer		Increased intake of isothiocyanates was associated with cancer-protective effect in GSTM1-positive individuals.	(56)
			Increased intake of cruciferous vegetables was associated with cancer risk reduction in GTSM-Null individuals.	(57)
			Increased intake of isothiocyanate-rich cruciferous vegetables was associated with cancer risk reduction in individuals with the GSTM1-Null and GSTT1-Null combination.	(58)
	Colorectal adenomas		Protective effect of broccoli was observed in subjects with GSTM1-Null genotype.	(59)
	Prostate cancer		Men with GSTM1-positive genotype had the greatest reduction of cancer risk.	(60)
	Head and neck cancer		Consumption of raw cruciferous vegetables was associated with cancer incidence reduction only in GSTM1-Null individuals.	(61)
	Breast cancer		Consumption of cruciferous vegetables, particularly broccoli, was marginally protective, but risk was unaffected by GSTM1 genotype.	(62)
Glutathione S-transferase P1 (GSTP1)	Lung cancer	Red meat	Among smokers with high animal fat and protein intake and low carbohydrate and fiber intake ("unhealthy" dietary pattern) individuals with Ile/Ile 105 homozygosity were at significantly higher lung cancer risk.	(52)
Glutathione S-transferase T1 (GSTT1)	Lung cancer	Intake of isothiocyanate-rich cruciferous vegetables (esp. broccoli)	Low intake of isothiocyanates was associated with marginally increased cancer risk in GSTT1-Null individuals.	(53)

TABLE 9.1 (CONTINUED)
Interactions between Common "Metabolic" Gene Variants and Dietary Factors in Cancer Risk Modulation

Gene	Tumor Site/Type	Dietary Factor(s)	Interactive Effects	Refs.
			Increased intake of isothiocyanates was associated with cancer-protective effect in individuals with simultaneous homozygous deletion of both GSTM1 and GSTT1.	(54, 55)
	Colorectal cancer		Increased intake of isothiocyanate-rich cruciferous vegetables was associated with cancer risk reduction in individuals with the GSTM1-Null and GSTT1-Null combination.	(58, 63, 64)
Manganese superoxide dismutase (MnSOD)	Breast cancer	Antioxidant-rich fruits and vegetables and dietary supplements	Women homozygous for the Ala(−9) allele (Val-9Ala polymorphism in the signal sequence of the MnSOD protein), especially those with lower antioxidant intake, were at higher risk of developing breast cancer.	(65, 66)
			No correlation of breast cancer risk with either MnSOD genotype or antioxidant intake.	(67)
	Prostate cancer	Beta-carotene treatment, antioxidants	Homozygosity for the Ala(−9) in combination with high antioxidant levels was associated with lower relative risk for both total and fatal prostate cancer.	(68)
Catalase (CAT)	Breast cancer	Fruit and vegetable consumption	The high-activity (wild type, CC) catalase homozygosity in combination with higher vegetable and, especially, fruit consumption was associated with breast cancer risk reduction.	(69)

interactions of food components with genetic variants of these enzymes were mostly approached from the point of view of nutritional cancer prevention. Efforts of investigators were concentrated predominantly on cancer-protective effects of isothiocyanate-rich cruciferous vegetables, which are believed to influence both Phase I and Phase II xenobiotic metabolism; in particular, through induction of GSTM1 and GSTT1.[78,79] Most of the cited studies revealed stronger protective effect of isothiocyanates in GST-deficient individuals (GSTM1-Null and GSTT1-Null genotypes); therefore, it can be suggested that this effect can be explained by compensatory activation of other GST family enzymes (e.g., GSTA1) providing an "overlapping" detoxifying effect.[80]

UDP-glucuronosyltransferases (UGTs) constitute another group of Phase II enzymes responsive to dietary effects.[81,82] Highly polymorphic UGTs exert conjugation of a variety of xenobiotics, including carcinogenic HCA and PAH, and complex dependence of enzyme activity of nutritional factors and polymorphisms in the genes encoding UGT1A181,[83–85] and UGT1A7[86] has already been reported.

Genes encoding enzymes that participate in the generation of reactive oxygen species (e.g., myeloperoxidase) and protection from its effects (superoxide dismutases, catalase, glutathione peroxidase) are considered here, together with those controlling Phase I and Phase II reactions, since oxidative stress is a known factor in carcinogenesis.[87] First studies linking variants of these genes with dietary factors indicate the importance of fruit- and vegetable-derived antioxidants in modulating cancer risk in a genotype-dependent manner (see Table 9.1).

It should be repeated that the modest size of Table 9.1 reflects the fact that, despite abundance of epidemiological studies approaching relationship between "metabolic" (i.e., Phase I and II metabolism-related) gene polymorphisms and cancer risk, relatively few authors have addressed the possible contribution of dietary factors to this relationship.

9.2.2 Folate Metabolism and DNA Methylation

Genes that encode enzymes of folate metabolism are especially interesting in view of their contribution to DNA methylation, which directly influences gene expression and, therefore, the processes of normal and neoplastic cell growth and differentiation.[88] At the same time, folate and related nutrients (group B vitamins, methionine, choline), being dietary constituents, provide a direct link to nutrition. Abundance of useful information regarding this metabolic pathway is not surprising. Considerable attention has been paid to the role of two common SNPs (C677T and A1298C) in the sequence of the methylenetetrahydrofolate reductase (MTHFR) gene in cancer susceptibility. It has been reported that interaction of folate status determined by dietary intake with the C677T polymorphism influences human DNA methylation,[89] whereas mechanisms behind possible effects of the A1298C SNP remain to be explored further.[90] This may depend generally on the genetic linkage between the two alleles,[91] since the MTHFR variant encoded by the C1298 (Ala429) appears to be functionally indistinguishable from the wild-type enzyme.[92]

There are numerous publications on colorectal cancer risks in relation to the T/T677 MTHFR homozygocity considered in detail in several recent reviews.[93–96] Briefly, the T/T677 genotype effect on colorectal cancer risk strongly depends on adequate folate status. The T/T homozygocity is associated with reduced risk of colorectal cancer in individuals with high folate intake and low alcohol consumption, whereas combination of low folate and high alcohol consumption increases colorectal cancer risk in this genotype group, even in comparison with individuals bearing the C/T or C/C677 allele combinations.[93–96] Essentially a similar pattern has been demonstrated in several breast cancer studies[97–99]; however, other investigators failed to reveal an effect of folate consumption, while observing reduction of breast cancer risk in postmenopausal women with T677 homozygocity and receiving hormone replacement therapy.[100] There are also reports indicating that the combination of T/T677 homozygocity and low folate intake may be regarded as a risk factor for cervical[101] and bladder[102] cancer.

It is likely that polymorphic variants of other genes encoding enzymes involved in folate metabolism (methionine synthase, methionine synthase reductase, cystathionine β-synthase, thymidylate synthase) can affect interaction between consumption of folate and associated nutrients and cancer risk,[95] but available information is not sufficient to allow arriving at firm conclusions. Nevertheless, a common polymorphism in methionine synthase gene (Asp919Gly) was shown to affect colorectal adenoma risk through interaction with methionine and alcohol intake.[103] Likewise, there are reports on the diet-dependent influence of thymidylate synthase gene promoter polymorphisms on colorectal adenoma[104] and lung cancer[105] risks, as well as of methionine synthase reductase A66G SNP on lung cancer risk.[106]

9.2.3 Alcohol Metabolism

Alcohol consumption is a common dietary habit repeatedly shown to be associated with tumors of several sites.[107] As it has already been mentioned, alcohol consumption is known to interact with folate intake and genotype of folate-metabolizing enzymes, presumably through alterations in one-carbon metabolism.[108] It is also known that polymorphic variants of alcohol dehydrogenases (ADHs) and aldehyde dehydrogenases (ALDHs), playing central roles in the metabolism of ethanol and its main metabolite, acetaldehyde, can influence risk levels for alcohol drinking-related cancers.[109] It is, however, difficult to distinguish between effects of different alleles of genes encoding these enzymes on carcinogenesis *per se* and their influence on drinking habits.[110] Indeed, ADH2*1 allele encoding less active variant of the enzyme is associated with increased risk for both alcohol dependence and upper gastrointestinal tract cancer.[111–113]

Similarly, the inactive ALDH2 allele (ALDH2*2), the presence of which greatly decreases tolerance to alcohol (homozygous individuals are normally unable to drink alcohol), is associated with excessive risk of esophageal and head and neck cancer in drinking heterozygote carriers.[110–114] It should be noted that these variants of the ADH2 and ALDH2 enzymes are especially common in

China, Japan, and other populations of East Asia. Studies of other genes of this group have shown that the presence of the low activity allele of the ADH3 (ADH3*2), in combination with alcohol drinking, appeared to result in elevated risk for the development of upper digestive tract tumors.[114–116] However, other investigators reported no effect.[117] Also, a higher risk of developing breast cancer[118] and colorectal adenomas[119] was observed in individuals homozygous for the ADH3*1, which is associated with increased activity of the enzyme. It was also found that the presence of ADH1C "rapid" allele ADH1C*1 in alcoholics was associated with increased risk of upper aerodigestive tract cancer.[120]

9.2.4 DNA Repair

It is generally accepted that insufficient or inadequate DNA repair is an important factor in cancer initiation. Interactions between dietary factors and DNA repair mechanisms are normally regarded from the point of view of effects of mutagenic derivatives of some food constituents at the level of DNA (e.g., DNA adduct formation) and their elimination by DNA repair systems. These mechanisms are often analyzed together with xenobiotic metabolism pathways discussed above. However, some authors directly addressed concerted influence of nutrients and polymorphic genes-encoding DNA repair enzymes on cancer risk, demonstrating, in particular, effects of variants of OGG1 (8-oxoguanine glycosylase I)[121] and XRCC3 (x-ray repair cross complementation group 3)[122] genes on colorectal cancer risk related to meat consumption.

Several groups tried to approach possible relationship of DNA repair enzyme genotypes and protective effects of antioxidant-rich fruits and vegetables. The presence of the Trp194 allele of XRCC1 gene was shown to enhance the breast cancer-protective action of high intake of fruits, fruit juices, vegetables, and antioxidant supplements,[123] whereas the presence of the XRCC1 Gln399 allele was associated with increased prostate cancer risk among men with low dietary intake of vitamin E or lycopene.[124] In a recent study, an inverse association between consumption of fruits and vegetables and breast cancer risk was observed among women homozygous for the Leu84 allele or bearing at least one Val143 allele of MGMT (O-6-methylguanine DNA methyltransferase) gene.[125]

Moreover, it has been shown that daily green tea consumption reduces lung cancer risk in individuals with the Cys326 allele of OGG1(8-oxoguanine-DNA glycosylase) gene[126] The latter group of studies highlights a possibility of interaction between DNA repair systems and dietary factors exerting protective influences against cancer. It is well established that calorie restriction inhibits experimental carcinogenesis and may be beneficial in humans.[127,128] Effects of calorie restriction include stimulation of nuclear DNA repair[129,130]; however, this phenomenon observed in experimental studies requires further investigation in humans. It is also likely that some dietary constituents can modulate DNA repair as it has already been demonstrated for selenomethionine *in vitro*.[131,132] The idea of active dietary interventions directed on DNA repair enhancement[133–135] appears to be very attractive, but its realization still belongs to the future.

9.2.5 ENERGY BALANCE REGULATION

There is no doubt that obesity and related disorders, especially metabolic syndrome,[9,136] may increase cancer risk. While caloric restriction is believed to be cancer-protective,[127] overeating is regarded as a major avoidable cause of cancer, and there is sufficient evidence linking obesity with cancer of the colon, breast, endometrium, kidney, and esophagus.[23,137] Although regulation of energy balance now attracts considerable attention of the scientific community,[9,138] the knowledge of its involvement in cancer pathogenesis remains at best fragmentary.

Recent studies of genes encoding factors regulating food/energy intake have revealed the existence of multiple polymorphic variants.[9] Publications suggesting impact of some of these variants in cancer risk determination are just starting to emerge. Among polymorphic genes encoding factors regulating food/energy intake leptin gene variants have been demonstrated to be associated with susceptibility to prostate cancer[139] and non-Hodgkin lymphomas;[139,140] in the latter case, a leptin receptor gene SNP has been shown to be interactive.[140,141] Polymorphisms in the ghrelin and neuropeptide Y genes also affected non-Hodgkin lymphoma risk.[142] Variation of the gene encoding melanocortin-1 receptor (an important factor in central regulation of energy intake) is proven to be a factor in skin cancer and melanoma risk,[143] but these links may reflect the key role of the gene in skin pigmentation regulation. Moreover, there is a growing body of evidence linking polymorphisms in the insulin and, especially, insulin-like growth factor pathway genes with colorectal,[144,145] breast,[146] lung,[147] prostate,[148,149] and oral cavity[150] cancers.

Modulation of cancer risk has also been reported for genes encoding proteins involved in energy expenditure control; however this effect may not be directly related to nutritional factors. Briefly, there were reports linking polymorphisms in the 2- and 3-adrenergic receptor genes with susceptibility to breast,[151] colorectal,[152] and endometrial[153] cancer. Multifunctional factors of the arachidonic acid pathway, in particular, peroxisome proliferator-activated receptor gamma (PPAR) can be mentioned here as well, since PPAR polymorphisms have been shown to affect risk of colorectal tumours,[154–156] bladder,[157] renal,[158] and endometrial[159] cancer. Interestingly, there appeared to be colorectal cancer risk-affecting interactions between polymorphic PPAR gene variants and diet[155,156]; however, these findings require confirmation.

Limits of this chapter do not allow extensive analysis of this complex field, ramifications of which expand far beyond the area of nutrigenetics and nutrigenomics.

9.2.6 OTHER PHYSIOLOGICAL PATHWAYS, GENES, AND RESEARCH PERSPECTIVES

Other regulatory and metabolic systems are certainly involved in cancer pathogenesis, but it is very difficult to analyze them in relation to gene–nutrient interactions due to the lack of available information. For instance, dietary approaches to cancer angiogenesis modulation definitely deserve intense development. It is known that plant-derived polyphenols can inhibit tumour angiogenesis in experimental conditions,[159,160] but adequate biomarkers (including relevant genes) of their effects for human studies remain to be identified despite discussions on developing strategies of dietary cancer prevention based on the use of products rich in these compounds.[160,161] Often mechanisms of dietary interventions are difficult to interpret, such as results indicating that calorie restriction inhibits tumor-associated endothelial growth in experimental mammary carcinogenesis, whereas specificity of its influence on tumor angiogenesis remains unclear.[162] It is also evident that effects of dietary factors almost always have multiple biological endpoints. Indeed, the same polyphenolic flavonoids exert their anticancer influence not only through angiogenesis inhibition, but also by increasing apoptosis rate, inhibiting cell proliferation and tumor invasion through multiple molecular mechanisms, including modulation of signal transduction pathways.[159–161,163]

This chapter does not specifically address the relationship of dietary influences with regulatory systems mediated by hormones and vitamins, which can strongly affect risk of some cancers, but the importance of genetic diversity in these systems should not be forgotten. For example, polymorphic variants of the vitamin D receptor gene have repeatedly been shown to be associated with altered susceptibility to several types of malignancies[164–167]; however, correct interpretation of these findings is difficult given apparent multiplicity of both external factors having effects on this system (intakes of calcium, vitamin D, dairy products, sun exposure) and its involvement in a wide variety of biological processes.[166] Likewise, mechanisms of action of potentially cancer-protective carotenoids[168] or ω-3 polyunsaturated fatty acids[169] are complex and not entirely understood. It is impossible to disagree with the conclusion that in the past many studies in the domain of diet and cancer research were hampered by inadequate design, use of invalid biomarkers, and problems with exposure monitoring.[13] Development of nutrigenomics of cancer on this shaky basis is hardly possible; thus, fundamental revision of research approaches is ongoing.

Complexity of dietary influences involving simultaneous diverse effects of multiple bioactive agents often makes their investigation a hard puzzle to solve. Therefore, a somewhat similar but much better defined field of cancer pharmacogenomics will be addressed in the next part of this chapter. Thorough investigation of interactions between well-characterized drugs and their biological targets, with a close view on the significance of genetic background in these interactions, has already resulted in much better understanding of both efficiency and complications of cancer chemotherapy. This experience can be used in the development of nutrigenomic approaches in cancer research. In addition, nutritional influences often interact with chemotherapeutic schemes; thus, analysis of recent developments in the field of pharmacogenetics/pharmacogenomics appears to be entirely justified.

9.3 ADVANCES IN CANCER PHARMACOGENOMICS AND LINKS TO NUTRIGENOMICS

Pharmacogenomics is a discipline that has recently arisen from pharmacogenetics after the groundbreaking event of human genome sequence determination. Although the main goal of revealing the genetic mechanisms behind interindividual variability of responses to pharmaceutical agents[10] remains the same, possibility of applying genome-wide research approaches can further accelerate the development of the field. However, efficient introduction of innovative research technologies requires time; therefore, pharmacogenetic approach remains dominant in the field. This section is devoted to characterization of the current state of pharmacogenomics of cancer with regard to possible links with nutrigenomics.

Cancer pharmacogenomics is understandably focused mostly on cytotoxic chemotherapy and, to some extent, radiotherapy of advanced tumors (including relatively early adjuvant therapy — see Figure 9.1), which commonly results in severe toxicity and side effects. For this reason, the main goal of pharmacogenomic studies in this field is the search for individual genetically determined patterns of sensitivity and responses to cytotoxic agents. This knowledge will allow the selection of the most efficient (in terms of their specific aggressiveness against malignancy) and, at the same time, the least harmful (in terms of general toxicity) schemes of treatment on the individual basis. Several authors reviewed main achievements in the field in general,[170–172] so it is logical to concentrate on the last advances.

Table 9.2 provides a more detailed outlook of recent studies in the area of cancer pharmacogenomics. It is remarkable that even superficial comparison of Table 9.1 and Table 9.2 shows considerable similarity of genes and metabolic pathways involved in control of nutrient and drug effects. Further discussion is subdivided into a few topics reflecting main biological mechanisms affected by genetic variability.

9.3.1 DRUG-METABOLIZING PHASE I AND PHASE II ENZYMES

Drug metabolism represents a particular case of xenobiotic metabolism, thus it is natural that Phase I and II enzymatic systems mentioned above are going to be discussed here. The reactions of Phase I mediated by cytochrome P450 family enzymes are very important for initial biotransformation of anticancer agents, often resulting in the activation of inactive prodrugs with production of highly cytotoxic (and, usually, generally toxic) active compounds. This mechanism has been described for such widely used medicines as cyclophosphamide, doxorubicine, thiotepa, and tegafur.[266] At the same time, P450s act as deactivators of other antitumor drugs, such as taxanes (paclitaxel, docetaxel), *Vinca* alkaloids (vinblastine, vincristine), camphotecins (irinotecan, topotecan), antiestrogens (tamoxifen), and some other agents.[266]

It is now established that the CYP3A subfamily of enzymes is especially important for Phase I drug metabolism, being the most abundant P450 in the human liver[73,267] and intestine.[74,268] Numerous anticancer drugs are known to be substrates of the widely expressed CYP3A4[266]; however, it is likely that the contribution of the CYP3A5 may be more important than previously suggested.[269] Although considerable interindividual variability in the expression of CYP3A subfamily enzymes is a well-known fact, and its implications for drug metabolism are difficult to underestimate, mechanisms of this variability are complex and not entirely clear. Recent studies have shown the presence of multiple polymorphisms in genes encoding CYP3A4[73,270–272] and CYP3A5,[73,273,274] the latter being increasingly regarded as a major polymorphic contributor to drug metabolism.[269,273] The role of the CYP3A family gene polymorphisms in relation to anticancer therapy remains poorly investigated; however, first studies in this direction are starting to emerge (see Table 9.2).

The CYP3A family is especially interesting in the context of this chapter because these enzymes are known to be targets of interaction with certain food components; in particular, grapefruit juice, oral intake of which selectively inhibits CYP3A4 activity in the small intestine[275,276] and liver[277] resulting in supression of the oxidative metabolism of relevant substrates. It is believed that furanocoumarins and isoflavones present in grapefruit juice act as CYP3A4 inhibitors (see Chapter 2, Hypolipidemic Therapy: Drugs, Diet and Interactive Effects). It is also intriguing that a popular herbal product, St. John's wort (*Hypericum perforatum*), has been shown to induce CYP3A4 expression.[278] Given the role of the CYP3A4 in transformation of a number of anticancer agents,[266] these interactions potentially may be important, especially in altering acute toxic reactions on the administration of cytotoxic drugs. It should be noted that information regarding possible influence of natural food components and common herbs on both efficiency and side effects of cancer chemothetapy is almost nonexistent. Only one pilot study described reduced bioavailability of the anticancer agent, etoposide, following grapefruit juice ingestion.[279]

Several other polymorphic Phase I enzymes are important for anticancer therapy. Pharmacogenomic approaches look promising for CYP1A2 and flutamide, CYP2A6 and tegafur, CYP2B6 and cyclophosphamide, CYP2C8 and paclitaxel, and CYP2D6 and tamoxifen,[266,280] but further studies are required for the identification of clinically relevant gene variants. Likewise, multiple polymorphisms have been identified in genes encoding carboxylesterases (CESs) 1 and 2[281]; however, their physiological significance remains to be explored. Polymorphic CESs participate in drug metabolism acting as Phase I enzymes participating in the activation of such anticancer agents as irinotecan (CPT-11), paclitaxel, and capecitabine[282]; therefore, information on the presence of CES variants may be used for the development of individualized chemotherapy schemes.

The importance of polymorphisms in genes encoding Phase II enzymes for cancer chemotherapy is well exemplified by the effects of variants of hepatic UDP-glucuronosyltransferase 1A1 (UGT1A1) in treatment of advanced solid (mostly colorectal) tumors with topoisomerase I inhibitor irinotecan. UGT1A1

TABLE 9.2
Polymorphic Genes Encoding Factors Affecting Outcome of Cancer Chemotherapy and Radiotherapy

Gene	Malignancy Site and Type	Therapeutic Agents (Chemo- or Radio-)	Reported Clinical Effects or Functional Importance (References given in parentheses)
	Polymorphic Genes Encoding Drug-Metabolizing Phase I and Phase II Enzymes		
CYP1A1	Childhood acute lymphoblastic leukemia (ALL)	Multiagent chemotherapy	The presence of the C6235 allele (T6235C SNP in the 3′ flanking region) was associated with increased risk of relapse (173).
CYP2B6	Haematological malignancies	Cyclophosphamide (CP)	The presence of the T516 allele (T516C SNP) was associated with increased rate of formation of CP-active metabolite,4-hydroxycyclophosphamide (174).
CYP3A4	Breast cancer	Anthracycline-based adjuvant chemotherapy followed by high-dose multiagent chemotherapy	Patients who carried the CYP3A4*1B in combination with CYP3A5*3 and functional variants of GSTM1 and GSTT1 had significantly lower probability of survival (175).
	Childhood acute lymphoblastic leukemia (ALL)	Multiagent chemotherapy	Patients with the CYP3A4*1B genotype had decreased risk of peripheral nephropathy caused by chemotherapy (176).
CYP3A5	Breast cancer	Anthracycline-based adjuvant chemotherapy followed by high-dose multiagent chemotherapy	Patients who carried the CYP3A5*3 in combination with CYP3A4*1B and functional variants of GSTM1 and GSTT1 had significantly lower probability of survival (175).
	Childhood acute lymphoblastic leukemia (ALL)	Multiagent chemotherapy	Patients with the CYP3A5*3 genotype had decreased risk of peripheral nephropathy caused by chemotherapy (176).

Gene (abbreviation)	Cancer type	Drug	Description
UDP-glucuronosyl-transferase 1A1 (UGT1A1)	Cancer of several sites, mostly advanced colorectal tumors	Irinotecan	The presence of the UGT1A1*28 (7 TA repeats instead of 6 in the promoter region) allele was associated with severe toxicity (177-180) and impaired glucuronidation of the active metabolite of irinotecan, SN-38 (178, 181, 182). The presence of the UGT1A1*27(Pro229Gln) alleles was associated with severe toxicity in a few cases (177). The presence of the A-3156 allele (G-3156A promoter SNP) was associated with the severe neutropenia (183). The presence of the G-3279 allele (T-3156G promoter region SNP) was associated with severe toxicity; this SNP was also shown to be linked to the UGT1A1*28 variant (184).
UDP-glucuronosyl-transferase 1A7 (UGT1A7)	Colorectal cancer	Irinotecan	Genotypes UGT1A7*2/*2 and UGT1A7*3/*3 encoding low activity variants of the enzyme were associated with better antitumor response and lower gastrointestinal toxicity; however, study size was small (185).
UDP-glucuronosyl-transferase 1A9 (UGT1A9)	Colorectal cancer	Irinotecan	UGT1A9 genotype 118 (dT)(9/9) was associated with better antitumor response and lower gastrointestinal toxicity; however, study size was small (185).
UDP-glucuronosyl-transferase 2B15 (UGT2B15)	Breast cancer	Tamoxifen	Tamoxifen-treated patients with high enzyme activity-associated UGT2B15 genotypes had increased risk of recurrence and poor survival (186).
Glutathione-S-transferase M1 (GSTM1)	Breast cancer	CP, 5-FU (5-fluorouracil), doxorubicin Anthracycline-based adjuvant chemotherapy plus high-dose multiagent chemotherapy	Combination of GSTM1-Null and GSTT1-Null genotypes was associated with better survival (187). Patients who carried the GSTM1-Null and GSTT1-Null in combination with low activity variants of CYP3A4 and CYP3A5 had significantly lower probability of treatment failure (175).

TABLE 9.2 (CONTINUED)
Polymorphic Genes Encoding Factors Affecting Outcome of Cancer Chemotherapy and Radiotherapy

Gene	Malignancy Site and Type	Therapeutic Agents (Chemo- or Radio-)	Reported Clinical Effects or Functional Importance (References given in parentheses)
	Ovarian cancer	Cisplatinum, alkylating agents	Combination of GSTM1-Null and GSTT1-Null was associated with better responses to chemotherapy (188).
		Paclitaxel, cisplatinum	The GSTM1-Null genotype was associated with significantly longer survival time (189).
		Several chemotherapy schemes	Patients carrying the GSTM1-Null were less likely to have disease progression (190).
	Malignant glioma	Nitrosoureas	The GSTM1-Null genotype was associated with better survival, but higher probability of adverse effects (191).
	Childhood acute lymphoblastic leukemia (ALL)	Multiagent chemotherapy	GSTM1-Null genotype was associated with a decreased risk of relapse following cytotoxic chemotherapy (192, 193).
			No evidence of GSTM1 genotype (alone or combined with GSTT1 genotype) effect was found (194).
		Multiagent chemotherapy	Simultaneous presence of GSTM1-Null and GSTT1-Null genotypes was associated with early relapses (195).
	Adult acute myeloid leukemia (AML)	Multiagent chemotherapy	The presence of either GSTM1-Null or its combination with GSTT1-Null was associated with poor survival following chemotherapy (196).
Glutathione-S-transferase T1 (GSTT1)	Breast cancer	CP, 5-FU, doxorubicin	Combination of GSTT1-Null and GSTM1-Null genotypes was associated with better survival (196).

Gene	Cancer type	Treatment	Findings
		Anthracycline-based adjuvant chemotherapy plus high-dose multiagent chemotherapy	Patients who carried the GSTT1-Null and GSTM1-Null in combination with low activity variants of CYP3A4 and CYP3A5 had significantly lower probability of treatment failure (175).
	Ovarian cancer	Cisplatinum, alkylating agents	Combination of GSTM1-Null and GSTT1-Null was associated with better responses to chemotherapy (188).
	Childhood acute lymphoblastic leukemia (ALL)	Multiagent chemotherapy	Combination of GSTT1-Null and GSTM1-Null genotypes was associated with a decreased risk of relapse following cytotoxic chemotherapy (189). Simultaneous presence of GSTT1-Null and GSTM1-Null genotypes was associated with early relapses (195).
	Childhood acute myeloid leukemia (AML)	Multiagent chemotherapy	Children with GSTT1-Null genotype had greater toxicity and reduced survival after chemotherapy (197).
	Adult acute myeloid leukemia (AML)	Multiagent chemotherapy	GSTT1-Null genotype was associated with an increased toxicity of combined chemotherapy and poor survival (198). The presence of either GSTT1-Null or its combination with GSTM1-Null was associated with poor survival following chemotherapy (196).
Glutathione-S-transferase P1 (GSTP1)	Breast cancer	Several chemotherapy schemes	Women homozygous for the Val105 allele (Ile105Val polymorphism) had a 60% reduction in mortality risk (199).
	Colorectal cancer	5-FU/oxaliplatin chemotherapy	The presence of the Val105/Val105 homozygocity was associated with increased survival (200, 201).
	Non-small lung carcinoma	Platinum-based chemotherapy	The presence of the Val105 allele was associated with significantly improved survival (202).
	Ovarian cancer	Several chemotherapy schemes	Patients carrying the Val105 allele were less likely to have disease progression (190).

TABLE 9.2 (CONTINUED)
Polymorphic Genes Encoding Factors Affecting Outcome of Cancer Chemotherapy and Radiotherapy

Gene	Malignancy Site and Type	Therapeutic Agents (Chemo- or Radio-)	Reported Clinical Effects or Functional Importance (References given in parentheses)
	Stomach cancer	5-FU/cisliplatinum chemotherapy	The presence of the Val105 allele was associated with significantly improved survival (203).
	Malignant glioma	Nitrosoureas	Homozygous simultaneous presence of Ile105 and Ala114 (Ala114Val) in combination with GSTM1-Null was associated with better survival, but higher probability of adverse effects (191).
	Childhood acute lymphoblastic leukemia (ALL)	Multiagent chemotherapy	The presence of the Val105 homozygocity was associated with a decreased risk of relapse following cytotoxic chemotherapy (192, 204).
	Therapy-related acute myeloid leukemia (t-AML)	Several chemotherapy schemes	The presence of the Val105 allele was associated with an increased risk of developing t-AML after cytotoxic chemotherapy (205).
Glutathione-S-transferase A1 (GSTA1)	Breast cancer	Cyclophosphamide-containing combined chemotherapy	The presence of the T-69 homozygocity (C−69T SNP in the promoter region) was associated with better survival following chemotherapy (206).
NAD(P)H: quinone oxidoreductase (NQO1)	Childhood acute lymphoblastic leukemia (ALL)	Multiagent chemotherapy	The presence of the NQO1*2 allele (609T allele of C609T SNP) was associated with increased risk of relapse (173).
	Superficial bladder cancer	Mitomycin C chemotherapy	The presence of the NQO1*2 allele was associated with reduced response to mitomycin C (207).
Sulfotransferase 1A1 (SULT1A1)	Breast cancer	Tamoxifen	The presence of the SULT1A1*2/*2 homozygocity (His/His of Arg213His polymorphism) was associated with poor survival following tamoxifen therapy (208).

Sulfotransferase 1E1 (SULT1E1)	Breast cancer	Several chemotherapy schemes	The presence of the C-1653 allele (T-1653C SNP in the promoter region) was associated with significantly higher risk of recurrence (209).
Polymorphic Genes Encoding Enzymes of Purine/Pyrimidine Metabolism			
Thiopurine S-methyltransferase (TPMT)	Acute lymphoblastic leukemia (ALL) and acute myeloid leukemia (AML) in children.	6-Mercaptopurine, 6-thioguanine, azathiopurine	The presence of alleles causing TPMT deficiency (TPMT*2, TPMT*3A, TPMT*3C, TPMT*7) was associated with intolerance of conventional therapeutic doses (170, 210–212). Genotype-dependent dose adjustment provided better chemotherapy tolerance (210, 212, 213).
Dihydro-pyrimidine dehydrogenase (DPD or DPYD)	Cancer of several sites	5-FU-based chemotherapy	The presence of the DPYD*2A allele causing a reduced DPD activity was associated with toxic effects of 5-fluorouracil (5-FU) chemotherapy (214–216).
Cytidine deaminase (CDA)	Cancer of several sites	Gemcitabine, cisplatin	Severe chemotherapy toxicity was observed in a patient homozygous for the Thr70 allele (Ala70Thr polymorphism); however, only a few patients were analyzed (217).
Deoxycytidine kinase (dCK)	Acute myeloid leukemia (AML)	1-β-arabinofuranosyl-cytosine (AraC)	The presence of the haplotype combining C-360 homozygocity (C-360G SNP in the 5' flanking region) with C-201 homozygocity (C-201T in the 5' flanking region) resulted in a poor response to chemotherapy (218).
Polymorphic Genes Encoding Enzymes and Regulatory Factors of Folate Metabolism			
Methylenetetrahydrofolate reductase (MTHFR)	Colorectal cancer	Fluoropyrimidine-based chemotherapy	The T677T homozygocity (C677T SNP) was associated with better chemotherapy response rates (219–221).
	Ovarian cancer	Methotrexate	The T677 homozygocity was associated with increased toxicity of methotrexate therapy (222).
	Acute leukemia	Methotrexate	The T677 homozygocity was associated with increased toxicity of methotrexate chemotherapy (223).

TABLE 9.2 (CONTINUED)
Polymorphic Genes Encoding Factors Affecting Outcome of Cancer Chemotherapy and Radiotherapy

Gene	Malignancy Site and Type	Therapeutic Agents (Chemo- or Radio-)	Reported Clinical Effects or Functional Importance (References given in parentheses)
	Childhood acute lymphoblastic leukemia (ALL)	Methotrexate	The presence of the T677T + A1298 (A1298G SNP) haplotype (especially in combination with TS high-activity genotype) was associated with reduced event-free survival (224).
			The presence of the T677 allele was associated with higher risk of relapse (225).
Thymidylate synthase (TS)	Colorectal cancer	5-FU-based chemotherapy schemes, capecitabine	The presence of TS genotypes associated with high activity of the enzyme (those with 3R or three 28-bp repeats in the 5′ promoter/enhancer region, G variant of the G12G SNP in the repeat sequence, and a 6bp insertion in the 3′-untranslated region) was associated with poorer prognosis and shorter survival (201, 203, 226–229).
		5-FU-based chemotherapy	Simultaneous presence of 2R (low activity-related) and 6bp ins in the 3′-UTR (high activity-related) was associated with severe side effects (230).
			The presence of high activity-related TS genotypes was associated with longer disease-free survival (231).
	Stomach cancer	5-FU-based chemotherapy	The presence of low activity-related TS genotypes was associated with longer disease-free and overall survival (232)
	Non-small-cell lung cancer	5-FU-based chemotherapy	The presence of TS genotypes associated with low activity of the enzyme was associated with better survival (233).

	Childhood acute lymphoblastic leukemia (ALL)	Methotrexate	The presence of TS genotypes associated with high activity of the enzyme in combination with either MTHFR T677A1298 haplotype or MTHFD1 A1958 allele was associated with reduced event-free survival (224).
Methylenetetra-hydrofolate dehydrogenase (MTHFD1)	Childhood acute lymphoblastic leukemia (ALL)	Methotrexate	The presence of the A1958 allele (G1958A SNP) in combination with TS high-activity genotype was associated with reduced event-free survival (224).
Methionine synthase (MTR)	Esophageal cancer	5-FU-based radiochemotherapy	The presence of the G2756 allele (A2756G SNP) was associated with significantly longer survival (234).
Reduced folate carrier (RFC1)	Childhood acute lymphoblastic leukemia (ALL)	Methotrexate	The A80 allele (G80A SNP) was associated with reduced event-free survival (235). No effect of RFC1 gene variants revealed (236).
Polymorphic Genes Encoding DNA Repair Enzymes			
Excision repair cross complementation group 1 (ERCC1)	Non-small-cell lung cancer	Cisplatin combination chemotherapy	The presence of the AAC codon 118 allele (Codon 118 AAC→AAT silent SNP) was associated with better survival (237).
		Docetaxel-cisplatin	The presence of the AAC codon 118 allele was associated with better survival (238).
		Platinim-based chemotherapy	The presence of the C8092 allele (C8092A SNP shown to be linked to the codon 118 SNP) was associated with better survival (239).
	Colorectal cancer	Platinum-based chemotherapy	The presence of the C8092 allele was associated with a significantly increased risk of grade 3 or 4 gastrointestinal toxicity. Codon 118 SNP did not affect toxicity (240). The presence of the AAC codon 118 allele was associated with better survival (241).

TABLE 9.2 (CONTINUED)
Polymorphic Genes Encoding Factors Affecting Outcome of Cancer Chemotherapy and Radiotherapy

Gene	Malignancy Site and Type	Therapeutic Agents (Chemo- or Radio-)	Reported Clinical Effects or Functional Importance (References given in parentheses)
Xeroderma pigmentosum group D (XPD or ERCC2)	Non-small-cell lung cancer	Oxaliplatin/5-FU	The presence of the AAT codon 118 allele was associated with higher chemotherapy response rate (242).
		Platinum-based chemotherapy	The presence of the Asn312 allele (Asp312Asn XPD polymorphism) was associated with reduced survival (243).
	Colorectal cancer	Oxaliplatin/5FU	The presence of the Lys751 homozygocity (Lys751Gln XPD polymorphism) was associated with better survival (244).
	Acute myeloid leukemia	Multiagent chemotherapy	The presence of the Lys751 homozygocity was associated with better survival (245).
Excision repair cross complementation group 6 (ERCC6)	Superficial bladder cancer	Bacillus Calmette–Guerin treatment	The presence of the Val1097 allele (Met1097Val ERCC6 polymorphism) was associated with reduced recurrence-free survival (246).
Xeroderma pigmentosum group A (XPA)	Superficial bladder cancer	Bacillus Calmette–Guerin treatment	The presence of the A-4 allele (G-4A SNP in the 5′ untranslated region) was associated with reduced recurrence-free survival (246).
X-ray repair cross complementation group 1 (XRCC1)	Colorectal cancer	Oxaliplatin/5-FU	The presence of the Gln399 allele (Arg399Gln XRCC1 polymorphism) was associated with resistance to chemotherapy and reduced survival (247).
	Breast cancer	Radiotherapy	The presence of the Trp(194) allele (Arg194Trp XRCC1 polymorphism) was associated with adverse responses to radiotherapy (248).

Gene	Cancer	Treatment	Finding
	Non-small-cell lung cancer	Radiotherapy	The presence of the Gln399 allele was associated with protection against adverse effects of radiotherapy (249). Combined analysis of polymorphisms at codons 194, 280, and 399 has shown correlations between XRCC1 haplotypes and survival (250).
Apurinic/apyrimidinic endonuclease 1 (APE1/APEX1)	Therapy-related acute myeloid leukemia (t-AML)	Radiotherapy	The presence of the Gln399 allele was associated with a decreased risk of developing t-AML (251).
	Breast cancer	Radiotherapy	The presence of the Glu148 allele (Asp148Glu APE1 polymorphism) was associated with protection against the development of acute adverse effects of radiotherapy (249).
DNA mismatch repair gene hMSH2	Therapy-related acute myeloid leukemia (t-AML)	Cyclophosphamide procarbazine	The presence of the (-6)C allele (T-6C SNP at the 3' splice acceptor site of exon 13) was associated with an increased risk of developing t-AML (252).
Polymorphic Genes Encoding ATP-Binding Cassette Transporters (ABC)			
Multi-drug resistance (MDR-1 or ABCB1)	Acute myeloid leukemia (AML)	Multiagent chemotherapy	The presence of the C3435 homozygocity (C3435T SNP) was associated with an increased probability of relapse and reduced overall survival (253).
	Breast cancer	Anthracyclines or anthracyclines combined with taxanes	The presence of the T3435 homozygocity was associated with an increased probability of favorable clinical response to preoperative chemotherapy (254).
	Cancer of several sites	Irinotecan	The presence of the C1236 allele (C1236T SNP) was associated with significantly increased exposure to irinotecan and its active metabolite SN-38 (178).
	Childhood acute lymphoblastic leukemia (ALL)	Multiagent chemotherapy	The presence of the T3435 allele was associated with reduced probability of CNS relapse (204).

TABLE 9.2 (CONTINUED)
Polymorphic Genes Encoding Factors Affecting Outcome of Cancer Chemotherapy and Radiotherapy

Gene	Malignancy Site and Type	Therapeutic Agents (Chemo- or Radio-)	Reported Clinical Effects or Functional Importance (References given in parentheses)
	Nasopharyngeal carcinoma	Irinotecan	The presence of the C3435 homozygocity was associated with reduced event-free survival and overall survival (255).
			Irinotecan clearance was lower in patients homozygous for the C3435 allele (256).
Breast cancer resistance protein (BCRP or ABCG2)	Cancer of several sites	Irinotecan	Extensive accumulation of SN-38 was observed in a patient homozygous for the A421 allele (C421A SNP) (257).
	Nasopharyngeal carcinoma	Irinotecan	Higher irinotecan to SN-38 conversion of was related to the absence of CTCA deletion in the 5' flanking region (256).
Polymorphic Genes Encoding Other Drug Targets (Receptors, Regulatory Factors, etc.)			
Epidermal growth factor receptor (EGFR or HER-1)	Colorectal cancer (rectum)	Adjuvant and neoadjuvant chemoradiation	Patients with Arg497 homozygocity (Arg497Lys SNP) or lower number (<20) of CA repeats (Inthron 1 CA_n repeat polymorphism) had a higher recurrence risk (258).
	Colorectal cancer	5-FU/oxaliplatin	Patients with less than 20 CA repeats were more likely to show disease progression (259).
HER-2 receptor (HER-2, c-erb-B2 or neu)	Ovarian cancer	Cisplatin, paclitaxel	The presence of Val655 homozygocity (Ile655Val polymorphism) was associated with reduced overall survival (260).

Immunoglobulin G F_c receptor II (FcRIIa, CD32)	Follicular lymphoma	Rituximab	The presence of His131 homozygocity (Arg131His polymorphism) was associated with better response rate and freedom from progression (261).
Immunoglobulin G F_c receptor III (FcRIIIa, CD16)	Follicular lymphoma	Rituximab	The presence of Val158 homozygocity (Phe158Val polymorphism) was associated with better response rate and freedom from progression (261).
		Id vaccination	The presence of Val158 homozygocity was associated with longer progression-free survival (262).
Interleukin-1β (IL-1B)	Stomach cancer	Palliative chemotherapy	The presence of T-511 (C-511T SNP) and C-31 (T-31C SNP) was associated with reduced progression-free and overall survival, but only in patients with wild-type genotype of interleukin-1 receptor antagonist (IL-RN) (263).
Interleukin-6 (IL-6)	Breast cancer	Anthracycline-based adjuvant chemotherapy and multiagent high-dose chemotherapy	The presence of the C-174 allele (G-174C SNP) was associated with better disease-free and overall survival (264).
Interleukin 8 receptor CXCR1	Colorectal cancer	5-FU/oxaliplatin	Patients with CXCR1 2607 heterozygocity (G2607C SNP) were more likely to show disease progression (254).
Interferon-γ (IFN-γ)	Melanoma	Cisplatin, vinblastine, and dacarbazine combined with interleukin-2 and interferon-α and in some cases tamoxifen	The presence of T834 allele (A874T SNP) was associated with better response, progression-free, and overall survival (265).

exerts glucuronidation of SN-38, the active metabolite of irinotecan, producing an inactive and nontoxic glucuronic acid conjugate SN-38G (178). It has repeatedly been shown that impaired activity of the enzyme caused by the presence of variant alleles, in particular the UGT1A1*28 causing reduced gene expression and enzyme activity, can result in severe toxicity (see Table 9.2). Although little is known about interactions between nutritional factors and UGTs, there are reports indicating that isothiocyanate-rich cruciferous vegetables can affect enzyme activity in individuals with the UGT1A1*28 variant,[84] and that curcumin transiently inhibits UGT activities in cell culture.[82]

Enzymes of the glutathione-S-transferase family have also been shown to be involved in Phase II drug metabolism, detoxifying drugs and their toxic derivatives by glutathione conjugation.[76] The presence of homozygous-long deletions in GSTM1 and GSTT1 genes ("Null" variants) is often associated with higher chemotherapy efficiency for solid tumors (breast, ovary); however, controversial results were obtained for leukemias (see Table 9.2). The presence of the Val105 allele of the GSTP1 gene was also associated with better outcomes of chemotherapy and improved survival in most studies. It is important to remember that activities of the GST family enzymes can be modulated by dietary intake of cruciferous vegetables; however, this type of diet–gene interaction has not been investigated in relation to anticancer chemotherapy.

9.3.2 ENZYMES OF PURINE/PYRIMIDINE METABOLISM

Thiopurine-S-methyltransferase (TPMT) is one of the key enzymes in the biotransformation of aromatic and heterocyclic sulfhydril compounds, including anileukemia agents 6-mercaptopurine, 6-thioguanine, and azathioprine. The TPMT is the catalyst for the S-methylation of these drugs leading to the formation of inactive metabolites.[170] It is now evident that several variants of the highly polymorphic TPMT gene encode the enzyme molecules with decreased stability and lower specific activity (especially TPMT*3A, TPMT*3C, TPMT*5).[283] Individuals homozygous for these variants as well as compound heterozygotes are TPMT-deficient and application of conventional doses of thiopurine chemotherapy can cause severe hematopoietic toxicity in such patients.[170,210–212] It has already been shown by several studies that prospective genetic screening can identify patients requiring lower thiopurine doses, thus increasing therapy tolerance.[210,212,213] Although influence of genetic variation on TPMT expression is well established, a possibility of contribution of other factors, including those of dietary origin, remains to be investigated.

Numerous studies have been devoted to the characterization of genetic factors affecting 5-fluorouracil (5-FU)-based chemotherapy. Dihydropyrimidine dehydrogenase (DPD) is the initial rate-limiting enzyme in the degradation of 5-FU. The enzyme activity is highly variable and its partial loss is observed in at least 3% of individuals.[170] DPD is encoded by a highly polymorphic DPYD gene and the DPYD*2 allele is associated with a reduced enzyme activity and high risk of 5-FU toxicity.[214–216] Nevertheless, other factors (in particular, aberrant methylation of the DPYD gene promoter region[284] and transcription regulation by a specific activator protein[285]) appear to be involved in variations in DPD activity; thus, the predictive value of DPYD genotype determination remains unclear. Nothing is known about effects of dietary factors on DPD activity.

9.3.3 ENZYMES AND REGULATORY FACTORS OF FOLATE METABOLISM

The folate system has already been briefly considered in this chapter as a good example of diet–gene interactions modulating cancer risk. Several cytotoxic agents employed in cancer chemotherapy schemes, including fluoropyrimidines (5-FU, capecitabine) and methotrexate, inhibit folate metabolism acting at its different stages.[171] For this reason polymorphic genes encoding enzymes of this metabolic pathway attracted considerable attention of investigators. Analysis of the effects of the methylenetetrahydrofolate reductase (MTHFR) gene variants revealed different response patterns in different malignancies. Several studies in colorectal cancer patients show that the presence of the T667 (Val222) allele was associated with better responses to fluoropyrimidine therapy,[219–221] whereas the same allele appeared to be linked with excessive toxicity and poor response during methotrexate therapy of ovarian cancer[222] and leukemias.[223–225]

Thymidylate synthase (TS) is another key polymorphic enzyme of folate metabolism. TS is one of the main targets of fluoropyrimidines, which inhibit its activity.[286] It is known that genetic variation (variable number of 28-bp repeats) in the promoter/enhancer region of the TS gene results in two- to fourfold changes in gene expression defining "rapid" and "slow" alleles (see Table 9.2). In most clinical studies, the presence of the rapid genotype was associated with poor prognosis in fluoropyrimidine-treated patients (see Table 9.2).

Several reports describe possible effects of other polymorphic genes encoding factors participating in folate metabolism regulation (methylenetetrahydrofolate dehydrogenase, methionine synthase, reduced folate carrier), but all of this information requires confirmation by further studies.

Antifolate chemotherapeutic agents are widely used in cancer treatment, but the role of dietary folate in these conditions is not completely clear. It could be assumed that high folate intake may decrease the effectiveness of this type of chemotherapy, but this assumption has not been corroborated in studies of breast cancer patients.[287] In contrast, folate supplementation has recently been suggested as a way to increase chemotherapy efficiency[288]; however, the problem still requires further research.

9.3.4 DNA REPAIR EFFECTS ON CANCER TREATMENT

Most cytostatic therapies are based on inducing irreversible lethal damage in tumor cell DNA; therefore, DNA repair systems, which serve as a protective mechanism at initial stages of carcinogenesis, may contribute to intrinsic drug resistance during anticancer chemotherapy. This phenomenon appears to be especially graphic in relation to platinum-based cytotoxic therapy, the treatment of choice for lung and ovarian cancer, and some colorectal tumors.[289] Platinum derivatives exert their cytotoxic effect through formation of platinum DNA adducts, which then become legitimate targets of the system of nucleotide excision repair.[289,290] Successful removal of platinum adducts can lead to reduced efficiency of the therapy and is believed to be the main mechanism responsible for the development of resistance to platinum therapy.

The excision repair, cross-complementation group 1 (ERCC1) gene plays the leading role in the nucleotide excision repair system, and the presence of a silent SNP (AACAAT, both coding for asparagine) in codon 118 of this gene has been found to cause reduced ERCC1 expression.[291,292] Several recent studies clearly show that this variant is also associated with higher response rate to platinum-based chemotherapy and better survival (see Table 9.2). These observations can be regarded as the most convincing evidence linking polymorphisms in DNA repair genes with the effectiveness of cytotoxic anticancer chemotherapy. Although numerous polymorphic variants are described for other genes encoding factors of DNA repair systems (XPD, ERCC2, XPA, XRCC1, APE1, hMSH2), and some of these variants have been associated with gene expression changes, their clinical importance needs to be confirmed.

Little is known about possible dietary effects on DNA repair with regard to anticancer chemotherapy. Recent discovery of DNA repair modulation by seleno-methionine,[131,132] abundantly present in Brazil nuts,[293] suggests that interactions are not excluded, but investigation of this area, again, belongs to the future.

9.3.5 ATP-Binding Cassette Transporters

Membrane-bound transporter proteins have recently emerged as a major defensive system that exerts protection from toxic influences through control of xenobiotic uptake and excretion.[170,294] The ATP-binding cassette transporter (ABC) gene superfamily appears to be the most important from the point of view of cancer chemotherapy since expression of its members has been implicated in tumor cell resistance to cytostatic agents, altered drug disposition, and toxic effects of drugs.[294] P-glycoprotein encoded by the MDR-1 (ABCB1) gene is the most extensively studied among ABC transporters. P-glycoprotein is closely involved in the regulation of drug bioavailability through interplay with CYP3A4.[295] Multiple polymorphisms have been determined in the sequence of the MDR-1 gene,[296,297] and their functional significance is now being investigated. Attempts to assess the role of some of these SNPs in response to cancer chemotherapy have been undertaken, but results of several studies published so far look conflicting (see Table 9.2). Although information on numerous polymorphisms in other ABC transporter genes (ABCC1, ABCC2, ABCC3, ABCC4, ABCC5, ABCC6, ABCG2) is now available,[294] their potential validity as biomarkers predicting response to drugs remains to be clarified.

ABC transporters are very intriguing as a known target for diet–drug interactions. Grapefruit juice components have already been mentioned as potent inhibitors of CYP3A4; however, they have also been shown to suppress P-glycoprotein transporter activity.[298] Another recent report describes inhibition of P-glycoprotein-mediated transport by curcuminoids.[299] On the other hand, induction of P-glycoprotein by St. John's wort has been demonstrated as well.[300] These facts again highlight the necessity of thorough investigation of diet–drug interactions in the context of anticancer treatment.

9.3.6 OTHER DRUG TARGETS AND RECENT ADVANCES

Table 9.2 indicates several reports implicating other polymorphic drug targets, including receptors and cytokines on the effects of anticancer chemotherapy. Some of these targets appear to be especially interesting due to their significance for innovative anticancer treatment methods based on the use of monoclonal antibodies[301,302] or small molecule inhibitors of the epidermal growth factor receptor (EGFR) tyrosine kinase activity.[302,303] Recently introduced monoclonal antibodies include anti-HER2/neu trastuzumab (Herceptin®), anti-VEGF bevacizumab (Avastin®), anti-EGFR cetuximab (Erbitux®), and anti-CD20 rituximab (Rituxan®).[301,302] Tyrosine kinase inhibitors comprise imatinib (Gleevec™), gefitinib (Iressa™), and erlotinib (Tarceva®).[302,303] The importance of pharmacogenomic approaches to these new therapeutic strategies is already highlighted by the association between polymorphisms of immunoglobulin GF_c receptors and clinical response to rituximab (see Table 9.2). It is very likely that variants of highly polymorphic targets of other new agents[304] will be found to be important for therapeutic efficiency as well. These modern directions of antitumor therapy have emerged very recently, so it is not surprising that information regarding possible impact of dietary factors is not yet available.

Pharmacogenomics of cancer is often related to later stages of the disease, when malignant process becomes irreversible and can be only temporarily contained by chemotherapy. At these stages, oncological patients are at a very high risk of developing cachexia, which is characterized by weight loss with depletion of host resources of adipose tissue and skeletal muscle.[305] About half of all cancer patients suffer from this syndrome.[305] It is known that the development of cachexia is related to profound deregulation of the central control of energy homeostasis followed by cytokine production, release of lipid-mobilizing and proteolysis-inducing factors, and eventually severe general metabolic alterations.[305–308] Given the presence of numerous polymorphic genes encoding regulatory proteins controlling these pathways,[9] it is impossible to exclude that the genetic background may determine predisposition or resistance to cachexia. Correlations of the presence of polymorphisms in the genes encoding interleukin-1β,[263,309] interleukin-1 receptor antagonist,[263] and interferon-γ[310] with survival of patients with advanced gastric[263] and pancreatic[309,310] tumors, which are typically aggravated by fatal cachexia, have already been reported suggesting that this is another nutrition-related problem requiring urgent investigation.

9.4 CONCLUSION

The presented overview of pharmacogenomic studies highlights a few impressive examples of successful utilization of information regarding genetic profiles of oncological patients in the development of individual-oriented ("tailored") chemotherapeutic strategies. These examples include interactions between UGT1A1 polymorphisms and treatment with irinotecan as well as TPMT variants and thiopurine chemotherapy. Furthermore, promising results have already emerged from studies of the effects of thymydilate synthase alleles on fluoropyrimidine-based chemotherapy, influence of ERCC1 genotype on platinum resistance, and effects of GST-family gene genotypes in different schemes of cytostatic treatment. This chapter was focused predominantly on the role of inherited structural DNA variations (polymorphisms); however, it should be understood that other mechanisms, especially changes in gene expression in the malignant tissue, are not less important in terms of the development of individually tailored schemes of cancer therapy. There is no doubt that clinical significance of pharmacogenomic information is going to increase rapidly with introduction of modern genome-wide analytical approaches.

In contrast, nutrigenomics of cancer is only starting to come into existence. Although serious attempts to reveal links between carcinogenesis and nutrition have been undertaken for decades, making firm conclusions remains difficult. Cooked red meat consumption appears to be the only dietary influence, which can be regarded as a proven risk factor for several types of cancer. A number of nutrients have been shown to have cancer-preventive potential, but further studies are needed to develop reliable strategies for their wide application. Introduction of nutrigenomic approaches into this area has brought little clarification so far; thus, full realization of potential strengths of this approach belongs to the future.

Parallel analysis of genetic factors involved in the metabolism of nutritional agents and anticancer drugs reveals a striking similarity, which is not surprising, given the plant-derived nature of many anticancer agents.[266] This similarity results in multiple opportunities for drug–nutrient interactions that is further modulated by variants of gene structure and expression (see schematic representation in Figure 9.2). Some situations of nutrient–drug interactions are recognized and partially investigated, which is exemplified by studies on modulation of drug transport and metabolism (MDR-1 and P-glycoprotein system and CYP3A enzymes, respectively) by bioactive substances present in grapefruit juice or St. John's wort. However, significance of these known interactions for anticancer therapy remains obscure. Only further studies in this direction will help to elucidate their importance.

Although it is obvious that successful development of nutrigenomics is complicated by many unsolved problems, the breathtaking speed of the technical progress introduces numerous new powerful research tools in the field. This innovation, along with the revision of some inefficient old investigative approaches in nutritional science, brings expectations that serious breakthroughs await us in the near future.

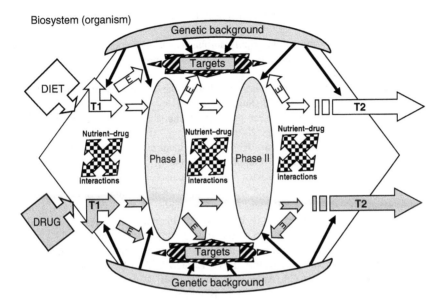

FIGURE 9.2 Diet–drug interactions and their genetic modulation. Abbreviations: **T1** — systems of initial transport of xenobiotics including drugs, also providing some reverse transport of unmetabolized agents: "Phase 0"; **Phase I** — Phase I metabolism of xenobiotics and drugs; **Phase II** — Phase II metabolism of xenobiotics and drugs; **T2** — systems of eventual transport (secretion/excretion) of xenobiotic end metabolites (conjugates): "Phase III"; **E** — effects of drugs; **Targets** — biomolecular targets of drugs and food-derived bioactive substances and their metabolites; symbols representing genetic background and targets are duplicated to simplify the scheme. It should be understood that in reality drugs and food-derived substances interact with the same targets regulated by the same genes.

REFERENCES

1. Peltonen L, McKusick VA. Genomics and medicine. Dissecting human disease in the postgenomic era. *Science* 2001; 291: 1224–1229.
2. Guttmacher AE, Collins FS. Genomic medicine — a primer. *N Engl J Med* 2002; 347: 1512–1520.
3. Elliott R, Ong TJ. Nutritional genomics. *BMJ.* 2002; 324: 1438–1442.
4. Müller M, Kersten S. Nutrigenomics: goals and strategies. *Nat Rev Genet* 2003; 3: 912–920.
5. German JB, Roberts MA, Watkins SM. Genomics and metabolomics as markers for the interaction of diet and health: lessons from lipids. *J Nutr* 2003; 133 (Suppl 1): 2078S–2083S.
6. Kaput J, Rodriguez RL. Nutritional genomics: the next frontier in the postgenomic era. *Physiol Genomics* 2004; 16: 166–177.
7. Nagy R, Sweet K, Eng C. Highly penetrant hereditary cancer syndromes. *Oncogene* 2004; 23: 6445–6470.

8. de la Chapelle A. Genetic predisposition to colorectal cancer. *Nat Rev Cancer* 2004; 4: 769–780.

9. Loktionov A. Common gene polymorphisms and nutrition: emerging links with pathogenesis of multifactorial chronic diseases (review). *J Nutr Biochem* 2003; 14: 426–451.

10. Evans WE. Pharmacogenomics: marshalling the human genome to individualise drug therapy. *Gut* 2003; 52 (Suppl 2): ii10–ii18.

11. Willett WC. Diet and cancer: one view at the start of the millennium. *Cancer Epidemiol Biomarkers Prev* 2001; 10: 3–8.

12. Wargovich MJ, Cunningham JE. Diet, individual responsiveness and cancer prevention. *J Nutr* 2003; 133 (Suppl): 2400S–2403S.

13. Milner JA. Incorporating basic nutrition science into health interventions for cancer prevention. *J Nutr* 2003; 133 (Suppl): 3820S–3826S

14. Hung HC, Joshipura KJ, Jiang R, Hu FB, Hunter D, Smith-Warner SA, Colditz GA, Rosner B, Spiegelman D, Willett WC. Fruit and vegetable intake and risk of major chronic disease. *J Natl Cancer Inst* 2004; 96: 1577–1584.

15. van Gils CH, Peeters PH, Bueno-de-Mesquita HB, Boshuizen HC, Lahmann PH, Clavel-Chapelon F, Thiebaut A, Kesse E, Sieri S, Palli D, Tumino R, Panico S, Vineis P, Gonzalez CA, Ardanaz E, Sanchez MJ, Amiano P, Navarro C, Quiros JR, Key TJ, Allen N, Khaw KT, Bingham SA, Psaltopoulou T, Koliva M, Trichopoulou A, Nagel G, Linseisen J, Boeing H, Berglund G, Wirfalt E, Hallmans G, Lenner P, Overvad K, Tjonneland A, Olsen A, Lund E, Engeset D, Alsaker E, Norat T, Kaaks R, Slimani N, Riboli E. Consumption of vegetables and fruits and risk of breast cancer. *JAMA* 2005; 293: 183–193.

16. English DR, MacInnis RJ, Hodge AM, Hopper JL, Haydon AM, Giles GG. Red meat, chicken, and fish consumption and risk of colorectal cancer. *Cancer Epidemiol Biomarkers Prev* 2004; 13: 1509–1514.

17. Chao A, Thun MJ, Connell CJ, McCullough ML, Jacobs EJ, Flanders WD, Rodriguez C, Sinha R, Calle EE. Meat consumption and risk of colorectal cancer. *JAMA* 2005; 293: 172–182.

18. Larsson SC, Rafter J, Holmberg L, Bergkvist L, Wolk A. Red meat consumption and risk of cancers of the proximal colon, distal colon and rectum: the Swedish Mammography Cohort. *Int J Cancer* 2005; 113: 829–834.

19. Schatzkin A, Kipnis V. Could exposure assessment problems give us wrong answers to nutrition and cancer questions? *J Natl Cancer Inst* 2004; 96: 1564–1565.

20. Bingham SA, Luben R, Welch A, Wareham N, Khaw KT, Day N. Are imprecise methods obscuring a relation between fat and breast cancer? *Lancet* 2003; 362: 212–214.

21. Calle EE, Rodriguez C, Walker-Thurmond K, Thun MJ. Overweight, obesity, and mortality from cancer in a prospectively studied cohort of U.S. adults. *N Engl J Med* 2003; 348: 1625–1638.

22. McCullough ML, Giovannucci EL. Diet and cancer prevention. *Oncogene* 2004; 23: 6349–6364.

23. Calle EE, Kaaks R. Overweight, obesity and cancer: epidemiological evidence and proposed mechanisms. *Nat Rev Cancer* 2004; 4: 579–591.

24. Prentice RL, Willett WC, Greenwald P, Alberts D, Bernstein L, Boyd NF, Byers T, Clinton SK, Fraser G, Freedman L, Hunter D, Kipnis V, Kolonel LN, Kristal BS, Kristal A, Lampe JW, McTiernan A, Milner J, Patterson RE, Potter JD, Riboli E, Schatzkin A, Yates A, Yetley E. Nutrition and physical activity and chronic disease prevention: research strategies and recommendations. *J Natl Cancer Inst* 2004; 96: 1276–1287.

25. Vineis P, Malats N, Lang M, d'Errico A, Caporaso N, Cuzick J, Boffetta P. (Eds.) *Metabolic Polymorpisms and Susceptibility to Cancer.* International Agency for Research on Cancer (IARC) Scientific Publication 148. Lyon: IARC, 2000.

26. Nebert DW, Russell DW. Clinical importance of the cytochromes P450. *Lancet* 2002; 360: 1155–1162.

27. Guengerich FP. Cytochrome P450: what have we learned and what are the future issues? *Drug Metab Rev* 2004; 36: 159–197.

28. Ingelman-Sundberg M. Polymorphism of cytochrome P450 and xenobiotic toxicity. *Toxicology* 2002; 181–182: 447–452.

29. Terry KL, Titus-Ernstoff L, Garner EO, Vitonis AF, Cramer DW. Interaction between CYP1A1 polymorphic variants and dietary exposures influencing ovarian cancer risk. *Cancer Epidemiol Biomarkers Prev* 2003; 12: 187–190.

30. Murtaugh MA, Sweeney C, Ma K, Caan BJ, Slattery ML. The CYP1A1 genotype may alter the association of meat consumption patterns and preparation with the risk of colorectal cancer in men and women. *J Nutr* 2005; 135: 179–186.

31. Le Marchand L, Hankin JH, Wilkens LR, Pierce LM, Franke A, Kolonel LN, Seifried A, Custer LJ, Chang W, Lum-Jones A, Donlon T. Combined effects of well-done red meat, smoking, and rapid N-acetyltransferase 2 and CYP1A2 phenotypes in increasing colorectal cancer risk. *Cancer Epidemiol Biomarkers Prev* 2001; 10: 1259–1266.

32. Sachse C, Brockmöller J, Bauer S, Roots I. Functional significance of CA polymorphism in intron 1 of the cytochrome P450 1A2 (CYP1A2) gene tested with caffeine. *Br J Clin Pharmacol* 1999; 47: 445–449.

33. Goodman MT, Tung KH, McDuffie K, Wilkens LR, Donlon TA. Association of caffeine intake and CYP1A2 genotype with ovarian cancer. *Nutr Cancer* 2003; 46: 23–29.

34. Sweeney C, Coles BF, Nowell S, Lang NP, Kadlubar FF. Novel markers of susceptibility to carcinogens in diet: associations with colorectal cancer. *Toxicology* 2002; 181–182: 83–87.

35. Nowell S, Coles B, Sinha R, MacLeod S, Luke Ratnasinghe D, Stotts C, Kadlubar FF, Ambrosone CB, Lang NP. Analysis of total meat intake and exposure to individual heterocyclic amines in a case-control study of colorectal cancer: contribution of metabolic variation to risk. *Mutat Res* 2002; 30: 175–185.

36. Sachse C, Smith G, Wilkie MJ, Barrett JH, Waxman R, Sullivan F, Forman D, Bishop DT, Wolf CR; Colorectal Cancer Study Group. A pharmacogenetic study to investigate the role of dietary carcinogens in the etiology of colorectal cancer. *Carcinogenesis* 2002; 23: 1839–1849.

37. Le Marchand L, Donlon T, Seifried A, Wilkens LR. Red meat intake, CYP2E1 genetic polymorphisms, and colorectal cancer risk. *Cancer Epidemiol Biomarkers Prev* 2002; 11: 1019–1024.

38. Chen SY, Liu TY, Shun CT, Wu MS, Lu TH, Lin JT, Sheu JC, Santella RM, Chen CJ. Modification effects of GSTM1, GSTT1 and CYP2E1 polymorphisms on associations between raw salted food and incomplete intestinal metaplasia in a high-risk area of stomach cancer. *Int J Cancer* 2004; 108: 606–612.

39. Bouchardy C, Hirvonen A, Coutelle C, Ward PJ, Dayer P, Benhamou S. Role of alcohol dehydrogenase 3 and cytochrome P-4502E1 genotypes in susceptibility to cancers of the upper aerodigestive tract. *Int J Cancer* 2000; 87: 734–740.

40. Ahn J, Gammon MD, Santella RM, Gaudet MM, Britton JA, Teitelbaum SL, Terry MB, Neugut AI, Josephy PD, Ambrosone CB. Myeloperoxidase genotype, fruit and vegetable consumption, and breast cancer risk. *Cancer Res* 2004; 64: 7634–7639.

41. Zheng W, Deitz AC, Campbell DR, Wen WQ, Cerhan JR, Sellers TA, Folsom AR, Hein DW. N-acetyltransferase 1 genetic polymorphism, cigarette smoking, well-done meat intake, and breast cancer risk. *Cancer Epidemiol Biomarkers Prev* 1999; 8: 233–239.

42. Krajinovic M, Ghadirian P, Richer C, Sinnett H, Gandini S, Perret C, Lacroix A, Labuda D, Sinnett D. Genetic susceptibility to breast cancer in French-Canadians: role of carcinogen-metabolizing enzymes and gene-environment interactions. *Int J Cancer* 2001; 92: 220–225.

43. Ishibe N, Sinha R, Hein DW, Kulldorff M, Strickland P, Fretland AJ, Chow WH, Kadlubar FF, Lang NP, Rothman N. Genetic polymorphisms in heterocyclic amine metabolism and risk of colorectal adenomas. *Pharmacogenetics* 2002; 12: 145–150.

44. Tiemersma EW, Voskuil DW, Bunschoten A, Hogendoorn EA, Witteman BJ, Nagengast FM, Glatt H, Kok FJ, Kampman E. Risk of colorectal adenomas in relation to meat consumption, meat preparation, and genetic susceptibility in a Dutch population. *Cancer Causes Control* 2004; 15: 225–236.

45. Deitz AC, Zheng W, Leff MA, Gross M, Wen WQ, Doll MA, Xiao GH, Folsom AR, Hein DW. N-Acetyltransferase-2 genetic polymorphism, well-done meat intake, and breast cancer risk among postmenopausal women. *Cancer Epidemiol Biomarkers Prev* 2000; 9: 905–910.

46. Delfino RJ, Sinha R, Smith C, West J, White E, Lin HJ, Liao SY, Gim JS, Ma HL, Butler J, Anton-Culver H. Breast cancer, heterocyclic aromatic amines from meat and N-acetyltransferase 2 genotype. *Carcinogenesis* 2000; 21: 607–615.

47. Huang YS, Chern HD, Wu JC, Chao Y, Huang YH, Chang FY, Lee SD. Polymorphism of the N-acetyltransferase 2 gene, red meat intake, and the susceptibility of hepatocellular carcinoma. *Am J Gastroenterol* 2003; 98: 1417–1422.

48. Zheng W, Xie D, Cerhan JR, Sellers TA, Wen W, Folsom AR. Sulfotransferase 1A1 polymorphism, endogenous estrogen exposure, well-done meat intake, and breast cancer risk. *Cancer Epidemiol Biomarkers Prev* 2001; 10: 89–94.

49. Nowell S, Ratnasinghe DL, Ambrosone CB, Williams S, Teague-Ross T, Trimble L, Runnels G, Carrol A, Green B, Stone A, Johnson D, Greene G, Kadlubar FF, Lang NP. Association of SULT1A1 phenotype and genotype with prostate cancer risk in African-Americans and Caucasians. *Cancer Epidemiol Biomarkers Prev* 2004; 13: 270–276.

50. Cortessis V, Siegmund K, Chen Q, Zhou N, Diep A, Frankl H, Lee E, Zhu QS, Haile R, Levy D. A case-control study of microsomal epoxide hydrolase, smoking, meat consumption, glutathione *S*-transferase M3, and risk of colorectal adenomas. *Cancer Res* 2001; 61: 2381–2385.

51. Ulrich CM, Bigler J, Whitton JA, Bostick R, Fosdick L, Potter JD. Epoxide hydrolase Tyr113His polymorphism is associated with elevated risk of colorectal polyps in the presence of smoking and high meat intake. *Cancer Epidemiol Biomarkers Prev* 2001; 10: 875–882.

52. Tsai YY, McGlynn KA, Hu Y, Cassidy AB, Arnold J, Engstrom PF, Buetow KH. Genetic susceptibility and dietary patterns in lung cancer. *Lung Cancer* 2003; 41: 269–281.

53. Spitz MR, Duphorne CM, Detry MA, Pillow PC, Amos CI, Lei L, de Andrade M, Gu X, Hong WK, Wu X. Dietary intake of isothiocyanates: evidence of a joint effect with glutathione *S*-transferase polymorphisms in lung cancer risk. *Cancer Epidemiol Biomarkers Prev* 2000; 9: 1017–1020.

54. London SJ, Yuan JM, Chung FL, Gao YT, Coetzee GA, Ross RK, Yu MC. Isothiocyanates, glutathione *S*-transferase M1 and T1 polymorphisms, and lung-cancer risk: a prospective study of men in Shanghai, China. *Lancet* 2000; 356: 724–729.

55. Zhao B, Seow A, Lee EJ, Poh WT, Teh M, Eng P, Wang YT, Tan WC, Yu MC, Lee HP. Dietary isothiocyanates, glutathione *S*-transferase -M1, -T1 polymorphisms and lung cancer risk among Chinese women in Singapore. *Cancer Epidemiol Biomarkers Prev* 2001; 10: 1063–1067.

56. Wang LI, Giovannucci EL, Hunter D, Neuberg D, Su L, Christiani DC. Dietary intake of cruciferous vegetables, Glutathione *S*-transferase (GST) polymorphisms and lung cancer risk in a Caucasian population. *Cancer Causes Control* 2004; 15: 977–985.

57. Slattery ML, Kampman E, Samowitz W, Caan BJ, Potter JD. Interplay between dietary inducers of GST and the GSTM-1 genotype in colon cancer. *Int J Cancer* 2000; 87: 728–733.

58. Seow A, Yuan JM, Sun CL, Van Den Berg D, Lee HP, Yu MC. Dietary isothiocyanates, glutathione *S*-transferase polymorphisms and colorectal cancer risk in the Singapore Chinese Health Study. *Carcinogenesis* 2002; 23: 2055–2061.

59. Lin HJ, Probst-Hensch NM, Louie AD, Kau IH, Witte JS, Ingles SA, Frankl HD, Lee ER, Haile RW. Glutathione transferase null genotype, broccoli, and lower prevalence of colorectal adenomas. *Cancer Epidemiol Biomarkers Prev* 1998; 7: 647–652.

60. Joseph MA, Moysich KB, Freudenheim JL, Shields PG, Bowman ED, Zhang Y, Marshall JR, Ambrosone CB. Cruciferous vegetables, genetic polymorphisms in glutathione *S*-transferases M1 and T1, and prostate cancer risk. *Nutr Cancer* 2004; 50: 206–213.

61. Gaudet MM, Olshan AF, Poole C, Weissler MC, Watson M, Bell DA. Diet, GSTM1 and GSTT1 and head and neck cancer. *Carcinogenesis* 2004; 25: 735–740.

62. Ambrosone CB, McCann SE, Freudenheim JL, Marshall JR, Zhang Y, Shields PG. Breast cancer risk in premenopausal women is inversely associated with consumption of broccoli, a source of isothiocyanates, but is not modified by GST genotype. *J Nutr* 2004; 134: 1134–1138.

63. Yeh CC, Hsieh LL, Tang R, Chang-Chieh CR, Sung FC. Vegetable/fruit, smoking, glutathione *S*-transferase polymorphisms and risk for colorectal cancer in Taiwan. *World J Gastroenterol* 2005; 11: 1473–1480.

64. Turner F, Smith G, Sachse C, Lightfoot T, Garner RC, Wolf CR, Forman D, Bishop DT, Barrett JH. Vegetable, fruit and meat consumption and potential risk modifying genes in relation to colorectal cancer. *Int J Cancer* 2004; 112: 259–264.

65. Ambrosone CB, Freudenheim JL, Thompson PA, Bowman E, Vena JE, Marshall JR, Graham S, Laughlin R, Nemoto T, Shields PG. Manganese superoxide dismutase (MnSOD) genetic polymorphisms, dietary antioxidants, and risk of breast cancer. *Cancer Res* 1999; 59: 602–606.

66. Cai Q, Shu XO, Wen W, Cheng JR, Dai Q, Gao YT, Zheng W. Genetic polymorphism in the manganese superoxide dismutase gene, antioxidant intake, and breast cancer risk: results from the Shanghai Breast Cancer Study. Breast *Cancer Res* 2004; 6: R647–R655.

67. Tamimi RM, Hankinson SE, Spiegelman D, Colditz GA, Hunter DJ. Manganese superoxide dismutase polymorphism, plasma antioxidants, cigarette smoking, and risk of breast cancer. *Cancer Epidemiol Biomarkers Prev* 2004; 13: 989–996.

68. Li H, Kantoff PW, Giovannucci E, Leitzmann MF, Gaziano JM, Stampfer MJ, Ma J. Manganese superoxide dismutase polymorphism, prediagnostic antioxidant status, and risk of clinical significant prostate cancer. *Cancer Res* 2005; 65: 2498–2504.

69. Ahn J, Gammon MD, Santella RM, Gaudet MM, Britton JA, Teitelbaum SL, Terry MB, Nowell S, Davis W, Garza C, Neugut AI, Ambrosone CB. Associations between breast cancer risk and the catalase genotype, fruit and vegetable consumption, and supplement use. *Am J Epidemiol* 2005; 162: 943–952.

70. Roberts-Thomson IC, Butler WJ, Ryan P. Meat, metabolic genotypes and risk for colorectal cancer. *Eur J Cancer Prev* 1999; 8: 207–211.

71. Le Marchand L. Meat intake, metabolic genes and colorectal cancer. *IARC Sci Publ.* 2002; 156: 481–485.

72. Cross AJ, Sinha R. Meat-related mutagens/carcinogens in the etiology of colorectal cancer. *Environ Mol Mutagen* 2004; 44: 44–55.

73. Lamba JK, Lin YS, Schuetz EG, Thummel KE. Genetic contribution to variable human CYP3A-mediated metabolism. *Adv Drug Deliv Rev* 2002; 54: 1271–1294.

74. Kaminsky LS, Zhang QY. The small intestine as a xenobiotic-metabolizing organ. *Drug Metab Dispos* 2003; 31: 1520–1525.

75. Keshava C, McCanlies EC, Weston A. CYP3A4 polymorphisms—potential risk factors for breast and prostate cancer: a HuGE review. *Am J Epidemiol* 2004; 160: 825–841.

76. Strange RC, Spiteri MA, Ramachandran S, Fryer AA. Glutathione-*S*-transferase family of enzymes. *Mutat Res* 2001; 482: 21–26.

77. Cotton SC, Sharp L, Little J, Brockton N. Glutathione *S*-transferase polymorphisms and colorectal cancer: a HuGE review. *Am J Epidemiol* 2000; 151: 7–32.

78. Lampe JW, Peterson S. Brassica, biotransformation and cancer risk: genetic polymorphisms alter the preventive effects of cruciferous vegetables. *J Nutr* 2002; 132: 2991–2994.

79. Seow A, Vainio H, Yu MC. Effect of glutathione-*S*-transferase polymorphisms on the cancer preventive potential of isothiocyanates: an epidemiological perspective. *Mutat Res* 2005; 592: 58–67.

80. Lampe JW, Chen C, Li S, Prunty J, Grate MT, Meehan DE, Barale KV, Dightman DA, Feng Z, Potter JD. Modulation of human glutathione *S*-transferases by botanically defined vegetable diets. *Cancer Epidemiol Biomarkers Prev* 2000; 9: 787–793.

81. Wells PG, Mackenzie PI, Chowdhury JR, Guillemette C, Gregory PA, Ishii Y, Hansen AJ, Kessler FK, Kim PM, Chowdhury NR, Ritter JK. Glucuronidation and the UDP-glucuronosyltransferases in health and disease. *Drug Metab Dispos* 2004; 32: 281–290.
82. Basu NK, Ciotti M, Hwang MS, Kole L, Mitra PS, Cho JW, Owens IS. Differential and special properties of the major human UGT1-encoded gastrointestinal UDP-glucuronosyltransferases enhance potential to control chemical uptake. *J Biol Chem* 2004; 279: 1429–1441.
83. Fang JL, Lazarus P. Correlation between the UDP-glucuronosyltransferase (UGT1A1) TATAA box polymorphism and carcinogen detoxification phenotype: significantly decreased glucuronidating activity against benzo(a)pyrene-7,8-dihydrodiol(-) in liver microsomes from subjects with the UGT1A1*28 variant. *Cancer Epidemiol Biomarkers Prev* 2004; 13: 102–109.
84. Peterson S, Bigler J, Horner NK, Potter JD, Lampe JW. Cruciferae interact with the UGT1A1*28 polymorphism to determine serum bilirubin levels in humans. *J Nutr* 2005; 135: 1051–1055.
85. Girard H, Thibaudeau J, Court MH, Fortier LC, Villeneuve L, Caron P, Hao Q, von Moltke LL, Greenblatt DJ, Guillemette C. UGT1A1 polymorphisms are important determinants of dietary carcinogen detoxification in the liver. *Hepatology* 2005; 42: 448–457.
86. Butler LM, Duguay Y, Millikan RC, Sinha R, Gagne JF, Sandler RS, Guillemette C. Joint effects between UDP-glucuronosyltransferase 1A7 genotype and dietary carcinogen exposure on risk of colon cancer. *Cancer Epidemiol Biomarkers Prev* 2005; 14: 1626–1632.
87. Klaunig JE, Kamendulis LM. The role of oxidative stress in carcinogenesis. *Annu Rev Pharmacol Toxicol* 2004; 44: 239–267.
88. Friso S, Choi SW. Gene-nutrient interactions and DNA methylation. *J Nutr* 2002; 132(Suppl): 2382S–2387S.
89. Friso S, Choi SW, Girelli D, Mason JB, Dolnikowski GG, Bagley PJ, Olivieri O, Jacques PF, Rosenberg IH, Corrocher R, Selhub J. A common mutation in the 5,10-methylenetetrahydrofolate reductase gene affects genomic DNA methylation through an interaction with folate status. *Proc Natl Acad Sci USA* 2002; 99: 5606–5611.
90. Friso S, Girelli D, Trabetti E, Olivieri O, Guarini P, Pignatti PF, Corrocher R, Choi SW. The MTHFR 1298A>C polymorphism and genomic DNA methylation in human lymphocytes. *Cancer Epidemiol Biomarkers Prev* 2005; 14: 938–943.
91. Chen J, Gammon MD, Chan W, Palomeque C, Wetmur JG, Kabat GC, Teitelbaum SL, Britton JA, Terry MB, Neugut AI, Santella RM. One-carbon metabolism, MTHFR polymorphisms, and risk of breast cancer. *Cancer Res* 2005; 65: 1606–1614.
92. Yamada K, Chen Z, Rozen R, Matthews RG. Effects of common polymorphisms on the properties of recombinant human methylenetetrahydrofolate reductase. *Proc Natl Acad Sci USA* 2001; 98: 14853–14858.
93. Potter JD. Methyl supply, methyl metabolizing enzymes and colorectal neoplasia. *J Nutr* 2002; 132(Suppl): 2410S–2412S.
94. Bailey LB. Folate, methyl-related nutrients, alcohol, and the MTHFR 677C–>T polymorphism affect cancer risk: intake recommendations. *J Nutr* 2003; 133 (Suppl): 3748S–3753S.

95. Sharp L, Little J. Polymorphisms in genes involved in folate metabolism and colorectal neoplasia: a HuGE review. *Am J Epidemiol* 2004; 159: 423–443.

96. Kim YI. Folate and DNA methylation: a mechanistic link between folate deficiency and colorectal cancer? *Cancer Epidemiol Biomarkers Prev* 2004; 13: 511–519.

97. Sharp L, Little J, Schofield AC, Pavlidou E, Cotton SC, Miedzybrodzka Z, Baird JO, Haites NE, Heys SD, Grubb DA. Folate and breast cancer: the role of polymorphisms in methylenetetrahydrofolate reductase (MTHFR). *Cancer Lett* 2002; 181: 65–71.

98. Shrubsole MJ, Gao YT, Cai Q, Shu XO, Dai Q, Hebert JR, Jin F, Zheng W. MTHFR polymorphisms, dietary folate intake, and breast cancer risk: results from the Shanghai Breast Cancer Study. *Cancer Epidemiol Biomarkers Prev* 2004; 13: 190–196.

99. Lee SA, Kang D, Nishio H, Lee MJ, Kim DH, Han W, Yoo KY, Ahn SH, Choe KJ, Hirvonen A, Noh DY. Methylenetetrahydrofolate reductase polymorphism, diet, and breast cancer in Korean women. *Exp Mol Med* 2004; 36: 116–121.

100. Le Marchand L, Haiman CA, Wilkens LR, Kolonel LN, Henderson BE. MTHFR polymorphisms, diet, HRT, and breast cancer risk: the multiethnic cohort study. *Cancer Epidemiol Biomarkers Prev* 2004; 13: 2071–2077.

101. Goodman MT, McDuffie K, Hernandez B, Wilkens LR, Bertram CC, Killeen J, Le Marchand L, Selhub J, Murphy S, Donlon TA. Association of methylenetetrahydrofolate reductase polymorphism C677T and dietary folate with the risk of cervical dysplasia. *Cancer Epidemiol Biomarkers Prev* 2001; 10: 1275–1280.

102. Lin J, Spitz MR, Wang Y, Schabath MB, Gorlov IP, Hernandez LM, Pillow PC, Grossman HB, Wu X. Polymorphisms of folate metabolic genes and susceptibility to bladder cancer: a case-control study. *Carcinogenesis* 2004; 25: 1639–1647.

103. Goode EL, Potter JD, Bigler J, Ulrich CM. Methionine synthase D919G polymorphism, folate metabolism, and colorectal adenoma risk. *Cancer Epidemiol Biomarkers Prev* 2004; 13: 157–162.

104. Ulrich CM, Bigler J, Bostick R, Fosdick L, Potter JD. Thymidylate synthase promoter polymorphism, interaction with folate intake, and risk of colorectal adenomas. *Cancer Res* 2002; 62: 3361–3364.

105. Shi Q, Zhang Z, Neumann AS, Li G, Spitz MR, Wei Q. Case-control analysis of thymidylate synthase polymorphisms and risk of lung cancer. *Carcinogenesis* 2005; 26: 649–656.

106. Shi Q, Zhang Z, Li G, Pillow PC, Hernandez LM, Spitz MR, Wei Q. Polymorphisms of methionine synthase and methionine synthase reductase and risk of lung cancer: a case-control analysis. *Pharmacogenet Genomics* 2005; 15: 547–555.

107. Poschl G, Stickel F, Wang XD, Seitz HK. Alcohol and cancer: genetic and nutritional aspects. *Proc Nutr Soc* 2004; 63: 65–71.

108. Giovannucci E. Alcohol, one-carbon metabolism, and colorectal cancer: recent insights from molecular studies. *J Nutr* 2004; 134: 2475S–2481S.

109. Crabb DW, Matsumoto M, Chang D, You M. Overview of the role of alcohol dehydrogenase and aldehyde dehydrogenase and their variants in the genesis of alcohol-related pathology. *Proc Nutr Soc* 2004; 63: 49–63.

110. Lewis SJ, Smith GD. Alcohol, ALDH2, and esophageal cancer: a meta-analysis, which illustrates the potentials and limitations of a Mendelian randomization approach. *Cancer Epidemiol Biomarkers Prev* 2005; 14: 1967–1971.

111. Yokoyama A, Kato H, Yokoyama T, Tsujinaka T, Muto M, Omori T, Haneda T, Kumagai Y, Igaki H, Yokoyama M, Watanabe H, Fukuda H, Yoshimizu H. Genetic polymorphisms of alcohol and aldehyde dehydrogenases and glutathione S-transferase M1 and drinking, smoking, and diet in Japanese men with esophageal squamous cell carcinoma. *Carcinogenesis* 2002; 23: 1851–1859.

112. Higuchi S, Matsushita S, Masaki T, Yokoyama A, Kimura M, Suzuki G, Mochizuki H. Influence of genetic variations of ethanol-metabolizing enzymes on phenotypes of alcohol-related disorders. *Ann N Y Acad Sci* 2004; 1025: 472–480.

113. Wu CF, Wu DC, Hsu HK, Kao EL, Lee JM, Lin CC, Wu MT. Relationship between genetic polymorphisms of alcohol and aldehyde dehydrogenases and esophageal squamous cell carcinoma risk in males. *World J Gastroenterol* 2005; 11: 5103–5108.

114. Muto M, Takahashi M, Ohtsu A, Ebihara S, Yoshida S, Esumi H. Risk of multiple squamous cell carcinomas both in the esophagus and the head and neck region. *Carcinogenesis* 2005; 26: 1008–1012.

115. Schwartz SM, Doody DR, Fitzgibbons ED, Ricks S, Porter PL, Chen C. Oral squamous cell cancer risk in relation to alcohol consumption and alcohol dehydrogenase-3 genotypes. *Cancer Epidemiol Biomarkers Prev* 2001; 10: 1137–1144.

116. Zavras AI, Wu T, Laskaris G, Wang YF, Cartsos V, Segas J, Lefantzis D, Joshipura K, Douglass CW, Diehl SR. Interaction between a single nucleotide polymorphism in the alcohol dehydrogenase 3 gene, alcohol consumption and oral cancer risk. *Int J Cancer* 2002; 97: 526–530.

117. Sturgis EM, Dahlstrom KR, Guan Y, Eicher SA, Strom SS, Spitz MR, Wei Q. Alcohol dehydrogenase 3 genotype is not associated with risk of squamous cell carcinoma of the oral cavity and pharynx. *Cancer Epidemiol Biomarkers Prev* 2001; 10: 273–275.

118. Terry MB, Gammon MD, Zhang FF, Knight JA, Wang Q, Britton JA, Teitelbaum SL, Neugut AI, Santella RM. ADH3 genotype, alcohol intake, and breast cancer risk. *Carcinogenesis* 2006; 27 (in press).

119. Tiemersma EW, Wark PA, Ocke MC, Bunschoten A, Otten MH, Kok FJ, Kampman E. Alcohol consumption, alcohol dehydrogenase 3 polymorphism, and colorectal adenomas. *Cancer Epidemiol Biomarkers Prev* 2003; 12: 419–425.

120. Visäpää JP, Götte K, Benesova M, Li J, Homann N, Conradt C, Inoue H, Tisch M, Horrmann K, Väkeväinen S, Salaspuro M, Seitz HK. Increased cancer risk in heavy drinkers with the alcohol dehydrogenase 1C*1 allele, possibly due to salivary acetaldehyde. *Gut* 2004; 53: 871–876.

121. Kim JI, Park YJ, Kim KH, Kim JI, Song BJ, Lee MS, Kim CN, Chang SH. hOGG1 Ser326Cys polymorphism modifies the significance of the environmental risk factor for colon cancer. *World J Gastroenterol* 2003; 9: 956–960.

122. Yeh CC, Hsieh LL, Tang R, Chang-Chieh CR, Sung FC. MS-920: DNA repair gene polymorphisms, diet and colorectal cancer risk in Taiwan. *Cancer Lett* 2005; 224: 279–288.

123. Shen J, Gammon MD, Terry MB, Wang L, Wang Q, Zhang F, Teitelbaum SL, Eng SM, Sagiv SK, Gaudet MM, Neugut AI, Santella RM. Polymorphisms in XRCC1 modify the association between polycyclic aromatic hydrocarbon-DNA adducts, cigarette smoking, dietary antioxidants, and breast cancer risk. *Cancer Epidemiol Biomarkers Prev* 2005; 14: 336–342.

124. van Gils CH, Bostick RM, Stern MC, Taylor JA. Differences in base excision repair capacity may modulate the effect of dietary antioxidant intake on prostate cancer risk: an example of polymorphisms in the XRCC1 gene. *Cancer Epidemiol Biomarkers Prev* 2002; 11: 1279–1284.

125. Shen J, Terry MB, Gammon MD, Gaudet MM, Teitelbaum SL, Eng SM, Sagiv SK, Neugut AI, Santella RM. MGMT genotype modulates the associations between cigarette smoking, dietary antioxidants and breast cancer risk. *Carcinogenesis* 2005; 26: 2131–2137.

126. Bonner MR, Rothman N, Mumford JL, He X, Shen M, Welch R, Yeager M, Chanock S, Caporaso N, Lan Q. Green tea consumption, genetic susceptibility, PAH-rich smoky coal, and the risk of lung cancer. *Mutat Res* 2005; 582: 53–60.

127. Hursting SD, Lavigne JA, Berrigan D, Perkins SN, Barrett JC. Calorie restriction, aging, and cancer prevention: mechanisms of action and applicability to humans. *Annu Rev Med* 2003; 54: 131–152.

128. Patel AC, Nunez NP, Perkins SN, Barrett JC, Hursting SD. Effects of energy balance on cancer in genetically altered mice. *J Nutr* 2004; 134 (Suppl): 3394S–3398S.

129. Rao KS. Dietary calorie restriction, DNA-repair and brain aging. *Mol Cell Biochem* 2003; 253: 313–318.

130. Stuart JA, Karahalil B, Hogue BA, Souza-Pinto NC, Bohr VA. Mitochondrial and nuclear DNA base excision repair are affected differently by caloric restriction. *FASEB J* 2004; 18: 595–597.

131. Seo YR, Sweeney C, Smith ML. Selenomethionine induction of DNA repair response in human fibroblasts. *Oncogene* 2002; 21: 3663–3669.

132. Seo YR, Kelley MR, Smith ML. Selenomethionine regulation of p53 by a ref1-dependent redox mechanism. *Proc Natl Acad Sci USA* 2002; 99: 14548–14553.

133. Collins AR, Harrington V, Drew J, Melvin R. Nutritional modulation of DNA repair in a human intervention study. *Carcinogenesis* 2003; 24: 511–515.

134. Moller P, Loft S. Interventions with antioxidants and nutrients in relation to oxidative DNA damage and repair. *Mutat Res* 2004; 551: 79–89.

135. Kotsopoulos J, Narod SA. Towards a dietary prevention of hereditary breast cancer. *Cancer Causes Control* 2005; 16: 125–138.

136. Ukkola O, Bouchard C. Clustering of metabolic abnormalities in obese individuals: the role of genetic factors. *Ann Med* 2001; 33: 79–90.

137. Calle EE, Thun MJ. Obesity and cancer. *Oncogene* 2004; 23: 6365–6378.

138. Broberger C. Brain regulation of food intake and appetite: molecules and networks. *J Intern Med* 2005; 258: 301–327.

139. Ribeiro R, Vasconcelos A, Costa S, Pinto D, Morais A, Oliveira J, Lobo F, Lopes C, Medeiros R. Overexpressing leptin genetic polymorphism (-2548 G/A) is associated with susceptibility to prostate cancer and risk of advanced disease. *Prostate* 2004; 59: 268–274.

140. Skibola CF, Holly EA, Forrest MS, Hubbard A, Bracci PM, Skibola DR, Hegedus C, Smith MT. Body mass index, leptin and leptin receptor polymorphisms, and non-hodgkin lymphoma. *Cancer Epidemiol Biomarkers Prev* 2004; 13: 779–786.

141. Willett EV, Skibola CF, Adamson P, Skibola DR, Morgan GJ, Smith MT, Roman E. Non-Hodgkin's lymphoma, obesity and energy homeostasis polymorphisms. *Br J Cancer* 2005; 93: 811–816.

142. Skibola DR, Smith MT, Bracci PM, Hubbard AE, Agana L, Chi S, Holly EA. Polymorphisms in ghrelin and neuropeptide Y genes are associated with non-Hodgkin lymphoma. *Cancer Epidemiol Biomarkers Prev* 2005; 14: 1251–1256.

143. Sturm RA. Skin colour and skin cancer — MC1R, the genetic link. *Melanoma Res* 2002; 12: 405–416.

144. Morimoto LM, Newcomb PA, White E, Bigler J, Potter JD. Insulin-like growth factor polymorphisms and colorectal cancer risk. *Cancer Epidemiol Biomarkers Prev* 2005; 14: 1204–1211.

145. Slattery ML, Murtaugh M, Caan B, Ma KN, Neuhausen S, Samowitz W. Energy balance, insulin-related genes and risk of colon and rectal cancer. *Int J Cancer* 2005; 115: 148–154.

146. Fletcher O, Gibson L, Johnson N, Altmann DR, Holly JM, Ashworth A, Peto J, Silva Idos S. Polymorphisms and circulating levels in the insulin-like growth factor system and risk of breast cancer: a systematic review. *Cancer Epidemiol Biomarkers Prev* 2005; 14: 2–19.

147. Moon JW, Chang YS, Ahn CW, Yoo KN, Shin JH, Kong JH, Kim YS, Chang J, Kim SK, Kim HJ, Kim SK. Promoter -202 A/C polymorphism of insulin-like growth factor binding protein-3 gene and non-small cell lung cancer risk. *Int J Cancer* 2006; 118: 353–356.

148. Ho GY, Melman A, Liu SM, Li M, Yu H, Negassa A, Burk RD, Hsing AW, Ghavamian R, Chua SC Jr. Polymorphism of the insulin gene is associated with increased prostate cancer risk. *Br J Cancer* 2003; 88: 263–269.

149. Tsuchiya N, Wang L, Horikawa Y, Inoue T, Kakinuma H, Matsuura S, Sato K, Ogawa O, Kato T, Habuchi T. CA repeat polymorphism in the insulin-like growth factor-I gene is associated with increased risk of prostate cancer and benign prostatic hyperplasia. *Int J Oncol* 2005; 26: 225–231.

150. Zavras AI, Pitiphat W, Wu T, Cartsos V, Lam A, Douglass CW, Diehl SR. Insulin-like growth factor II receptor gene-167 genotype increases the risk of oral squamous cell carcinoma in humans. *Cancer Res* 2003; 63: 296–297.

151. Huang XE, Hamajima N, Saito T, Matsuo K, Mizutani M, Iwata H, Iwase T, Miura S, Mizuno T, Tokudome S, Tajima K. Possible association of beta-2 and beta-3 adrenergic receptor gene polymorphisms with susceptibility to breast cancer. *Breast Cancer Res* 2001; 3: 264–269.

152. Takezaki T, Hamajima N, Matsuo K, Tanaka R, Hirai T, Kato T, Ohashi K, Tajima K. Association of polymorphisms in the beta-2 and beta-3 adrenoceptor genes with risk of colorectal cancer in Japanese. *Int J Clin Oncol* 2001; 6: 117–122.

153. Babol K, Przybylowska K, Lukaszek M, Pertynski T, Blasiak J. An association between the Trp64Arg polymorphism in the beta3-adrenergic receptor gene and endometrial cancer and obesity. *J Exp Clin Cancer Res* 2004; 23: 669–674.

154. Gong Z, Xie D, Deng Z, Bostick RM, Muga SJ, Hurley TG, Hebert JR. The PPAR{gamma} Pro12Ala polymorphism and risk for incident sporadic colorectal adenomas. *Carcinogenesis* 2005; 26: 579–585.

155. Siezen CL, van Leeuwen AI, Kram NR, Luken ME, van Kranen HJ, Kampman E. Colorectal adenoma risk is modified by the interplay between polymorphisms in arachidonic acid pathway genes and fish consumption. *Carcinogenesis* 2005; 26: 449–457.

156. Murtaugh MA, Ma KN, Caan BJ, Sweeney C, Wolff R, Samowitz WS, Potter JD, Slattery ML. Interactions of peroxisome proliferator-activated receptor {gamma} and diet in etiology of colorectal cancer. *Cancer Epidemiol Biomarkers Prev* 2005; 14: 1224–1229.

157. Leibovici D, Grossman HB, Dinney CP, Millikan RE, Lerner S, Wang Y, Gu J, Dong Q, Wu X. Polymorphisms in inflammation genes and bladder cancer: from initiation to recurrence, progression, and survival. *J Clin Oncol* 2005; 23: 5746–5756.

158. Smith WM, Zhou XP, Kurose K, Gao X, Latif F, Kroll T, Sugano K, Cannistra SA, Clinton SK, Maher ER, Prior TW, Eng C. Opposite association of two PPARG variants with cancer: overrepresentation of H449H in endometrial carcinoma cases and underrepresentation of P12A in renal cell carcinoma cases. *Hum Genet* 2001; 109: 146–151.

159. Cao Y, Cao R, Brakenhielm E. Antiangiogenic mechanisms of diet-derived polyphenols. *J Nutr Biochem* 2002; 13: 380–390.

160. Kanadaswami C, Lee LT, Lee PP, Hwang JJ, Ke FC, Huang YT, Lee MT. The antitumor activities of flavonoids. *In Vivo* 2005; 19: 895–909.

161. Hoensch HP, Kirch W. Potential role of flavonoids in the prevention of intestinal neoplasia: a review of their mode of action and their clinical perspectives. *Int J Gastrointest Cancer* 2005; 35: 187–195.

162. Thompson HJ, McGinley JN, Spoelstra NS, Jiang W, Zhu Z, Wolfe P. Effect of dietary energy restriction on vascular density during mammary carcinogenesis. *Cancer Res* 2004; 64: 5643–5650.

163. Lambert JD, Hong J, Yang GY, Liao J, Yang CS. Inhibition of carcinogenesis by polyphenols: evidence from laboratory investigations. *Am J Clin Nutr* 2005; 81(Suppl): 284S–291S.

164. Guy M, Lowe LC, Bretherton-Watt D, Mansi JL, Peckitt C, Bliss J, Wilson RG, Thomas V, Colston KW. Vitamin D receptor gene polymorphisms and breast cancer risk. *Clin Cancer Res* 2004; 10: 5472–5481.

165. Slattery ML, Neuhausen SL, Hoffman M, Caan B, Curtin K, Ma KN, Samowitz W. Dietary calcium, vitamin D, VDR genotypes and colorectal cancer. *Int J Cancer* 2004; 111: 750–756.

166. Uitterlinden AG, Fang Y, Van Meurs JB, Pols HA, Van Leeuwen JP. Genetics and biology of vitamin D receptor polymorphisms. *Gene* 2004; 338: 143–156.

167. Chen WY, Bertone-Johnson ER, Hunter DJ, Willett WC, Hankinson SE. Associations between polymorphisms in the vitamin D receptor and breast cancer risk. *Cancer Epidemiol Biomarkers Prev* 2005; 14: 2335–2339.

168. Chew BP, Park JS. Carotenoid action on the immune response. *J Nutr* 2004; 134: 257S–261S.

169. Roynette CE, Calder PC, Dupertuis YM, Pichard C. n-3 polyunsaturated fatty acids and colon cancer prevention. *Clin Nutr* 2004; 23: 139–151.

170. Nagasubramanian R, Innocenti F, Ratain MJ. Pharmacogenetics in cancer treatment. *Annu Rev Med* 2003; 54: 437–452.

171. Ulrich CM, Robien K, McLeod HL. Cancer pharmacogenetics: polymorphisms, pathways and beyond. *Nat Rev Cancer* 2003; 3: 912–920.

172. Loktionov A. Common gene polymorphisms, cancer progression and prognosis. *Cancer Lett* 2004; 208: 1–33.

173. Krajinovic M, Labuda D, Mathonnet G, Labuda M, Moghrabi A, Champagne J, Sinnett D. Polymorphisms in genes encoding drugs and xenobiotic metabolizing enzymes, DNA repair enzymes, and response to treatment of childhood acute lymphoblastic leukemia. *Clin Cancer Res* 2002; 8: 802–810.

174. Xie H, Griskevicius L, Stahle L, Hassan Z, Yasar U, Rane A, Broberg U, Kimby E, Hassan M. Pharmacogenetics of cyclophosphamide in patients with hematological malignancies. *Eur J Pharm Sci* 2006; 27: 54–61.

175. DeMichele A, Aplenc R, Botbyl J, Colligan T, Wray L, Klein-Cabral M, Foulkes A, Gimotty P, Glick J, Weber B, Stadtmauer E, Rebbeck TR. Drug-metabolizing enzyme polymorphisms predict clinical outcome in a node-positive breast cancer cohort. *J Clin Oncol* 2005; 23: 5552–5559.

176. Aplenc R, Glatfelter W, Han P, Rappaport E, La M, Cnaan A, Blackwood MA, Lange B, Rebbeck T. CYP3A genotypes and treatment response in paediatric acute lymphoblastic leukaemia. *Br J Haematol* 2003; 122: 240–244.

177. Ando Y, Saka H, Ando M, Sawa T, Muro K, Ueoka H, Yokoyama A, Saitoh S, Shimokata K, Hasegawa Y. Polymorphisms of UDP-glucuronosyltransferase gene and irinotecan toxicity: a pharmacogenetic analysis. *Cancer Res* 2000; 60: 6921–6926.

178. Mathijssen RH, Marsh S, Karlsson MO, Xie R, Baker SD, Verweij J, Sparreboom A, McLeod HL. Irinotecan pathway genotype analysis to predict pharmacokinetics. *Clin Cancer Res* 2003; 9: 3246–3253.

179. Rouits E, Boisdron-Celle M, Dumont A, Guerin O, Morel A, Gamelin E. Relevance of different UGT1A1 polymorphisms in irinotecan-induced toxicity: a molecular and clinical study of 75 patients. *Clin Cancer Res* 2004; 10: 5151–5159.

180. Marcuello E, Altes A, Menoyo A, Del Rio E, Gomez-Pardo M, Baiget M. UGT1A1 gene variations and irinotecan treatment in patients with metastatic colorectal cancer. *Br J Cancer* 2004; 91: 678–682.

181. Sai K, Saeki M, Saito Y, Ozawa S, Katori N, Jinno H, Hasegawa R, Kaniwa N, Sawada J, Komamura K, Ueno K, Kamakura S, Kitakaze M, Kitamura Y, Kamatani N, Minami H, Ohtsu A, Shirao K, Yoshida T, Saijo N. UGT1A1 haplotypes associated with reduced glucuronidation and increased serum bilirubin in irinotecan-administered Japanese patients with cancer. *Clin Pharmacol Ther* 2004; 75: 501–515.

182. Paoluzzi L, Singh AS, Price DK, Danesi R, Mathijssen RH, Verweij J, Figg WD, Sparreboom A. Influence of genetic variants in UGT1A1 and UGT1A9 on the *in vivo* glucuronidation of SN-38. *J Clin Pharmacol* 2004; 44: 854–860.

183. Innocenti F, Undevia SD, Iyer L, Chen PX, Das S, Kocherginsky M, Karrison T, Janisch L, Ramirez J, Rudin CM, Vokes EE, Ratain MJ. Genetic variants in the UDP-glucuronosyltransferase 1A1 gene predict the risk of severe neutropenia of irinotecan. *J Clin Oncol* 2004; 22: 1382–1388.

184. Kitagawa C, Ando M, Ando Y, Sekido Y, Wakai K, Imaizumi K, Shimokata K, Hasegawa Y. Genetic polymorphism in the phenobarbital-responsive enhancer module of the UDP-glucuronosyltransferase 1A1 gene and irinotecan toxicity. *Pharmacogenet Genomics* 2005; 15: 35–41.

185. Carlini LE, Meropol NJ, Bever J, Andria ML, Hill T, Gold P, Rogatko A, Wang H, Blanchard RL. UGT1A7 and UGT1A9 polymorphisms predict response and toxicity in colorectal cancer patients treated with capecitabine/irinotecan. *Clin Cancer Res* 2005; 11: 1226–1236.

186. Nowell SA, Ahn J, Rae JM, Scheys JO, Trovato A, Sweeney C, MacLeod SL, Kadlubar FF, Ambrosone CB. Association of genetic variation in tamoxifen-metabolizing enzymes with overall survival and recurrence of disease in breast cancer patients. *Breast Cancer Res Treat* 2005; 91: 249–258.

187. Ambrosone CB, Sweeney C, Coles BF, Thompson PA, McClure GY, Korourian S, Fares MY, Stone A, Kadlubar FF, Hutchins LF. Polymorphisms in glutathione *S*-transferases (GSTM1 and GSTT1) and survival after treatment for breast cancer. *Cancer Res* 2001; 61: 7130–7135.

188. Howells RE, Holland T, Dhar KK, Redman CW, Hand P, Hoban PR, Jones PW, Fryer AA, Strange RC. Glutathione *S*-transferase GSTM1 and GSTT1 genotypes in ovarian cancer: association with p53 expression and survival. *Int J Gynecol Cancer* 200; 11: 107–112.

189. Medeiros R, Pereira D, Afonso N, Palmeira C, Faleiro C, Afonso-Lopes C, Freitas-Silva M, Vasconcelos A, Costa S, Osorio T, Lopes C. Platinum/paclitaxel-based chemotherapy in advanced ovarian carcinoma: glutathione *S*-transferase genetic polymorphisms as predictive biomarkers of disease outcome. *Int J Clin Oncol* 2003; 8: 156–161.

190. Beeghly A, Katsaros D, Chen H, Fracchioli S, Zhang Y, Massobrio M, Risch H, Jones B, Yu H. Glutathione *S*-transferase polymorphisms and ovarian cancer treatment and survival. *Gynecol Oncol* 2006; 100: 330–337.

191. Okcu MF, Selvan M, Wang LE, Stout L, Erana R, Airewele G, Adatto P, Hess K, Ali-Osman F, Groves M, Yung AW, Levin VA, Wei Q, Bondy M. Glutathione *S*-transferase polymorphisms and survival in primary malignant glioma. *Clin Cancer Res* 2004; 10: 2618–2625.

192. Stanulla M, Schrappe M, Brechlin AM, Zimmermann M, Welte K. Polymorphisms within glutathione *S*-transferase genes (GSTM1, GSTT1, GSTP1) and risk of relapse in childhood B-cell precursor acute lymphoblastic leukemia: a case-control study. *Blood* 2000; 95: 1222–1228.

193. Rocha JC, Cheng C, Liu W, Kishi S, Das S, Cook EH, Sandlund JT, Rubnitz J, Ribeiro R, Campana D, Pui CH, Evans WE, Relling MV. Pharmacogenetics of outcome in children with acute lymphoblastic leukemia. *Blood* 2005; 105: 4752–4758.

194. Davies SM, Bhatia S, Ross JA, Kiffmeyer WR, Gaynon PS, Radloff GA, Robison LL, Perentesis JP. Glutathione *S*-transferase genotypes, genetic susceptibility, and outcome of therapy in childhood acute lymphoblastic leukemia. *Blood* 2002; 100: 67–71.

195. Takanashi M, Morimoto A, Yagi T, Kuriyama K, Kano G, Imamura T, Hibi S, Todo S, Imashuku S. Impact of glutathione *S*-transferase gene deletion on early relapse in childhood B-precursor acute lymphoblastic leukemia. *Haematologica* 2003; 88: 1238–1244.

196. Voso MT, D'Alo' F, Putzulu R, Mele L, Scardocci A, Chiusolo P, Latagliata R, Lo-Coco F, Rutella S, Pagano L, Hohaus S, Leone G. Negative prognostic value of glutathione *S*-transferase (GSTM1 and GSTT1) deletions in adult acute myeloid leukemia. *Blood* 2002; 100: 2703–2707.

197. Davies SM, Robison LL, Buckley JD, Tjoa T, Woods WG, Radloff GA, Ross JA, Perentesis JP. Glutathione *S*-transferase polymorphisms and outcome of chemo-therapy in childhood acute myeloid leukaemia. *J Clin Oncol* 2001; 19: 1279–1287.

198. Naoe T, Tagawa Y, Kiyoi H, Kodera Y, Miyawaki S, Asou N, Kuriyama K, Kusumoto S, Shimazaki C, Saito K, Akiyama H, Motoji T, Nishimura M, Shinagawa K, Ueda R, Saito H, Ohno R. Prognostic significance of the null genotype of glutathione S-transferase-T1 in patients with acute myeloid leukemia: increased early death after chemotherapy. *Leukemia* 2002; 16: 203–208.

199. Yang G, Shu XO, Ruan ZX, Cai QY, Jin F, Gao YT, Zheng W. Genetic polymorphisms in glutathione-S-transferase genes (GSTM1, GSTT1, GSTP1) and survival after chemotherapy for invasive breast carcinoma. *Cancer* 2005; 103: 52–58.

200. Stoehlmacher J, Park DJ, Zhang W, Groshen S, Tsao-Wei DD, Yu MC, Lenz HJ. Association between glutathione S-transferase P1, T1, and M1 genetic polymorphism and survival of patients with metastatic colorectal cancer. *J Natl Cancer Inst* 2002; 94: 936–942.

201. Stoehlmacher J, Park DJ, Zhang W, Yang D, Groshen S, Zahedy S, Lenz HJ. A multivariate analysis of genomic polymorphisms: prediction of clinical outcome to 5-FU/oxaliplatin combination chemotherapy in refractory colorectal cancer. *Br J Cancer* 2004; 91: 344–354.

202. Lu C, Spitz MR, Zhao H, Dong Q, Truong M, Chang JY, Blumenschein GR Jr, Hong WK, Wu X. Association between glutathione S-transferase pi polymorphisms and survival in patients with advanced nonsmall cell lung carcinoma. *Cancer* 2006; 105: 441–447.

203. Goekkurt E, Hoehn S, Wolschke C, Wittmer C, Stueber C, Hossfeld DK, Stoehlmacher J. Polymorphisms of glutathione S-transferases (GST) and thymidylate synthase (TS) — novel predictors for response and survival in gastric cancer patients. *Br J Cancer* 2006; 94: 281–286.

204. Stanulla M, Schaffeler E, Arens S, Rathmann A, Schrauder A, Welte K, Eichelbaum M, Zanger UM, Schrappe M, Schwab M. GSTP1 and MDR1 genotypes and central nervous system relapse in childhood acute lymphoblastic leukemia. *Int J Hematol* 2005; 81: 39–44.

205. Allan JM, Wild CP, Rollinson S, Willett EV, Moorman AV, Dovey GJ, Roddam PL, Roman E, Cartwright RA, Morgan GJ. Polymorphism in glutathione S-transferase P1 is associated with susceptibility to chemotherapy-induced leukemia. *Proc Natl Acad Sci USA* 2001; 98: 11592–11597.

206. Sweeney C, Ambrosone CB, Joseph L, Stone A, Hutchins LF, Kadlubar FF, Coles BF. Association between a glutathione S-transferase A1 promoter polymorphism and survival after breast cancer treatment. *Int J Cancer* 2003; 103: 810–814.

207. Basu S, Brown JE, Flannigan GM, Gill JH, Loadman PM, Martin SW, Naylor B, Puri R, Scally AJ, Seargent JM, Shah T, Phillips RM. NAD(P)H:Quinone oxidoreductase-1 C609T polymorphism analysis in human superficial bladder cancers: relationship of genotype status to NQO1 phenotype and clinical response to Mitomycin C. *Int J Oncol* 2004; 25: 921–927.

208. Nowell S, Sweeney C, Winters M, Stone A, Lang NP, Hutchins LF, Kadlubar FF, Ambrosone CB. Association between sulfotransferase 1A1 genotype and survival of breast cancer patients receiving tamoxifen therapy. *J Natl Cancer Inst* 2002; 94: 1635–1640.

209. Choi JY, Lee KM, Park SK, Noh DY, Ahn SH, Chung HW, Han W, Kim JS, Shin SG, Jang IJ, Yoo KY, Hirvonen A, Kang D. Genetic polymorphisms of SULT1A1 and SULT1E1 and the risk and survival of breast cancer. *Cancer Epidemiol Biomarkers Prev* 2005; 14: 1090–1095.

210. Relling MV, Hancock ML, Rivera GK, Sandlund JT, Ribeiro RC, Krynetski EY, Pui CH, Evans WE. Mercaptopurine therapy intolerance and heterozygosity at the thiopurine S-methyltransferase gene locus. *J Natl Cancer Inst* 1999; 91: 2001–2008.

211. Ando M, Ando Y, Hasegawa Y, Sekido Y, Shimokata K, Horibe K. Genetic polymorphisms of thiopurine S-methyltransferase and 6-mercaptopurine toxicity in Japanese children with acute lymphoblastic leukaemia. *Pharmacogenetics* 2001; 11: 269–273.

212. Evans WE, Hon YY, Bomgaars L, Coutre S, Holdsworth M, Janco R, Kalwinsky D, Keller F, Khatib Z, Margolin J, Murray J, Quinn J, Ravindranath Y, Ritchey K, Roberts W, Rogers ZR, Schiff D, Steuber C, Tucci F, Kornegay N, Krynetski EY, Relling MV. Preponderance of thiopurine S-methyltransferase deficiency and heterozygosity among patients intolerant to mercaptopurine or azathioprine. *J Clin Oncol* 2001; 19: 2293–2301.

213. Stanulla M, Schaeffeler E, Flohr T, Cario G, Schrauder A, Zimmermann M, Welte K, Ludwig WD, Bartram CR, Zanger UM, Eichelbaum M, Schrappe M, Schwab M. Thiopurine methyltransferase (TPMT) genotype and early treatment response to mercaptopurine in childhood acute lymphoblastic leukemia. *JAMA* 2005; 293: 1485–1489.

214. van Kuilenburg AB, Haasjes J, Richel DJ, Zoetekouw L, Van Lenthe H, De Abreu RA, Maring JG, Vreken P, van Gennip AH. Clinical implications of dihydropyrimidine dehydrogenase (DPD) deficiency in patients with severe 5-fluorouracil-associated toxicity: identification of new mutations in the DPD gene. *Clin Cancer Res* 2000; 6: 4705–4712.

215. Raida M, Schwabe W, Hausler P, Van Kuilenburg AB, Van Gennip AH, Behnke D, Hoffken K. Prevalence of a common point mutation in the dihydropyrimidine dehydrogenase (DPD) gene within the 5'-splice donor site of intron 14 in patients with severe 5-fluorouracil (5-FU)- related toxicity compared with controls. *Clin Cancer Res* 2001; 7: 2832–2839.

216. Van Kuilenburg AB, Meinsma R, Zoetekouw L, Van Gennip AH. High prevalence of the IVS14 + 1G>A mutation in the dihydropyrimidine dehydrogenase gene of patients with severe 5-fluorouracil-associated toxicity. *Pharmacogenetics* 2002 Oct; 12(7): 555–558.

217. Yonemori K, Ueno H, Okusaka T, Yamamoto N, Ikeda M, Saijo N, Yoshida T, Ishii H, Furuse J, Sugiyama E, Kim SR, Kikura-Hanajiri R, Hasegawa R, Saito Y, Ozawa S, Kaniwa N, Sawada J. Severe drug toxicity associated with a single-nucleotide polymorphism of the cytidine deaminase gene in a Japanese cancer patient treated with gemcitabine plus cisplatin. *Clin Cancer Res* 2005; 11: 2620–2624.

218. Shi JY, Shi ZZ, Zhang SJ, Zhu YM, Gu BW, Li G, Bai XT, Gao XD, Hu J, Jin W, Huang W, Chen Z, Chen SJ. Association between single nucleotide polymorphisms in deoxycytidine kinase and treatment response among acute myeloid leukaemia patients. *Pharmacogenetics* 2004; 14: 759–768.

219. Cohen V, Panet-Raymond V, Sabbaghian N, Morin I, Batist G, Rozen R. Methylenetetrahydrofolate reductase polymorphism in advanced colorectal cancer: a novel genomic predictor of clinical response to fluoropyrimidine-based chemotherapy. *Clin Cancer Res* 2003; 9: 1611–1615.

220. Etienne MC, Formento JL, Chazal M, Francoual M, Magne N, Formento P, Bourgeon A, Seitz JF, Delpero JR, Letoublon C, Pezet D, Milano G. Methylene-tetrahydrofolate reductase gene polymorphisms and response to fluorouracil-based treatment in advanced colorectal cancer patients. *Pharmacogenetics* 2004; 14: 785–792.

221. Jakobsen A, Nielsen JN, Gyldenkerne N, Lindeberg J. Thymidylate synthase and methylenetetrahydrofolate reductase gene polymorphism in normal tissue as predictors of fluorouracil sensitivity. *J Clin Oncol* 2005; 23: 1365–1369.

222. Toffoli G, Russo A, Innocenti F, Corona G, Tumolo S, Sartor F, Mini E, Boiocchi M. Effect of methylenetetrahydrofolate reductase 677 C–>T polymorphism on toxicity and homocysteine plasma level after chronic methotrexate treatment of ovarian cancer patients. *Int J Cancer* 2003; 103: 294–299.

223. Chiusolo P, Reddiconto G, Casorelli I, Laurenti L, Sora F, Mele L, Annino L, Leone G, Sica S. Preponderance of methylenetetrahydrofolate reductase C677T homozygosity among leukemia patients intolerant to methotrexate. *Ann Oncol* 2002; 13: 1915–1918.

224. Krajinovic M, Lemieux-Blanchard E, Chiasson S, Primeau M, Costea I, Moghrabi A. Role of polymorphisms in MTHFR and MTHFD1 genes in the outcome of childhood acute lymphoblastic leukemia. *Pharmacogenomics J* 2004; 4: 66–72.

225. Aplenc R, Thompson J, Han P, La M, Zhao H, Lange B, Rebbeck T. Methylene-tetrahydrofolate reductase polymorphisms and therapy response in pediatric acute lymphoblastic leukemia. *Cancer Res* 2005; 65: 2482–2487.

226. Villafranca E, Okruzhnov Y, Dominguez MA, Garcia-Foncillas J, Azinovic I, Martinez E, Illarramendi JJ, Arias F, Martinez Monge R, Salgado E, Angeletti S, Brugarolas A. Polymorphisms of the repeated sequences in the enhancer region of the thymidylate synthase gene promoter may predict downstaging after preoperative chemoradiation in rectal cancer. *J Clin Oncol* 2001; 19: 1779–1786.

227. Iacopetta B, Grieu F, Joseph D, Elsaleh H. A polymorphism in the enhancer region of the thymidylate synthase promoter influences the survival of colorectal cancer patients treated with 5-fluorouracil. *Br J Cancer* 2001; 85: 827–830.

228. Park DJ, Stoehlmacher J, Zhang W, Tsao-Wei D, Groshen S, Lenz HJ. Thymidylate synthase gene polymorphism predicts response to capecitabine in advanced colorectal cancer. *Int J Colorectal Dis* 2002; 17: 46–49.

229. Marcuello E, Altes A, del Rio E, Cesar A, Menoyo A, Baiget M. Single nucleotide polymorphism in the 5' tandem repeat sequences of thymidylate synthase gene predicts for response to fluorouracil-based chemotherapy in advanced colorectal cancer patients. *Int J Cancer* 2004; 112: 733–737.

230. Lecomte T, Ferraz JM, Zinzindohoue F, Loriot MA, Tregouet DA, Landi B, Berger A, Cugnenc PH, Jian R, Beaune P, Laurent-Puig P. Thymidylate synthase gene polymorphism predicts toxicity in colorectal cancer patients receiving 5-fluorouracil-based chemotherapy. *Clin Cancer Res* 2004; 10: 5880–5888.

231. Hitre E, Budai B, Adleff V, Czegledi F, Horvath Z, Gyergyay F, Lovey J, Kovacs T, Orosz Z, Lang I, Kasler M, Kralovanszky J. Influence of thymidylate synthase gene polymorphisms on the survival of colorectal cancer patients receiving adjuvant 5-fluorouracil. *Pharmacogenet Genomics* 2005; 15: 723–730.

232. Kawakami K, Graziano F, Watanabe G, Ruzzo A, Santini D, Catalano V, Bisonni R, Arduini F, Bearzi I, Cascinu S, Muretto P, Perrone G, Rabitti C, Giustini L, Tonini G, Pizzagalli F, Magnani M. Prognostic role of thymidylate synthase polymorphisms in gastric cancer patients treated with surgery and adjuvant chemotherapy. *Clin Cancer Res* 2005; 11: 3778–3783.

233. Shintani Y, Ohta M, Hirabayashi H, Tanaka H, Iuchi K, Nakagawa K, Maeda H, Kido T, Miyoshi S, Matsuda H. New prognostic indicator for non-small-cell lung cancer, quantitation of thymidylate synthase by real-time reverse transcription polymerase chain reaction. *Int J Cancer* 2003; 104: 790–795.

234. Sarbia M, Stahl M, von Weyhern C, Weirich G, Puhringer-Oppermann F. The prognostic significance of genetic polymorphisms (Methylenetetrahydrofolate Reductase C677T, Methionine Synthase A2756G, Thymidilate Synthase tandem repeat polymorphism) in multimodally treated oesophageal squamous cell carcinoma. *Br J Cancer* 2006; 94: 203–207.

235. Laverdiere C, Chiasson S, Costea I, Moghrabi A, Krajinovic M. Polymorphism G80A in the reduced folate carrier gene and its relationship to methotrexate plasma levels and outcome of childhood acute lymphoblastic leukemia. *Blood* 2002; 100: 3832–3834.

236. Kaufman Y, Drori S, Cole PD, Kamen BA, Sirota J, Ifergan I, Arush MW, Elhasid R, Sahar D, Kaspers GJ, Jansen G, Matherly LH, Rechavi G, Toren A, Assaraf YG. Reduced folate carrier mutations are not the mechanism underlying methotrexate resistance in childhood acute lymphoblastic leukemia. *Cancer* 2004; 100: 773–782.

237. Park DJ, Zhang W, Stoehlmacher J, Tsao-Wei D, Groshen S, Gil J, Yun J, Sones E, Mallik N, Lenz HJ. ERCC1 gene polymorphism as a predictor for clinical outcome in advanced colorectal cancer patients treated with platinum-based chemotherapy. *Clin Adv Hematol Oncol* 2003; 1: 162–166.

238. Ryu JS, Hong YC, Han HS, Lee JE, Kim S, Park YM, Kim YC, Hwang TS. Association between polymorphisms of ERCC1 and XPD and survival in non-small-cell lung cancer patients treated with cisplatin combination chemotherapy. *Lung Cancer* 2004; 44: 311–316.

239. Isla D, Sarries C, Rosell R, Alonso G, Domine M, Taron M, Lopez-Vivanco G, Camps C, Botia M, Nunez L, Sanchez-Ronco M, Sanchez JJ, Lopez-Brea M, Barneto I, Paredes A, Medina B, Artal A, Lianes P. Single nucleotide polymorphisms and outcome in docetaxel-cisplatin-treated advanced non-small-cell lung cancer. *Ann Oncol* 2004; 15: 1194–1203.

240. Zhou W, Gurubhagavatula S, Liu G, Park S, Neuberg DS, Wain JC, Lynch TJ, Su L, Christiani DC. Excision repair cross-complementation group 1 polymorphism predicts overall survival in advanced non-small cell lung cancer patients treated with platinum-based chemotherapy. *Clin Cancer Res* 2004; 10: 4939–4943.

241. Suk R, Gurubhagavatula S, Park S, Zhou W, Su L, Lynch TJ, Wain JC, Neuberg D, Liu G, Christiani DC. Polymorphisms in ERCC1 and grade 3 or 4 toxicity in non-small cell lung cancer patients. *Clin Cancer Res* 2005; 11: 1534–1538.

242. Viguier J, Boige V, Miquel C, Pocard M, Giraudeau B, Sabourin JC, Ducreux M, Sarasin A, Praz F. ERCC1 codon 118 polymorphism is a predictive factor for the tumor response to oxaliplatin/5-fluorouracil combination chemotherapy in patients with advanced colorectal cancer. *Clin Cancer Res* 2005; 11: 6212–6217.

243. Gurubhagavatula S, Liu G, Park S, Zhou W, Su L, Wain JC, Lynch TJ, Neuberg DS, Christiani DC. XPD and XRCC1 genetic polymorphisms are prognostic factors in advanced non-small-cell lung cancer patients treated with platinum chemotherapy. *J Clin Oncol* 2004; 22: 2594–2601.
244. Park DJ, Stoehlmacher J, Zhang W, Tsao-Wei DD, Groshen S, Lenz HJ. A xeroderma pigmentosum group D gene polymorphism predicts clinical outcome to platinum-based chemotherapy in patients with advanced colorectal cancer. *Cancer Res* 2001; 61: 8654–8658.
245. Allan JM, Smith AG, Wheatley K, Hills RK, Travis LB, Hill DA, Swirsky DM, Morgan GJ, Wild CP. Genetic variation in XPD predicts treatment outcome and risk of acute myeloid leukemia following chemotherapy. *Blood* 2004; 104: 3872–3877.
246. Gu J, Zhao H, Dinney CP, Zhu Y, Leibovici D, Bermejo CE, Grossman HB, Wu X. Nucleotide excision repair gene polymorphisms and recurrence after treatment for superficial bladder cancer. *Clin Cancer Res* 2005; 11: 1408–1415.
247. Stoehlmacher J, Ghaderi V, Iobal S, Groshen S, Tsao-Wei D, Park D, Lenz HJ. A polymorphism of the XRCC1 gene predicts for response to platinum-based treatment in advanced colorectal cancer. *Anticancer Res* 2001; 21: 3075–3079.
248. Moullan N, Cox DG, Angele S, Romestaing P, Gerard JP, Hall J. Polymorphisms in the DNA repair gene XRCC1, breast cancer risk, and response to radiotherapy. *Cancer Epidemiol Biomarkers Prev* 2003; 12: 1168–1174.
249. Chang-Claude J, Popanda O, Tan XL, Kropp S, Helmbold I, von Fournier D, Haase W, Sautter-Bihl ML, Wenz F, Schmezer P, Ambrosone CB. Association between polymorphisms in the DNA repair genes, XRCC1, APE1, and XPD and acute side effects of radiotherapy in breast cancer patients. *Clin Cancer Res* 2005; 11: 4802–4809.
250. Yoon SM, Hong YC, Park HJ, Lee JE, Kim SY, Kim JH, Lee SW, Park SY, Lee JS, Choi EK. The polymorphism and haplotypes of XRCC1 and survival of non-small-cell lung cancer after radiotherapy. *Int J Radiat Oncol Biol Phys.* 2005; 63: 885–891.
251. Seedhouse C, Bainton R, Lewis M, Harding A, Russell N, Das-Gupta E. The genotype distribution of the XRCC1 gene indicates a role for base excision repair in the development of therapy-related acute myeloblastic leukemia. *Blood* 2002; 100: 3761–3766.
252. Worrillow LJ, Travis LB, Smith AG, Rollinson S, Smith AJ, Wild CP, Holowaty EJ, Kohler BA, Wiklund T, Pukkala E, Roman E, Morgan GJ, Allan JM. An intron splice acceptor polymorphism in hMSH2 and risk of leukemia after treatment with chemotherapeutic alkylating agents. *Clin Cancer Res* 2003; 9: 3012–3020.
253. Illmer T, Schuler US, Thiede C, Schwarz UI, Kim RB, Gotthard S, Freund D, Schakel U, Ehninger G, Schaich M. MDR1 gene polymorphisms affect therapy outcome in acute myeloid leukemia patients. *Cancer Res* 2002; 62: 4955–4962.
254. Kafka A, Sauer G, Jaeger C, Grundmann R, Kreienberg R, Zeillinger R, Deissler H. Polymorphism C3435T of the MDR-1 gene predicts response to preoperative chemotherapy in locally advanced breast cancer. *Int J Oncol* 2003; 22: 1117–1121.
255. Jamroziak K, Mlynarski W, Balcerczak E, Mistygacz M, Trelinska J, Mirowski M, Bodalski J, Robak T. Functional C3435T polymorphism of MDR1 gene: an impact on genetic susceptibility and clinical outcome of childhood acute lymphoblastic leukemia. *Eur J Haematol* 2004; 72: 314–321.

256. Zhou Q, Sparreboom A, Tan EH, Cheung YB, Lee A, Poon D, Lee EJ, Chowbay B. Pharmacogenetic profiling across the irinotecan pathway in Asian patients with cancer. *Br J Clin Pharmacol* 2005; 59: 415–424.

257. de Jong FA, Marsh S, Mathijssen RH, King C, Verweij J, Sparreboom A, McLeod HL. ABCG2 pharmacogenetics: ethnic differences in allele frequency and assessment of influence on irinotecan disposition. *Clin Cancer Res* 2004; 10: 5889–5894.

258. Zhang W, Park DJ, Lu B, Yang DY, Gordon M, Groshen S, Yun J, Press OA, Vallbohmer D, Rhodes K, Lenz HJ. Epidermal growth factor receptor gene polymorphisms predict pelvic recurrence in patients with rectal cancer treated with chemoradiation. *Clin Cancer Res* 2005; 11: 600–605.

259. Zhang W, Stoehlmacher J, Park DJ, Yang D, Borchard E, Gil J, Tsao-Wei DD, Yun J, Gordon M, Press OA, Rhodes K, Groshen S, Lenz HJ. Gene polymorphisms of epidermal growth factor receptor and its downstream effector, interleukin-8, predict oxaliplatin efficacy in patients with advanced colorectal cancer. *Clin Colorectal Cancer* 2005; 5: 124–131.

260. Pinto D, Pereira D, Portela C, da Silva JL, Lopes C, Medeiros R. The influence of HER2 genotypes as molecular markers in ovarian cancer outcome. *Biochem Biophys Res Commun* 2005; 335: 1173–1178.

261. Weng WK, Levy R. Two immunoglobulin G fragment C receptor polymorphisms independently predict response to rituximab in patients with follicular lymphoma. *J Clin Oncol* 2003; 21: 3940–3947.

262. Weng WK, Czerwinski D, Timmerman J, Hsu FJ, Levy R. Clinical outcome of lymphoma patients after idiotype vaccination is correlated with humoral immune response and immunoglobulin G Fc receptor genotype. *J Clin Oncol* 2004; 22: 4717–4724.

263. Graziano F, Ruzzo A, Santini D, Humar B, Tonini G, Catalano V, Berardi R, Pizzagalli F, Arduini F, Bearzi I, Scartozzi M, Cascinu S, Testa E, Ficarelli R, Magnani M. Prognostic role of interleukin-1beta gene and interleukin-1 receptor antagonist gene polymorphisms in patients with advanced gastric cancer. *J Clin Oncol* 2005; 23: 2339–2345.

264. DeMichele A, Martin AM, Mick R, Gor P, Wray L, Klein-Cabral M, Athanasiadis G, Colligan T, Stadtmauer E, Weber B. Interleukin-6 -174G–>C polymorphism is associated with improved outcome in high-risk breast cancer. *Cancer Res* 2003; 63: 8051–8056.

265. Liu D, O'Day SJ, Yang D, Boasberg P, Milford R, Kristedja T, Groshen S, Weber J. Impact of gene polymorphisms on clinical outcome for stage IV melanoma patients treated with biochemotherapy: an exploratory study. *Clin Cancer Res* 2005; 11: 1237–1246.

266. McFadyen MC, Melvin WT, Murray GI. Cytochrome P450 enzymes: novel options for cancer therapeutics. *Mol Cancer Ther* 2004; 3: 363–371.

267. Shimada T, Yamazaki H, Mimura M, Inui Y, Guengerich FP. Interindividual variations in human liver cytochrome P-450 enzymes involved in the oxidation of drugs, carcinogens and toxic chemicals: studies with liver microsomes of 30 Japanese and 30 Caucasians. *J Pharmacol Exp Ther* 1994; 270: 414–423.

268. Kivisto KT, Niemi M, Fromm MF. Functional interaction of intestinal CYP3A4 and P-glycoprotein. *Fundam Clin Pharmacol* 2004; 18: 621–626.

269. Williams JA, Cook J, Hurst SI. A significant drug-metabolizing role for CYP3A5? *Drug Metab Dispos* 2003; 31: 1526–1530.

270. Lamba JK, Lin YS, Thummel K, Daly A, Watkins PB, Strom S, Zhang J, Schuetz EG. Common allelic variants of cytochrome P4503A4 and their prevalence in different populations. *Pharmacogenetics* 2002; 12: 121–132.

271. Schuetz EG. Lessons from the CYP3A4 promoter. *Mol Pharmacol* 2004; 65: 279–281.

272. Matsumura K, Saito T, Takahashi Y, Ozeki T, Kiyotani K, Fujieda M, Yamazaki H, Kunitoh H, Kamataki T. Identification of a novel polymorphic enhancer of the human CYP3A4 gene. *Mol Pharmacol* 2004; 65: 326–334.

273. Xie HG, Wood AJ, Kim RB, Stein CM, Wilkinson GR. Genetic variability in CYP3A5 and its possible consequences. *Pharmacogenomics* 2004; 5: 243–272.

274. Roy JN, Lajoie J, Zijenah LS, Barama A, Poirier C, Ward BJ, Roger M. CYP3A5 genetic polymorphisms in different ethnic populations. *Drug Metab Dispos* 2005; 33: 884–887.

275. Fujita K. Food-drug interactions via human cytochrome P450 3A (CYP3A). *Drug Metabol Drug Interact* 2004; 20: 195–217.

276. Paine MF, Criss AB, Watkins PB. Two major grapefruit juice components differ in time to onset of intestinal CYP3A4 inhibition. *J Pharmacol Exp Ther* 2005; 312: 1151–1160.

277. Veronese ML, Gillen LP, Burke JP, Dorval EP, Hauck WW, Pequignot E, Waldman SA, Greenberg HE. Exposure-dependent inhibition of intestinal and hepatic CYP3A4 *in vivo* by grapefruit juice. *J Clin Pharmacol* 2003; 43: 831–839.

278. Markowitz JS, Donovan JL, DeVane CL, Taylor RM, Ruan Y, Wang JS, Chavin KD. Effect of St. John's wort on drug metabolism by induction of cytochrome P450 3A4 enzyme. *JAMA* 2003; 290: 1500–1504.

279. Reif S, Nicolson MC, Bisset D, Reid M, Kloft C, Jaehde U, McLeod HL. Effect of grapefruit juice intake on etoposide bioavailability. *Eur J Clin Pharmacol* 2002; 58: 491–494.

280. van Schaik RH. Implications of cytochrome P450 genetic polymorphisms on the toxicity of antitumor agents. *Ther Drug Monit* 2004; 26: 236–240.

281. Marsh S, Xiao M, Yu J, Ahluwalia R, Minton M, Freimuth RR, Kwok PY, McLeod HL. Pharmacogenomic assessment of carboxylesterases 1 and 2. *Genomics* 2004; 84: 661–668.

282. Rooseboom M, Commandeur JN, Vermeulen NP. Enzyme-catalyzed activation of anticancer prodrugs. *Pharmacol Rev* 2004; 56: 53–102.

283. Salavaggione OE, Wang L, Wiepert M, Yee VC, Weinshilboum RM. Thiopurine S-methyltransferase pharmacogenetics: variant allele functional and comparative genomics. *Pharmacogenet Genomics* 2005; 15: 801–815.

284. Noguchi T, Tanimoto K, Shimokuni T, Ukon K, Tsujimoto H, Fukushima M, Noguchi T, Kawahara K, Hiyama K, Nishiyama M. Aberrant methylation of DPYD promoter, DPYD expression, and cellular sensitivity to 5-fluorouracil in cancer cells. *Clin Cancer Res* 2004; 10: 7100–7107.

285. Ukon K, Tanimoto K, Shimokuni T, Noguchi T, Hiyama K, Tsujimoto H, Fukushima M, Toge T, Nishiyama M. Activator protein accelerates dihydropyrimidine dehydrogenase gene transcription in cancer cells. *Cancer Res* 2005; 65: 1055–1062.

286. Longley DB, Harkin DP, Johnston PG. 5-fluorouracil: mechanisms of action and clinical strategies. *Nat Rev Cancer* 2003; 3: 330–338.

287. Sellers TA, Alberts SR, Vierkant RA, Grabrick DM, Cerhan JR, Vachon CM, Olson JE, Kushi LH, Potter JD. High-folate diets and breast cancer survival in a prospective cohort study. *Nutr Cancer* 2002; 44: 139–144.

288. Hooijberg JH, de Vries NA, Kaspers GJ, Pieters R, Jansen G, Peters GJ. Multidrug resistance proteins and folate supplementation: therapeutic implications for anti-folates and other classes of drugs in cancer treatment. *Cancer Chemother Pharmacol* 2005; 1 (Online): 1–12.

289. Guminski AD, Harnett PR, deFazio A. Scientists and clinicians test their metal-back to the future with platinum compounds. *Lancet Oncol* 2002; 3: 312–318.

290. Altaha R, Liang X, Yu JJ, Reed E. Excision repair cross complementing-group 1: gene expression and platinum resistance. *Int J Mol Med* 2004; 14: 959–970.

291. Yu JJ, Mu C, Lee KB, Okamoto A, Reed EL, Bostick-Bruton F, Mitchell KC, Reed E. A nucleotide polymorphism in ERCC1 in human ovarian cancer cell lines and tumor tissues. *Mutat Res* 1997; 382: 13–20.

292. Yu JJ, Lee KB, Mu C, Li Q, Abernathy TV, Bostick-Bruton F, Reed E. Comparison of two human ovarian carcinoma cell lines (A2780/CP70 and MCAS) that are equally resistant to platinum, but differ at codon 118 of the ERCC1 gene. *Int J Oncol* 2000; 16: 555–560.

293. Vonderheide AP, Wrobel K, Kannamkumarath SS, B'Hymer C, Montes-Bayon M, Ponce De Leon C, Caruso JA. Characterization of selenium species in Brazil nuts by HPLC-ICP-MS and ES-MS. *J Agric Food Chem* 2002; 50: 5722–5728.

294. Lockhart AC, Tirona RG, Kim RB. Pharmacogenetics of ATP-binding cassette transporters in cancer and chemotherapy. *Mol Cancer Ther* 2003; 2: 685–698.

295. Benet LZ, Cummins CL, Wu CY. Unmasking the dynamic interplay between efflux transporters and metabolic enzymes. *Int J Pharm* 2004; 277: 3–9.

296. Schwab M, Eichelbaum M, Fromm MF. Genetic polymorphisms of the human MDR1 drug transporter. *Annu Rev Pharmacol Toxicol* 2003; 43: 285–307.

297. Sakaeda T, Nakamura T, Okumura K. Pharmacogenetics of MDR1 and its impact on the pharmacokinetics and pharmacodynamics of drugs. *Pharmacogenomics* 2003; 4: 397–410.

298. Dahan A, Altman H. Food-drug interaction: grapefruit juice augments drug bio-availability—mechanism, extent and relevance. *Eur J Clin Nutr* 2004; 58: 1–9.

299. Chearwae W, Wu CP, Chu HY, Lee TR, Ambudkar SV, Limtrakul P. Curcuminoids purified from turmeric powder modulate the function of human multidrug resistance protein 1 (ABCC1). *Cancer Chemother Pharmacol* 2006; 57: 376–388.

300. Dürr D, Stieger B, Kullak-Ublick GA, Rentsch KM, Steinert HC, Meier PJ, Fattinger K. St. John's Wort induces intestinal P-glycoprotein/MDR1 and intestinal and hepatic CYP3A4. *Clin Pharmacol Ther* 2000; 68: 598–604.

301. Adams GP, Weiner LM. Monoclonal antibody therapy of cancer. *Nat Biotechnol* 2005; 23: 1147–1157.

302. Zhang Z, Li M, Rayburn ER, Hill DL, Zhang R, Wang H. Oncogenes as novel targets for cancer therapy (part I): growth factors and protein tyrosine kinases. *Am J Pharmacogenomics* 2005; 5: 173–190.

303. Wakeling AE. Inhibitors of growth factor signalling. *Endocr Relat Cancer* 2005; 12 (Suppl): S183–S187.

304. Yan L, Beckman RA. Pharmacogenetics and pharmacogenomics in oncology therapeutic antibody development. *Biotechniques* 2005; 39: 565–568.

305. Tisdale MJ. Cachexia in cancer patients. *Nat Rev Cancer* 2002; 2: 862–871.

306. Zigman JM, Elmquist JK. From anorexia to obesity—the yin and yang of body weight control. *Endocrinology* 2003; 144: 3749–3756.

307. Inui A. Cancer anorexia-cachexia syndrome: current issues in research and management. *CA Cancer J Clin* 2002; 52: 72–91.

308. Rubin H. Cancer cachexia: its correlations and causes. *Proc Natl Acad Sci USA.* 2003; 100: 5384–5389.

309. Barber MD, Powell JJ, Lynch SF, Fearon KC, Ross JA. A polymorphism of the interleukin-1 beta gene influences survival in pancreatic cancer. *Br J Cancer* 2000; 83: 1443–1447.

310. Halma MA, Wheelhouse NM, Barber MD, Powell JJ, Fearon KC, Ross JA. Interferon-gamma polymorphisms correlate with duration of survival in pancreatic cancer. *Hum Immunol* 2004; 65: 1405–1408.

Index

A

9 780367 390655